CLINICAL ONCOLOGY
FOR STUDENTS
OF
RADIATION THERAPY TECHNOLOGY

CLINICAL ONCOLOGY
FOR STUDENTS
OF
RADIATION THERAPY TECHNOLOGY

By

JOHN A. STRYKER, MD
Department of Radiology
Division of Radiation Therapy
The Pennsylvania State University
Hershey, PA

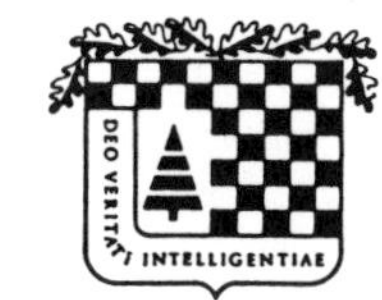

WARREN H. GREEN, INC.
St. Louis, Missouri U.S.A.

Published by

WARREN H. GREEN, INC.
8356 Olive Boulevard
St. Louis, Missouri 63132, U.S.A.

©1992 by WARREN H. GREEN, INC.

ISBN No. 87527-488-9

Printed in the United States of America

Acknowledgement

The author wishes to thank Gail Eberly for her assistance in the preparation of this book.

PREFACE

You have chosen a career field which has undergone phenomenal growth during the past 30 years. In 1964, following the first examination in radiation therapy technology given by the American Registry of Radiation Therapy Technology, there were only 88 registered technologists. Currently, there are more than 7,000 registered radiation therapy technologists. Furthermore, the field has grown in complexity and of necessity, the training programs have become more exacting. Therefore, the quality, as well as the quantity of trained radiation therapy technologists has increased dramatically. Nevertheless, there remains an acute shortage of trained people in the field in spite of the fact that there are now more than 100 certified training programs.

Radiation therapy technology is one of the most demanding and responsible careers in the entire paramedical field. For this reason, the highest quality trainees are needed and this book is dedicated, with appreciation to you. You have the opportunity, indeed the obligation to bring technical excellence, as well as emotional support and comfort to each and every patient that you treat. One could not ask for a higher calling. It is hoped that this book will be of assistance to you in reaching these high goals.

TABLE OF CONTENTS

CLINICAL ONCOLOGY
FOR STUDENTS
OF
RADIATION THERAPY TECHNOLOGY

Chapter 1

THE NATURE AND CAUSES OF CANCER

INTRODUCTION

The number of deaths from cancer in the U.S. currently exceeds 510,000 per year.[1] The death rate from cancer has doubled every 30 years in this century.[2] One in four persons will develop cancer during his or her lifetime and one in six will die from cancer. Mortality from cancer is exceeded only by death from cardiovascular diseases.

THE NATURE OF CANCER

Cancer is a general term for a wide variety of diseases that behave in a similar way. They are diseases of cells which are characterized by abnormal cell proliferation. The diseased cells have the capacity to transfer the abnormality to their descendants resulting in unceasing, excessive, and abnormal cell proliferation. The basic characteristics of cancer cell proliferations are autonomy (the abnormal cells do not respond to normal limitations of cell proliferation) and anaplasia (the abnormal cells have lost their normal organization and function). To date, biochemical studies have failed to revel the molecular basis for these alterations in cell growth and function.

The abnormal cell proliferation causes masses of cells to develop which, because of their increasing size and capacity for tissue invasion, induce structural changes and altered function in abnormal tissues. In addition, cancer cells usually have the ability to become detached from the main cell mass and to spread throughout the body so relentlessly that they cause death.

THE EPIDEMIOLOGY OF CANCER

Epidemiology is the study of the distribution of and causes of disease frequency in the population. Epidemiologic studies identify factors associated with a high risk of cancer and suggest possible causative agents requiring additional investigation. Epidemiologic studies are usually surveys of large population groups, but may be clinical investigations of small groups of patients with a particular form of cancer. Such studies have identified a number of factors which influence the occurrence of cancer in the population:

Age The incidence of most forms of cancer varies with age. In general, cancer develops more frequently in persons over 40, and 60% of cancer deaths occur in persons over 65.

Sex The incidence of cancer in the U.S. is higher for men than women and the specific types of cancer vary in frequency between the sexes (Table 1.1)[1]

Table 1.1 Estimated new cancer cases by sex and site in US, 1990[1]

Site	Male	Female
Oral Cavity and pharynx	20,400	10,100
Digestive organs	121,300	115,500
Stomach	13,900	3,200
Large intestine	52,000	58,000
Rectum	24,000	21,000
Pancreas	13,600	14,500
Respiratory System	115,000	58,700
Genital Organs	113,100	72,900
Prostate	106,000	----
Cervix	----	13,500
Endometrium	----	33,000
Ovary	----	20,500
Urinary Organs	51,000	22,000
Bone	1,200	900
Connective tissue	3,000	2,700
Skin	14,800	12,800
Breast	900	150,000
Eye	900	800
Brain & CNS	8,500	7,100
Endocrine glands	4,000	9,600
Leukemia	15,700	12,100
Other Blood & lymph tissue	28,900	25,900
Other sites	21,300	19,900

Race In American blacks the incidence of cancers of the lung, esophagus, prostate, pancreas, and large intestine has increased more than in whites in the past 30 years.

Family History Breast, colon, and stomach cancers occasionally develop more frequently in families called "cancer families."[3]

Marital Status The incidence of breast cancer is higher in unmarried women.

Religion Mormons tend to have a low incidence of most forms of cancer; Jewish women have low incidence of cervix cancer.

Personal Habits Smoking is the major cause of lung cancer and contributes to the development of cancer of the pancreas, esophagus and bladder.

Socioeconomic Status Low socioeconomic status is associated with cervix, lung, and stomach cancer, whereas high socioeconomic status tends to be associated with breast, endometrial, and colon cancer.

Occupation Excess lung cancer has been found in workers who handle asbestos, uranium, nickel, and arsenic, whereas bladder cancer rates are high in persons who work with leather, dyes, and rubber.

Geography Cancer rates vary by factors of as high as 30 between all countries.[4] In Italy, Japan, Federal Republic of Germany, England, Wales, and the USA, patterns of cancer mortality have shifted over the past two decades. Stomach cancer continues to decline, while brain and central nervous system cancer, breast cancer, multiple myeloma, kidney cancer, non-Hodgkin lymphoma, and melanoma have increased in persons aged 55 or older. Cancer of the lung is declining for men under age 85 and women under age 60 in England and Wales and men under 45 in the USA, but is still rising for men and women in other countries.

Sexual Activity Cervix cancer develops more frequently in females who begin sexual activity at a young age and have multiple sex partners.

Residence The incidence of prostate and many other cancers is higher in urban than rural dwellers.

Diet There is evidence that the typical American diet with its high meat, high fat and low fiber content is associated with the high incidence of colon carcinoma.[5]

Geophysical Factors Two physical agents, ionizing radiation and UV light, were among the first agents to be recognized as carcinogenic to humans.

Infection Statistical studies have shown that cancer is not an infectious disease. People who come into close contact with a patient do not have a higher risk of developing the disease.

The proportion of cancer deaths attributed to the various factors just mentioned have been estimated by Doll and Peto (See Table 1.2).[7]

THE GENETIC BASIS OF CANCER

There is strong evidence that cancer is a genetic disease of body cells.[8] Development of a tumor probably requires two or more mutations in the stem cells of the tissue of origin, but expression of the mutation as a tumor depends on the kinetics of cellular proliferation and numerous host factors. A few rare tumors, such as retinoblastoma and Wilms' tumor, are frequently heritable and in these, a precise chromosomal location has been established for genes where mutation leads to malignancy. Most forms of cancer probably have a heritable subgroup and studies of partially inbred populations, such as the Mormon population in Utah, suggest that the risk of developing most of the common cancers is associated with genetic factors.

VIRUSES AND CANCER

Some animal tumors have been shown to be caused by DNA- or RNA-containing tumor viruses.[9] An essential step in malignant transformation of normal cells by tumor viruses is union of all or part of the viral DNA or DNA copy of retroviral RNA with the host cell genome. Such viral DNA then acquires immortality as a chromosomal parasite.

Retroviruses are RNA viruses that reproduce through DNA intermediates.[10] A viral particle (viron) attaches to the cell surface and enters the cell. The viral

Table 1.2 Percentage of cancer deaths attributed to various factors (Doll and Peto)[7]

Factor	Percent of all cancer deaths
Tobacco	30
Alcohol	3
Diet	35
Food additives	<1
Sexual behavior	7
Occupation	4
Pollution	2
Industrial products	<1
Medicines	1
Geophysical factors	3
Infection	10
Unknown	?

RNA genome is reverse transcribed into DNA; this viral DNA then combines with the host chromosome forming a provirus. Host RNA polymerase II transcribes the provirus to produce viral RNA which is either translated to produce viral proteins or packaged as the viral genome. Virus is released from the cell by budding.

Expression of specific viral genes leads to the synthesis of new proteins which may cause malignant transformation of cells directly, or the viral genes or their protein product may act indirectly by activating a cellular oncogene. The outcome is a loss of regulation of cellular proliferation and changes on the cell surface which modify the cell's interaction with the immune system of the host.

In humans there is evidence that DNA containing viruses can cause the following diseases: (a) hepatitis B virus can cause a form of liver cancer called hepatocellular carcinoma (b) the human papilloma viruses cause benign warts and papillomas and are implicated in the etiology of cervix carcinoma (c) the Epstein-Barr herpes virus is the etiological agent of Burkitt's lymphoma and possibly nasopharyngeal carcinoma. Furthermore, there is evidence that retroviruses cause adult T-cell lympocytic leukemia and acquired immunodeficiency syndrome (AIDS).

ONCOGENES

Oncogenes are genes that are capable of causing cancer.[11] All mammalian cells contain genes, known as proto-oncogenes, which when activated to oncogenes may contribute to the development of malignancy. Proto-oncogenes are essential to normal cell functions such as cell division.[12] Mutations which change the levels of gene expression or the form of gene products in the normal pathways of cell division can activate their oncogenic potential. The first oncogenes were identified in studies of cancer causing retroviruses, but they have also been identified in DNA tumor viruses. Activated oncogenes have been detected in malignant cells of human origin such as colon carcinoma, breast carcinoma, and small cell lung carcinoma, but their role in the generation of human cancer is unknown.

CHEMICAL CARCINOGENESIS

In experimental animals, tumors can be induced by exposing them to certain chemical and physical agents called carcinogens. The process by which tumors are induced by such agents is called carcinogenesis. A list of industrial chemicals and drugs known to be carcinogenic for humans is seen in Table 1.3.[13, 14]

Carcinogenesis is a multistage process. The first stage is called initiation and the product is an initiated cell (Figure 1.1). Initiated cells are not tumor cells. In the second stage, called promotion, the initiated cells develop into tumor cells. Promotion requires a prolonged period of time and probably comprises more than one process. The third stage, called progression, results in measurable and/ or morphologically detectable alteration in the cell genome's structure and leads to the growth of altered cells, resulting in benign and/or malignant neoplasms. The initiation and progression stages appear to be irreversible whereas the promotion stage may be reversible.

RADIATION CARCINOGENESIS

Ionizing radiation is the most extensively studied human carcinogen. Epidemiologic studies conducted on populations exposed to radiation for military, occupational, or medical reasons and experimental studies on irradiated cultured cells and animals have yielded much information about radiation carcinogenesis. A number of generalizations can be made.[15]

1.   A single radiation exposure is sufficient to elevate cancer incidence many years later.

2.   Radiation-induced cancers cannot be distinguished from naturally occurring cancers.

3.   The incidence of nearly all cancers appear to be increased after radiation, except chronic lymphocytic leukemia, Hodgkin's disease and a few others.

4.   Breast tissue, thyroid gland and bone marrow appear to be the most susceptible to radiation carcinogenesis.

5.   Leukemia is the most common form of radiation-induced cancer. The time following exposure to development of leukemia (latent period) begins at two to four years, with a peak incidence at six to eight years.

6.   Solid tumors have a latent period of about ten years.

7.   Age at exposure is an important host factor influencing cancer risk following radiation, i.e., women who are irradiated at less than 20 years of age are at a higher relative risk for breast cancer than those who are irradiated later in life.

Table 1.3 Chemicals known to be carcinogenic for humans[13]

Chemical	Site
Industrial	
2-Napthylamine	Bladder
Benzidine	Bladder
4-Aminobiphenyl	Bladder
Bis (choloromethyl) ether	Lung
Bis (2-chlorethey) sulfide	Lung
Vinyl chloride	Liver
Certain tars, soot, oils	Skin, lung
Chromium compounds	Lung
Nickel compounds	Lung, sinuses
Asbestos	Pleura
Benzene	Lymph tissue
Medical	
Radioactive drugs (Phosphorus 32, radium, mesothorium, thorotrast)	Leukemia, bone, sinuses, liver
Chlornaphazine	Bladder
Arsenic	Skin
Methoxypsoralen	Skin
Alkylating agents	Acute leukemia
Societal	
Cigarette smoke	Lung, bladder
Betel nut and tobacco chewing	Oral cavity

8. The recent BEIR V report on the <u>Health Effects of Exposure to Low Levels of Ionizing Radiation</u> concluded that, on the basis of available evidence, the average life-time excess risk of death from cancer following an acute radiation dose to all body organs of 0.1 sievert (Sv) (0.1 Gy of low-LET radiation) is estimated to be 0.8%, although the risk varies with age at exposure.[16]

IMMUNITY AND CANCER

The nature and mechanisms of host resistance to cancer development are not well understood. In experimental animals and humans, humoral and cell, mediated immunity seem to be important in tumor growth and development and

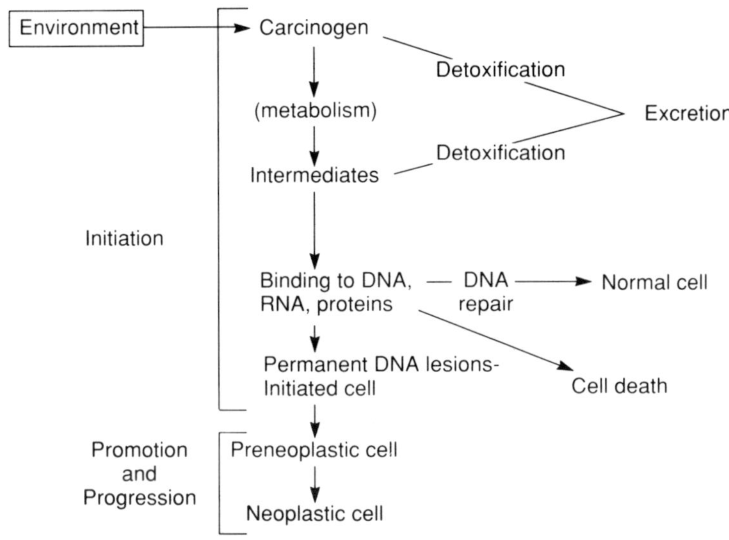

Figure 1.1 The stages of chemical carcinogenesis are initiation, promotion and progression.

research suggests that the lymphatic system controls the emergence of cancerous clones by a network of cellular surveillance.[17] The major role of the immune system is to distinguish between "self" and "nonself" and to actively eliminate "nonself".[18] The concept of immune surveillance postulates that all tumors are nonself and that it is the function of the immune system to destroy tumors as they arise. This theory assumes that tumor cells carry tumor-specific antigens that are recognized by the immune system. It appears that some tumors are immunogenic in the sense that they can be recognized by lymphocytes whereas others are not.

Support for the concept that altered immunity leads to cancer is suggested by the following clinical observations:

1. Patients who receive drugs which suppress the immune system for the purpose of preventing graft rejection have a greatly increased risk of developing cancer.

2. Patients who receive drugs for cancer treatment, which also suppress the immune system, have an increased risk of developing second and third malignancies.

3. There are a number of rare congenital diseases which are associated with deficient function of the immune system. Individuals with these diseases also have a high risk of developing cancer.

Table 1.4 Estimated cancer costs for all neoplasms and for malignant neoplasms only in 1990[19]

Cost Category	Cost, millions of dollars
Direct costs	
All neoplasms	35,256
Malignant neoplasms only	29,328
Morbidity costs	
All neoplasms	11,896
Malignant neoplasms only	9,895
Mortality costs	
All neoplasms	56,788
Malignant neoplasms only	55,127
Total	
All neoplasms	103,940
Malignant neoplasms only	94,350

4. Patients with AIDS, who have a severe immune deficiency, develop a wide spectrum of neoplasms, especially Kaposi's sarcoma and malignant lymphomas.

Cancer of the lymph system is the predominant tumor type seen in immunosuppressed individuals, but other tumor types also occur with increased frequency.

THE ECONOMIC BURDEN OF CANCER

The economic burden of cancer has been estimated by Brown.[19] In Table 1.4, direct costs are the national expenditures for services such as hospital care and physician services. This data was produced by the Health Care Financing Administration. Morbidity costs were estimated from data on work days lost due to illness (National Health Interview Study) and the mortality costs were estimated by calculation of person-years lost to premature cancer death (National Center for Health Statistics).

REFERENCES

1. Silverberg E, Boring CC, Squires TS. Cancer statistics, 1990. CA-A Cancer Journal for Clinicians 40:9-26, 1990.

2. Schottenfeld D. The epidemiology of cancer: An overview. Cancer 47:1095-1108, 1981.

3. Lynch HT, Albano WA, Shannon D, et al. Genetic predisposition to breast cancer. Cancer 53:612-622, 1984.

4. David DL, Hoel D, Lopez A. International trends in cancer mortality in France, West

Germany, Italy, Japan, England and Wales, and the USA. Lancet 336:474-481, 1990.

5. Trock B., Lanza E., Greenwald P., Dietary fiber, vegetables, and colon cancer: Critical review and meta-analyses of the epidemiologic evidence. J Natl Cancer Inst 82;650-661, 1990.

6. Howe GR, Horohata T, Hislop TG, et al, Dietary factors and risk of breast cancer: Combined analysis of 12 case-control studies. J Natl Cancer Inst 82:561-569, 1990.

7. Doll R, Peto R. The Causes of Cancer, Oxford University Press, New York, 1981.

8. Phillips RA. Chapter 3, The Genetic basis of cancer, in The Basic Science of Oncology, Eds. Tannock, IF, Hill RP, Pergamon Press, New York, 1987, pp 24-51.

9. Sheinin R., Tak WM, Clark SP. Viruses and cancer, in The Basic Science of Oncology, Eds. Tannock IF, Hill RP, Pergamon Press, New York, 1987, pp. 52-71.

10. Hu. WS, Temin HM. Retroviral recombination and reverse transcription . Science 250:1227-1233, 1990.

11. Minden M. Oncogenes, in The Basic Science of Oncology, Eds. Tannock IF, Hill RP, Pergamon Press, New York, 1987, pp. 72-88.

12. Park M, Vande Woude GF. Chapter 4, Principles of molecular cell biology of cancer: Oncogenes, in cancer: Principles and Practice of Oncology, 3rd Edition, Eds. DeVita VT, Hellman S. Rosenberg SA, J.B.Lippincott Company, Philadelphia, 1989, pp 45-66.

13. Miller EC, Miller JA. Mechanisms of Carcinogenesis. Cancer 47:1051-1064, 1981.

14. Pitot HC. Chapter 8, Principles of carcinogenesis: Chemical, in Cancer: Principles & Practice of Oncology, Eds. DeVita VT, Hellman S, Rosenberg SA, J.B.Lippincott Company, Philadelphia, 1989, pp. 116-135.

15. Boice JD. Cancer following medical irradiation. Cancer 47:1081-1090, 1982.

16. Health Effects of Exposure to Low Levels of Ionizing Radiation BEIR V, National Academy Press, Washington, D.C., 1990.

17. Merigan TC. Virology and immune mechanisms. Cancer 47:1091-1094, 1981

18. Miller RG. Immunology related to cancer, in The Basic Science of Oncology, Eds. Tannnock IF, Hill RP, Pergamon Press, New York, 1987, pp. 223-233.

19. Brown ML. The national economic burden of cancer: An update. J Natl Cancer Inst. 82:1811-1814, 1990.

Chapter 2

THE DIAGNOSIS OF CANCER

THE MEDICAL HISTORY

The medical history is the initial step in cancer diagnosis.[1] In patients presenting with symptoms, 80-90% of cancer diagnoses are suggested by the history. The components of the medical history are:

Chief Complaint The main symptom(s) that brought the patient to the physician.

History of the present illness Details of the illness such as time of onset, duration, severity, associated symptoms.

Review of systems Questions relating to the function of each organ system.

Past medical history Previous illnesses, operations, current and past medications, allergies.

Social history Past and present tobacco and alcohol use, and sexual activity.

Family history Illnesses and cause of death in parents, siblings and children.

Work history Occupation, possible exposure to carcinogens.

The history is important in revealing the patient's understanding of his or her illness, expectations of the disease and its treatment, coping ability and general level of maturity. It aids also in establishing the physician-patient relationship.

Reliance on early symptom reporting by patients is the mainstay of cancer detection. The seven warning signs of cancer published by the American Cancer Society are:

1.   Change in bowel or bladder habit-suggests presence of rectal, bladder, prostate cancer.

2.   Sore that does not heal-suggests presence of skin, oral cancer.

3.   Unusual bleeding or discharge-often seen with cancer of bladder, cervix, uterus, rectum, lung.

4.   Thickening or lump in breast or elsewhere-most common presenting complaint in breast cancer.

5.   Indigestion or difficulty swallowing-indigestion often occurs with cancer of stomach or pancreas. Difficulty swallowing is a common complaint with cancer of the pharynx or esophagus.

6.   Recent change in mole or wart-suggests presence of an aggressive form of skin cancer called malignant melanoma.

7.   Cough or hoarseness of voice-common complaints in cancer of the lung and larynx.

THE PHYSICAL EXAMINATION

The next important step in cancer diagnosis is the physical examination. The physical examination must be conducted systematically and thoroughly in a comfortable, well-illuminated, private examining room. Complete disrobing is imperative. Aids to examination are essential and include otoscope, opthalmoscope, plastic gloves, head lamp, tongue depressors, nasal speculum, laryngeal mirror, blood pressure cuff, vaginal speculum, and sigmoidoscope.

Each of the following organs should be inspected in any physical examination for cancer diagnosis:

Skin-Any ulcerated or pigmented lesion may be malignant.

Lymph nodes-Nodes greater than 2 cm in size usually contain cancer.

Oral cavity and pharynx-Ulcers or masses may be malignant.

Larynx-Suspicious lesions can be seen with a laryngeal mirror.

Breast- Any discrete mass present after completion of menstrual period may be malignant.

Testis-Masses suggest cancer.

Rectum-Masses or ulcers detected by digital rectal examination or sigmoidoscopy may be malignant.

Other aspects of the physical examination relating to specific tumor will be covered in later chapters.

The physical examination is also important in the follow-up of patients after completion of treatment. Locally recurrent and disseminated cancers can often be detected by physical examination.

BIOPSY FOR CANCER DIAGNOSIS

The biopsy is the most important step in the diagnosis of cancer. Biopsy is the removal of tissue for microscopic examination by the pathologist.

BIOPSY TECHNIQUES

Collection of body secretions-Collection of sputum or urine for examination by Papanicolaou techniques is the simplest form of biopsy.

Scraping or curettage of a tumor surface-Collection of cells from the surface of the cervix with a cotton-tipped swab or by scraping with a wooden spatula is a simple biopsy procedure. The collected cells are examined by Papanicolaou techniques. Dilation of the cervix and curettage of the uterine cavity is another example of this method.

Aspiration of fluid-Abnormal accumulations of body fluids in the chest or abdomen can be collected by needle drainage. The collected fluids are then examined by Papanicolaou techniques. Aspiration of dislodged cells from the uterine cavity is another example of this technique.

Needle Aspiration biopsy-In this technique, a needle is inserted into a fluid-filled tumor mass in the neck, breast, or other soft tissue and vacuum is applied to the attached syringe. The aspirated material is examined by Papanicolaou techniques.

Needle biopsy-A variety of special needles have been designed for obtaining a core of tissue for microscopic examination. Needle biopsies can be performed under local anesthesia. Masses in the breast, prostate, liver, pleura, lung, bone and bone marrow, kidney, muscles, or subcutaneous tissue can be biopsied in this way. Deeper tumors are biopsied with radiologic guidance to prevent injury to normal tissue.

Dermal punch-Accessible lesions of the skin or oral cavity can be biopsied with a special instrument which removes a small plug of tissue.

Scalpel incision or excision-Accessible lesions can be biopsied under local anesthesia with a scalpel. Small lesions are removed completely (excision), whereas for larger lesions, a small piece of the lesion is removed (incision).

Direct biopsy by endoscopy-Flexible fiberoptic instruments have improved the techniques of biopsy for inaccessible sites such as the gastrointestinal, genitourinary, and respiratory tracts. Lesions in such locations can be visualized and biopsied safely and simply with little patient discomfort.

Formal surgical procedure-A formal surgical procedure under general anesthesia is often necessary for masses in the lung, kidney, liver, breast, ovary, thyroid, parotid, brain, pancreas, testis, and retroperitoneal tissue.

APPROACHES TO EARLY CANCER DETECTION

In recent years, attempts have been made to detect cancers at an early stage before they cause symptoms. It is hoped that by early diagnosis cure rates will improve. Three general approaches to early cancer detection have been studied: 1. General population screening employs a screening test administered to asymptomatic members of the general population; 2. Selective screening employs the screening test only for members of the population known to be at high risk for developing a particular cancer because of exposure to carcinogens or personal characteristics associated with high risk; 3. Clinical case finding is usually initiated by the patient and the screening test administered as a part of routine medical care.

Cancer screening studies in the U.S. have focused on cancer of the breast, uterine cervix, colon and rectum, mouth, and lung. Analysis of data from these studies has resulted in the following recommendations (Table 2.1) for the use of screening tests in the population.

Table 2.1 Summary of American Cancer Society recommedations for the early detection of cancer in asymptomatic people[2]

Test	Sex	Age	Frequency
Stool guaiac	M & F	50 and over	Every year
Digital rectal exam	M & F	50 and over	Every year
Sigmoidoscpopy	M & F	50 and over	Every 3 to 5 years
Pap test	F	Women who are sexually active or are 18+ years of age should have annual Pap test and pelvic exam.	
Pelvic examination	F	After 3 consecutive negative exams the test can be performed less frequently.	
Breast self-exam	F	20 and over	Every month
Breast physical exam	F	20-40	Every 3 years.
Mammography	F	35-39	Baseline
		40-49	Every 1-2 years
		50 and over	Every year
Chest x-ray		Not recommended for screening	
Health counseling+	M & F	Over 20	Every 3 years

REFERENCES

1. Williams PA. A productive history and physical examination in the prevention and early detection of cancer. Cancer 47:1146-1150,, 1981.

2. 1989 survey of physicians' attitudes and practices in early cancer detection. CA-A Cancer Journal for Clinicians 40:77-101, 1990.

Chapter 3

PATHOLOGY OF CANCER

THE ROLE OF THE PATHOLOGIST

The role of the pathologist is to classify tumors according to histologic type behavior (benign versus malignant), degree of malignancy (grade), and extent (stage).[1]

TERMINOLOGY

Adenocarcinoma--malignant tumor of glandular epithelium

Adenoma--benign tumor of glandular epithelium

Anaplasia--loss of normal cellular organization or differentiation--synonym undifferentiation

Benign--mild or innocent type; refers to a neoplasm that grows slowly, remains localized and usually does little harm

Cachexia--severe wasting of body tissues due to a chronic disease such as cancer

Cancer--malignant tumor

Carcinogen--agent that produces carcinoma

Carcinoma--malignant tumor of epithelium

Carcinoma in-situ--malignant epithelial tumor showing no invasion

Cytology--study of cells; refers to study of cells by Papanicolaou technique

Differentiated--possession by a tumor of cellular maturity and organization similar to normal tissue of origin

Dysplasia--abnormal, atypical cell proliferation; not tumor

Epidermoid carcinoma--cancer of squamous epithelium, i.e., skin, oral mucous membranes

Grade--estimate of degree of malignancy based on microscopic appearance

Lymphoma--tumor arising from lymph tissue

Malignancy--state or quality of being malignant

Malignant--a neoplasm with the ability to invade, metastasize, and cause death

Metastasis--cancerous growth at a site distant from the original primary site

Mixed tumor--a tumor with mixed elements

Neoplasm--new growth, tumor

Occult--hidden; term used to describe a cancer not detected by clinical examination

Oncogenic--tumor producing; term applied mostly to tumor producing viruses

Oncology--the study of tumors

Papilloma--benign epithelial tumor in which neoplastic cells cover finger-like projections of stroma

Polyp--tumor or tumor-like mass projecting from a mucosal surface

Sarcoma--nonepithelial tumor; includes most malignant tumors of mesodermal origin such as connective tissue, muscle, lymph tissue

Squamous carcinoma--synonym for epidermoid carcinoma

Stage--estimate of extent of spread of a cancer

Teratoma--neoplasm composed of numerous types of tissues
Tumor--any swelling; currently used as a synonym for neoplasm
-oma--a suffix that implies tumor, i.e., adenoma, carcinoma, sarcoma

CLASSIFICATION OF TUMORS

Tumors are classified by a combination of two systems. They are classified according to the tissue from which the tumor arose (histogenic classification). The tissue of origin can usually be determined by microscopic examination. In addition, they are classified according to their anticipated biologic behavior. The biologic behavior of a tumor can be predicted from an analysis of microscopic and clinical features, allowing the pathologist to classify the tumor as benign or malignant. Some of the differences between benign and malignant tumors are listed in Table 3.1.

Table 3.1 Characteristics of benign and malignant tumors[1]		
	Benign	**Malignant**
Growth Rate	Slow	Rapid
Mitosis	Few	Many
Nuclear chromatin	Normal	Increased
Differentiation	Normal	Poor
Local growth	Expanding	Invasive
Encapsulation	Present	Absent
Destruction of tissue	Little	Much
Blood vessel invasion	None	Frequent
Metastasis	None	Frequent
Effect on host	Little	Significant

Some examples of tumors classified according to tissue of origin and predicted biologic behavior are shown in Table 3.2.

CHARACTERISTICS OF TUMOR CELLS AND TISSUES

Gross appearance Tumors tend to differ in color, texture, and consistency from the tissue of origin. Benign tumors are usually round or ovoid. They have sharply defined margins and are often encapsulated. They are freely moveable, firm, and uniform in appearance. Malignant tumors, on the other hand, are irregularly shaped with poorly defined margins and have projections from the main growth extending into adjacent tissue so as to make the entire mass fixed. Sarcomas are often fleshy in consistency (like fish flesh), whereas carcinomas are usually hard (like raw potato).

Microscopic appearance The growth patterns and arrangement of cells, compared to the tissue of origin, are important in the recognition and classfication of tumors. The orientation and alignment of the cells of benign tumors are usually similar to that of the tissue of origin. Malignant tumors usually have a microscopic pattern that is considerably different from the tissue of origin. In malignancy, orderly orientation and alignment of the cells are disrupted. In addition, there is often invasion by tumor cells of the supporting connective tissue and blood vessels in malignancy.

Table 3.2 Tumor Classification

Tissue of origin	Benign tumor	Malignant tumor
Connective tissue		
Cartilage	Chondroma	Chondrosarcoma
Bone	Osteoma	Osteosarcoma
Fat	Lipoma	Liposarcoma
Fibrous tissue	Fibroma	Fibrosarcoma
Muscle		
Smooth muscle	Leiomyoma	Leiomyosarcoma
Striated muscle	Rhabdomyoma	Rhabdomyosarcoma
Endothelium		
Lymph vessels	Lymphangioma	Lymphangiosarcoma
Blood vessels	Hemangioma	Hemangiosarcoma
Lymph tissue	None recognized	Lymphoma
Bone marrow	None recognized	Leukemia
Neural tissue		
Glial tissue	Glioma	Malignant glioma
Nerve cells	None recognized	Neuroblastoma
Nerve sheath	Neurilemmoma	Neurogenic sarcoma
Epithelium		
Squamous epithelium	Papilloma	Squamous cell carcinoma
Transitional epithelium	Papilloma	Transitional cell carcinoma
Glandular epithelium	Adenoma	Adenocarcinoma

The appearance of the cytoplasm and nuclei of the cells of benign tumors also differs from malignant tumors. Cells of benign tumors differ from the tissue of origin, whereas malignant cells tend to be larger than normal, have irregular borders, and vary in size and shape (pleomorphism). The nuclei of malignant cells are usually larger and more irregularly shaped and the chromatin (DNA fixed to protein) is more densely staining. The nuceloli are more prominent and mitosis is more frequent. The cytoplasm of malignant cells often lacks the characteristic features of the normal cells of the tissue of origin such as mucus, keratin, or cross striations, and it may have more open space (vacuoles) than normal.

The microscopic appearance of individual malignant cells differs so markedly from normal cells that they can be recognized individually as malignant. This fact is the basis of the technique known as exfoliative cytology (Papanicolaou technique). Malignant cells are less cohesive than normal cells and are readily shed (exfoliated) from the surface of the tumor. These can be collected, stained and recognized by the pathologist as malignant. The Papanicolaou technique has allowed tumors to be diagnosed at an early stage, often before they are detectable clinically. This technique has found its greatest application in the early diagnosis of cervix cancer.

Tumor stroma In addition to tumor cells, tumors consist of a supporting network of blood vessels and connective tissue. The stroma originates from the normal tissues of the host and may vary greatly in amount. In general, rapidly growing tumors such as sarcomas have a large number of blood vessels with little connective tissue, whereas slowly growing tumors tend to be less vascular. Some tumors contain a large amount of connective tissue (desmoplasia) and are called scirrhous cancers.

Biochemistry and function of tumor cells Attempts to detect basic biochemical differences between tumor cells and normal cells have been unsuccessful. Furthermore, most tumor cells do not produce specific enzymes, proteins, or metabolic alterations which would be of value in tumor diagnosis.

Tumor cells usually use their energy for proliferation, but often produce intracellular substances such as keratin in squamous cell carcinoma or mucin in adenocarcinoma. Extracellular material such as osteoid in osteosarcoma and cartilage matrix in chondrosarcoma can also be produced.

Neoplastic cells can also produce excessive amounts of enzymes. For example, prostate cancers often produce acid phosphatase which is detected in the serum of patients with disseminated prostate cancer. Also, serum amylase is often elevated in patients with pancreatic carcinoma.

Tumors of endocrine organs can produce excessive amounts of hormones. For example, in acromegaly the pituitary tumor produces excessive amounts of growth hormone, and in hyperparathyroidism excessive parathyroidhormone is produced by the parathyroid tumor. Hormones can also be produced by nonendocrine tumors. For example, small cell lung cancers occasionally produce antidiuretic hormone (ADH) or adrenocorticotrophic hormone (ACTH).

PRECANCEROUS CONDITIONS

Precancerous states are those in which cancer has not yet developed, but the risk of future cancer development is great. Precancerous changes can often be recognized histologically and are called dysplasia or atypical hyperplasia. In dysplasia, the pathologist sees disorderly maturation of cells with irregular shapes and sizes. Dysplasia can be recognized microscopically in tissue preparations and in Papanicolaou smears. It is a reversible process which can be induced by chronic inflammation. Dysplasia can precede by many years, cancers of the cervix, mouth and lung.

TUMOR BEHAVIOR

Growth rate Benign tumors usually grow slowly and may require many years to reach large size. Malignant tumors usually grow rapidly and reach a large size within weeks or months. An estimate of the growth rate of a tumor can be obtained microscopically by counting the number of mitoses per 1000 cells. Twenty or more mitoses per 1000 cells is common in malignant tumors, whereas in benign tumors and normal tissues there is usually less than one mitosis per 1000 cells.

An estimate of the growth rate of a tumor can also be made from measurements of its doubling time (the time required for a tumor to double in size). For some rapidly growing tumors, i.e., Burkitt's lymphoma, the doubling time may be only five days whereas other tumors have doubling times as long as 200 days. Other factors, in addition to cell division, can influence the growth rate of a tumor including hemorrhage, edema, death of cells due to insufficient blood supply and the presence of bacterial infection.

Local growth and invasion All tumors grow by expansion resulting in increased bulk with compression of surrounding tissues. Most benign tumors push the surrounding tissue aside and the compressed tissue forms a capsule around the tumor with well-defined margins. Malignant tumors usually invade and destroy the surrounding tissues yielding margins that are ill-defined and irregular. Invasiveness is a characteristic of malignant cells, but the mechanism of the invasiveness is not understood. It is thought that cancer cells produce substances such as enzymes or other factors which modify the stroma at the margins of the tumor making the tissues more vulnerable to invasion. The capacity of tumor cells to invade tissues at a distance from the main tumor mass is a problem for the surgeons and radiotherapists. Surgical excision of a malignant tumor must include a wide margin of normal tissues to ensure removal of cells which have invaded beyond the mass of tumor. Likewise, the margins of radiation fields around a tumor must be great enough to include these cells. If all such extensions of the tumor are not removed or irradiated a local recurrence is certain.

Metastasis Metastasis is the process by which malignant cells (1) invade blood vessels and tissue spaces, (2) detach and migrate or be transported to a distant site, and (3) settle in the new site to grow into a secondary tumor mass. The most common route for metastatic spread of cancer is through lymphatic vessels. Carcinomas tend to favor this route whereas sarcomas tend to metastasize via the venous system. Metastatic spread can take place by continuous growth along lymphatic vessels which is known as lymphatic permeation. Lymphatic permeation along nerves can also occur.

The most common method of lymphatic metastasis is embolization of detached cancer cells in lymph vessels to regional lymph nodes. The cancer cells then grow in the lymph nodes resulting in lymph node enlargement and eventual replacement of the entire lymph node by the secondary tumor growth. Tumors usually metastasize initially to regional lymph nodes, so that with a knowledge of the primary site one can predict the probable routes of lymphatic spread. For example, carcinoma of the breast usually metastasizes to axillary lymph nodes and carcinoma of the lower lip metastasizes to submental lymph nodes.

Metastasis via blood vessels is common for sarcomas but carcinomas also frequently metastasize in this way. Carcinomas of the lung, breast, kidney, prostate, and thyroid are particularly likely to metastasize via blood vessels. Since it is easier for tumor cells to invade veins than arteries, the venous route is the usual pathway of tumor embolization. Blood-borne emboli of single cells or aggregates of tumor cells can occur

Metastasis through serous cavities is common with some cancers. For example, in carcinoma of the ovary, cancer cells become detached from the surface of the tumor to spread throughout the peritoneal cavity. Metastasis via the cerebrospinal fluid can also occur. This route is particularly common with a rare brain tumor of childhood called medulloblastoma.

GRADING OF TUMORS

The pathologist can make an estimate of the degree of malignancy or grade of a tumor by evaluating certain microscopic characteristics of the tumor. Two factors are considered in the microscopic grading of a tumor: (1) the degree of anaplasia or undifferentiation and (2) an estimate of the rate of growth. Customarily, tumors are graded on a scale of 1 to 3 or 4 where the lower numbers signify a lesser degree of malignancy.

Estimation of the degree of differentiation is based on how much the tumor resembles the tissue of origin. For example, a well-differentiated grade 1 tumor arising from squamous epithelium forms large amounts of keratin and intercellular bridges, whereas a poorly differentiated grade 3 tumor has very little keratin and no intercellular bridges.

Evidence of rapidity of growth is based on the number of mitoses per unit of tissue i.e., per one microscopic field of view at high power. For example, a grade 1 squamous cell carcinoma has less than two mitoses per high-power field, whereas a grade 3 tumor has more than four mitoses per high-power field. The main value of determining the grade of a tumor is in predicting outcome or prognosis. However, for some cancers, i.e., endometrial carcinoma, it is also used in choosing therapy.

THE EFFECT OF TUMORS ON THE HOST

Benign tumors primarily affect the host because of their size and location. A large benign tumor may be a cosmetic problem or it may compress important structures. Some benign tumors are also harmful to the host because they produce excessive amounts of hormone, i.e., adenomas of the pituitary gland can produce excessive growth hormone.

Malignant tumors also affect the host because of their size and location. In addition, malignant tumors are more likely than benign tumors to become necrotic (dead cells) and ulcerated leading to hemorrhage and anemia. Furthermore, when cancer becomes disseminated the patient becomes weakened and susceptible to infections such as pneumonia.

Many patients with cancer develop extreme wasting and malnutrition, a condition called cachexia. Cachexia is caused by a number of factors including infection, hemorrhage, necrosis of tissue with release of toxins, reduced immunity, poor appetite, sleeplessness and anxiety. Usually a number of these factors are present in patients with disseminated disease.

The mechanisms of host resistance to the development and growth of tumors are not well understood. There is a wide range of virulence or aggressiveness of cancers of the same clinical and histologic type. Some seem to behave more aggressively in the young, whereas others are more aggressive in the elderly. Hormones can influence the behavior of certain cancers. The adequacy of blood supply is also important for tumor growth. Furthermore, host immunity can influence the rate of tumor growth.

Finally, there is a wide range of other systemic affects of cancer which are only rarely seen. In some patients, the tumor cells produce substances which cause characteristic alterations in the blood and blood-forming organs, skin, brain and peripheral nerves, or muscles and skeletal system.

REFERENCES

1. Diamandopoulos GT, Meissner WA. Chapter 15, Neoplasia, in Anderson's Pathology, Eighth Edition, Ed. Kissane JM, The C.V. Mosby Company, St. Louis, 1985, pp 514-559.

Chapter 4

STAGING OF CANCER

INTRODUCTION

Decisions regarding proper therapy for cancer are made only after a careful assessment of the anatomic extent of disease for each individual patient. This assessment of the extent of disease is called the stage of disease. Determination of the stage of disease, for some tumor types, can be made by simple methods such as the physical examination and routine radiographic studies. For most patients, however, specialized methods, such as surgical procedures or special radiographic investigations are required to accurately assess the extent of disease.

STAGING

Staging of cancer is based on the concept that each cancer has a life history that is definable in time from beginning to end. The early life is silent, but eventually the tumor becomes large enough to cause signs and symptoms and be diagnosed. The size and extent of the primary tumor, designated by the letter T in the staging system, increases continually throughout this time and the measurement of its size and extent is an important part of the staging classification. The description of the T stage system for each tumor type is published by the American Joint Committee on Cancer and will not be repeated here.[1] However, for each tumor type, the T stage is designated numerically from T1 to T4 depending on the extent of the tumor.

As the primary tumor increases in size, local invasion is followed by spread to regional lymph nodes draining the primary. The detection of regional lymph node spread is, therefore, another important part of the staging process. The status of disease in regional lymph nodes is designated by the letter N. The N stages increase from N1 to N3 depending on the extent of nodal disease.

Late in the life history of each cancer distant spread or metastasis becomes evident. Distant metastasis, the third part of the staging classifications, is designated by the letter M. In the staging system, the absence of distant metastasis is designated MO whereas the presence of distant metastasis is indicated as M1.

The TNM system provides a basis for categorizing disease extent and is the system used to classify most tumor types. The classification is extended by the following designations:

TUMOR
      TX   Tumor extent cannot be assessed
      TO   No evidence of a primary tumor
      T1, T2, T3,T4 Progressive increase in tumor size
NODES
      NX   Regional lymph nodes cannot be assessed
      NO   Regional lymph nodes normal
      N1, N2, N3 Increasing degrees of lymph node involvement
METASTASIS
      MX   Cannot be assessed
      MO   No known distant metastasis
      M1   Distant metastasis present. Specify sites of metastasis.

The final step in the staging process is the reduction of the TNM classification into a single numerical indicator of disease extent. In general, the stage I label indicates that the primary tumor is small and there are no nodal or distant metastasis. Stage II indicates that the primary tumor is still relatively small but there are early nodal metastasis and no distant metastasis. Stage III indicates that the primary and nodal disease are more extensive but there are still no distant metastasis. Stage IV indicates that either the primary and/or nodal disease is very advanced or there are distant metastasis present.

For cancer at sites which can be examined easily the extent of disease should be determined before treatment. Cancers of the cervix, larynx and oral cavity are customarily staged before treatment. For cancers at sites not easily examined such as ovary, stomach, colon, kidney and lung, it is customary to stage the disease after surgical exploration, resection of the diseased organ and histopathologic study of the involved tissues by the pathologist.

Staging classifications are based on the observation that survival time and cure rates for a particular cancer are greater for patients whose disease is of lesser extent than for those whose disease is of greater extent. Thus, the usefulness of a staging classification is primarily in predicting prognosis for each patient. The stage is also used in choosing therapy since treatment results for each modality often vary with disease extent. Another important reason for determining the stage for each patient is that treatment results for a particular treatment method can be compared with other methods only if the patients are uniformly staged according to an accepted, widely used classification system.

REFERENCE

1. Manual for Staging of Cancer, Third Edition, Eds. Beahrs OH, Henson DE, Hutter RV, Myers MH, J.B. Lippincott Company, Philadelphia, 1988.

Chapter 5

SURGERY FOR CANCER
GENERAL PRINCIPLES

INTRODUCTION

Surgery is the oldest cancer treatment modality and until recent years was the only curative modality. The surgeon has a central role in the diagnosis, staging and treatment of cancer and in the rehabilitation of the patient following successful treatment. The basic principles underlying each of these roles is discussed in this chapter.

DIAGNOSIS AND STAGING

The role of the surgeon in cancer management usually begins with obtaining tissue for histologic diagnosis. The surgeon can perform a biopsy as a small procedure or as part of a larger operation on the chest or abdomen. The surgeon's role in diagnosis does not end with the procedure itself, however, because consultation with the pathologist is often necessary in cases where the microscopic appearances of the tumor are ambiguous or in cases where the histologic diagnosis does not fit the clinical picture.

In recent years, surgery has played an increasingly important role in the staging of cancer. In some cases, operations are performed at a considerable distance from the known tumor for the purpose of obtaining biopsy specimens to find small foci of cancer undetectable by radiographic methods. For example, it is common for patients with Hodgkin's disease involving lymph nodes in the neck or chest to undergo an abdominal operation, called a staging laparotomy, to remove the spleen and obtain samples of lymph nodes, liver and bone for histologic study. The findings from the staging laparotomy are of critical importance in selecting proper therapy. If small foci of Hodgkin's disease are found in the liver, bone or spleen, chemotherapy may be needed, whereas if no foci of disease are found in the abdomen, radiotherapy may be the treatment of choice.

TREATMENT OF CANCER

The role of surgery in the treatment of cancer patients can be categorized as follows:[1]
1) Treatment for the primary cancer
2) Surgery to reduce the bulk of residual disease.

3) Resection of metastatic disease with intent to cure
4) Treatment of oncologic emergencies
5) Surgery for palliation
6) Reconstruction and rehabilitation

Surgery for primary cancer If the tumor is treatable by surgery, the surgeon must assess the patient to determine whether the tumor is operable or inoperable. A tumor might be considered inoperable for a number of reasons: 1) it may be so large that it is technically impossible to resect it; 2) it may be technically resectable, but of a type that is rarely cured by surgery; 3) the tumor may be situated anatomically in an area that cannot be approached surgically for cancer resection; 4) there is evidence of distant metastasis.

The surgeon must assess the patient's physiologic and psychologic status before proceeding with a cancer operation. For example, a patient with poor pulmonary function may not be able to withstand the removal of an entire lung. In this situation it might be better to use radiotherapy rather than surgery. In another example, a woman with major concerns about her body image might not be emotionally able to tolerate removal of an entire breast. In this case, a limited breast operation followed by radiotherapy to the entire breast may be preferable.

In most situations, therefore, a number of therapeutic options are available to the surgeon. These options should be presented to the patient so that his or her concerns can be taken into consideration in choosing an operation which is suited to the individual patient's needs.

An operation designed to remove all known tumor is called a curative resection. The basic principle of cancer surgery is that the primary tumor must be totally excised without cutting across the margins of the tumor, which would cause contamination of the wound by tumor cells, resulting in local recurrence. In many situations the regional lymph vessels and nodes are removed with the primary tumor to increase the likelihood that cancer cells are removed from the body.

Surgery to reduce tumor bulk. In some cases local spread of disease is so extensive that removal of all known disease is impossible. Surgical resection of bulky masses, called debulking, to reduce the body burden of cancer may lead to an improved response to chemotherapy. However, evidence that this approach improves treatment results is available for only a few tumor types such as ovarian carcinoma and a rare form of lymphoma called Burkitt's lymphoma.

Surgery for metastasis Soft tissue sarcomas, osteosarcomas, malignant melanoma, and testicular carcinomas frequently metastasize to lungs. Single lung metastasis, without demonstrable metastasis elsewhere in the body, can be removed for cure. Single metastasis to the brain from colon cancer, melanoma of the skin and other sites can occasionally be removed resulting in cure of the patient. Partial liver resection for single metastasis to the liver from colon cancer can result in cure.

Oncologic emergencies Emergencies may arise in cancer patients that require surgical treatment. Operations may be needed for the treatment of hemorrhage, bowel perforation or obstruction, bile duct obstruction, drainage of abscesses, or impending destruction of vital organs. An operation to remove bone surrounding the spinal cord, called laminectomy, may be needed to relieve spinal cord compression caused by metastatic tumor growth in the spinal canal.

Palliation Tumors that are considered to be resectable by preparative clinical assessment may be discovered to be unrsectable at the time of operation because of direct extension to near-by vital organs or detection of distant metastasis. In this situation, it may be desirable to proceed with the resection of the primary tumor to relieve present or prevent future symptoms. Such operations are called palliative resections because known residual cancer remains at the conclusion of the operation.

Indirect operations are often performed to remove endocrine organs for palliative treatment of hormonally sensitive tumors. For example, the ovaries are often removed in an operation called oophorectomy to treat metastatic breast cancer by removing the major source of estrogen. Furthermore, the testicles may be removed in an operation called orchiectomy to treat metastatic prostate cancer by removing the major androgen producing organs.

Reconstruction and rehabilitation Surgical operations have been developed to assist cancer patients in their rehabilitation following radical therapy. Surgeons can reconstruct anatomic defects using free flaps and microvascular techniques to bring fresh tissue to resected or heavily irradiated areas to improve function and cosmetic appearance.

RECURRENT CANCER

Operations may be required later in the course of the patient's disease and in some situations, such operations may be curative. For example, local recurrences of cancers of the oral cavity or uterine cervix developing after radiotherapy may occasionally be completely removed.

An operation to explore the abdomen in the absence of clinically apparent recurrent cancer is called a "second-look" operation. Second-look operations are performed for the purpose of removing recurrent cancer while it is still small. This practice assumes that it is much easier to resect a tumor before it becomes large enough to cause symptoms or be detectable by radiographic studies. Cancers of the colon and ovary are the tumors for which second-look procedures have been most frequently used. However, the value of second-look operations in improving the overall cure rates for these diseases has not been proven.

CONCLUSION

Surgery has a major role in the diagnosis and treatment of cancer. Surgeons must have broad experience in cancer treatment and be familiar with the results of other modalities and have a close working relationship with the other cancer specialists on the multidisciplinary team so that a balanced, well thought-out plan of treatment for each patient is arrived at.

REFERENCE

1. Rosenberg SA. Chapter 14, Principles of Surgical Oncology, in Cancer: Principles and Practice of Oncology, 3rd Edition, Eds. DeVita VT, Hellman S, Rosenberg SA. J.B. Lippincott Company, Philadelphia, 1989, pp. 236-246.

Chapter 6

BASIC PHYSICS OF RADIOTHERAPY

INTRODUCTION

The role of radiotherapy in oncology cannot be appreciated without a basic knowledge of physics. What follows, therefore, is background material designed to assist in comprehension of material presented in subsequent chapters. The reader is referred to the classic texts for a complete presentation of the role of physics in radiology. [1,2]

THE STRUCTURE OF MATTER

All matter consists of atoms.[1] There are more than 100 known kinds of atoms. Each atom has a small dense nucleus surrounded by electrons which circle in orbits around the nucleus. The electrons are small compared to the nucleus but they occupy a great deal of space. Atoms differ from one another in the make-up of their nuclei and in the number and arrangement of their electrons.

There are two fundamental particles within the nucleus of atoms (Table 6.1). They are called protons and neutrons. Protons and neutrons have nearly the

Table 6.1 Properties of fundamental particles			
Particle	Mass	Charge	Properties
Alpha	4.003	+2	The nucleus of the helium atom
Proton	1.007277	+1	The nucleus of the hydrogen atom
Neutron	1.008665	0	Difficult to stop and to detect
Electron	0.000548	-1	Abound in nature. Sometimes called beta particles
Positron	0.000548	+1	Exist in nature only while in motion
Photon	0	0	Photons are not particles but bundles of energy

same mass which is about 1900 times that of electrons. Protons carry a positive charge whereas neutrons carry no charge. Electrons carry a negative charge. Since atoms are electrically neutral, there must be one proton in the nucleus for every electron outside the nucleus. The atomic number (Z) of an atom corresponds to the number of protons in the nucleus and the number of electrons outside the nucleus. The mass number of an atom (A) corresponds to the total number of protons and neutrons in the nucleus. Atoms composed of the same number of protons but different number of neutrons are called isotopes. Isotopes have the same number of electrons and, therefore, cannot be separated by chemical methods. Since isotopes have different mass numbers, however, they can be separated by physical devices such as the mass spectrometer.

Isotopes may be stable or unstable. The nuclei of unstable isotopes have an uneven number of protons and neutrons. This unbalance eventually results in the ejection of a particle, a process which is called disintegration. Another term for disintegration is radioactivity. Nuclei will continue to eject particles until a stable isotope is formed.

EXTRANUCLEAR STRUCTURE

The electrons of atoms move about the nucleus in orbits or shells. The positively charged nucleus attracts the negatively charged electrons causing them to move in orbits much the same as the earth moves about the sun. The orbits or shells are designated with letters of the alphabet beginning with K. In general, chemical properties of atoms are determined by the number of electrons in the outermost shell. Atoms with completely filled outer shells tend to be very stable. If the outer shell of an atom is not filled the atom will react with any atom which can supply electrons to the outer shell. If there are excess electrons in the outer shell the atom will react with atoms which can accept the excess electrons.

ATOMIC ENERGY LEVELS

The orbits of electrons moving about the nucleus of an atom are characterized by having a definite energy. For example, the binding energies of the electrons in the K, L, and M shells of the metal tungsten are 70,000 ev, 11,000 ev, and 2500 ev respectively.

The electron volt (ev) is a unit of energy. It is the amount of energy released when an electron falls through a potential difference of 1 volt. In radiology, a unit 1 million times as large as the ev, the million electron volt (MeV) is more useful than the ev.

To remove an electron from the K shell of a tungsten atom at least 70,000 ev of energy are required. However, if an electron is removed from the K shell an electron from one of the outer orbits will fall into its space and when this happens energy in the form of electromagnetic radiation (an x-ray) is released.

ELECTROMAGNETIC RADIATION

Light waves, heat waves, radio waves, ultraviolet waves, x-rays, and gamma rays are all forms of electromagnetic radiation (Table 6.2). Electromagnetic radiations of all kinds are made up of small bundles of energy called

Table 6.2 The electromagnetic spectrum

Wave type	Frequency (cycles/ sec)	Wavelength (cm = centimeters) (A = Angstrom)	Photon Energy (ev = electron volts) (MeV = million ev)
Radio waves	1.0×10^5	3×10^5 cm	4×10^{-10} ev
Infrared radiation	3.0×10^{10}	.01 cm	.0124 ev
Visible light	4.3×10^{14}	7000A	1.77 ev
Ultraviolet light	7.5×10^{14}	4000A	3.1 ev
Diagnostic x-rays	3.0×10^{18}	1A	12,400 ev
Radium gamma rays	3.0×10^{20}	.01A	1.24 MeV
X-rays from linear accelerator	3.0×10^{21}	.001A	12.4 MeV

photons which travel in waves with a velocity of 3.0×10^8 meters/second or 186,000 miles per second in a vacuum. The electromagnetic waves of interest in radiology have a very short wavelength (distance between wave peaks) and the frequency is large (the number of waves passing a fixed point per second). As the wavelength becomes shorter the energy associated with one photon becomes larger.

RADIOACTIVITY

The protons and neutrons in the nuclei of atoms are in constant motion and energy is continually transfered between the particles. In stable nuclei, the particles never acquire sufficient energy to overcome the forces of attraction which holds the particles in the nuclei, but if a large number of radioactive nuclei of a given element are present, it can be predicted that a certain percentage will disintegrate per unit time. In the disintegration process alpha particles (helium atoms), beta particles (electrons), and /or gamma rays may be emitted.

For atoms with Z numbers less than 82 (lead), there is usually at least one stable isotope, but all elements with Z numbers greater than lead are radioactive. They decay through a series of disintegrations to form stable isotopes of lead. Some radioactive elements such as radium and uranium occur naturally, whereas others are produced artificially by bombarding stable nuclei with neutrons, protons, deuterons, alpha particles, or gamma rays in devices such as nuclear reactors, cyclotrons or linear accelerators.

The radioactivity of a radioactive source is defined as the number of disintegrations per unit time. The special SI unit of activity is the becquerel (Bq):

1 Bq = 1 distintegration per second. Another useful unit activity is the curie (Ci): 1 Ci = 3.7 X 1020 ^{Bq}. These units are named after the physicists who discovered radioactivity (Becquerel) and radium (Curie).

Radionuclides (radioactive isotopes) decay at a constant rate with half-lives ranging from microseconds to millions of years. For example, radium decays with a half-life of 1622 years to the radioactive gas, radon. Radon, in turn, decays with a half-life of 3.83 days by a complicated decay scheme to yield seven daughter products consisting of isotopes of lead, bismuth, and plutonium. During the decay process alpha and beta particles and gamma rays are emitted. The gamma ray spectrum is complicated consisting of 12 different energies, but for clinical purposes can be considered as consisting of two energy peaks at 0.55 and 1.65 MeV. For clinical use, the radium is encapsulated in platinum which absorbs the alpha and beta particles and allows the gamma rays to pass through. The half-lives and photon energies of a number of radionuclides which are used in radiotherapy are shown in Table 6.3.

WHAT IS IONIZING RADIATION?

The absorption of energy from a radiation beam by matter may result in excitation or ionization in the atoms of the irradiated material. If the electrons of the atoms in the irradiated material are merely raised to a higher energy level the process is called excitation. If, however, the radiation has sufficient energy to eject electrons from the atoms the process is referred to as ionization. The importance of ionization is that a relatively large amount of energy is released

Table 6.3 Half-life and photon energy for gamma ray sources used in radiotherapy

Radionuclide	Photon energy (MeV)	Half-life
Cesium ^{137}	0.662	30 years
Cobalt ^{60}	1.17-1.33	5.26 years
Gold ^{198}	0.41-1.06	2.70 days
Iodine ^{125}	0.035	60.25 days
Iridium ^{192}	0.14-1.06	74.20 days
Radium ^{226}	0.047-2.44	1622 years

locally (33 ev per ionizing event). As far as the radiobiological effects of radiation are concerned, electromagnetic radiation is considered ionizing if the energy of the photons exceeds 124 ev corresponding to a wavelength shorter than 10^{-6}cm.

ABSORPTION OF ELECTROMAGNETIC RADIATIONS

Photoelectric absorption is the predominate process by which energy is absorbed from an x-ray beam at energies used in diagnostic radiology (<100 KeV). By this process the x-ray photon interacts with one of the tightly bound

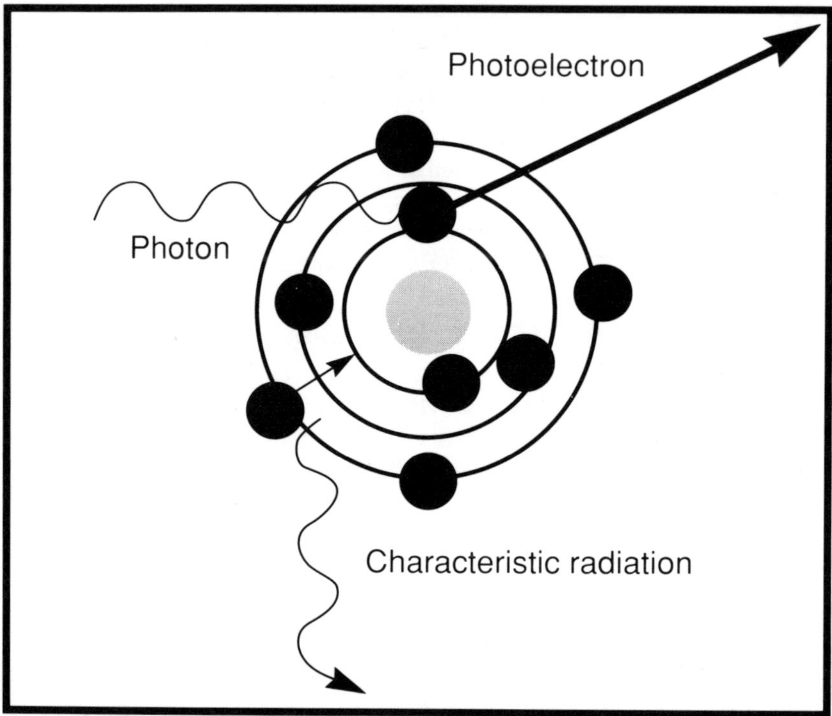

Figure 6.1 Photoelectric absorption results in emission of characteristic x-rays and photoelectrons from the ionized atoms. They, in turn, ionize other atoms.

electrons close to the nucleus of the atom (Figure 6.1). The photon gives up its energy entirely to the electron which is ejected with a kinetic energy equal to that of the photon, minus the binding energy which previously held the electron in the atom. The electron vacancy is filled by an electron from another electron orbit or by a free electron from outside the atom. When an electron changes energy levels the difference in energy is emitted as a low energy x-ray.

Compton absorption is the predominant process by which energy is absorbed from high energy beams used in radiotherapy. In Compton absorption the photon interacts with electrons in the outer orbits of the atom (Figure 6.2). These electrons have a low binding energy compared to that of the photon. Part of the photon energy is given to the electron as kinetic energy and the photon is

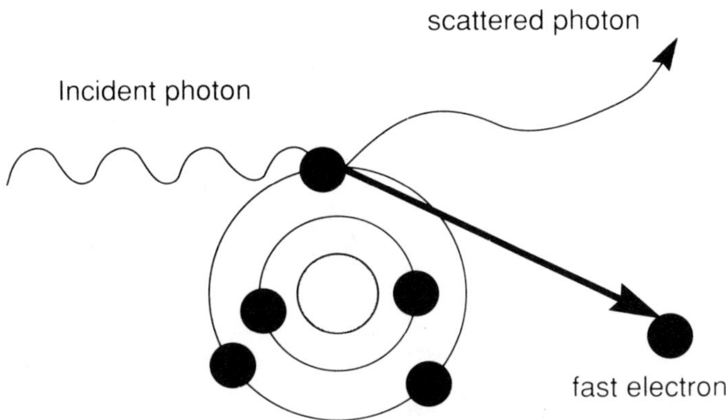

Figure 6.2 Compton absorption results in scattered photons and fast electrons which ionize other atoms.

deflected from its original path and continues at reduced energy. In place of the original photon, therefore, is a fast electron and a photon of reduced energy both of which can undergo additional interactions. The net result is the production of a large number of fast electrons which ionize other atoms of the absorbing material.

The photoelectric and Compton absorption processes differ from each other in one important way. The mass absorption coefficient (the proportion by which the intensity of an x-ray beam is reduced by an absorber) varies with the atomic number (Z) of the absorbing material. The Compton process of absorption is independent of the atomic number of the absorbing material. This has an important influence on clinical application of x-rays in the photoelectric and Compton energy ranges. For diagnostic radiology, x-rays in the photoelectric range are useful because increased absorption in high (Z) materials such as calcium in bone, yields radiographs with contrast between air, soft tissues and bone. On the other hand, in radiotherapy, high energy photons are preferred because in this range the Compton process predominates, resulting in relatively uniform absorption throughout the volume of tissue irradiated.

Pair production is the third process in radiation absorption. When the energy of the incident photon is greater than 1.02 MeV the photon may be absorbed through this mechanism. When the photon passes near the nucleus of the atom and is subjected to the strong field of the nucleus it may disappear as a photon and become a positively charged electron (positron) and a negatively charged electron pair (Figure 6.3). This is an excellent example of the conversion

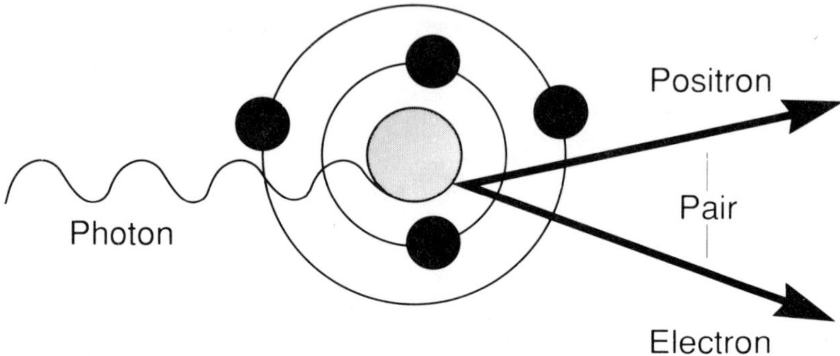

Figure 6.3 Pair production results in release of a positron and electron each with 1.022 MeV of energy.

of energy into matter. Although the threshold for pair production is 1.022 MeV, this mechanism is not the predominant type of absorption until energies of 50-100 MeV are reached.

If photoelectric absorption is present, bone will absorb six times more energy gram for gram than soft tissue. If Compton absorption alone is present bone and soft tissue will absorb equal amounts of energy gram for gram. If pair production alone is present, bone absorbs about two times as much energy gram for gram.

Although the differences between the absorption mechanisms have practical significance in radiology, the radiobiologic significance is minimal. Regardless of whether the absorption process is photoelectric, Compton or pair production, most of the absorbed photon energy is converted to the kinetic energy of fast electrons.

ABSORPTION OF NEUTRONS

Neutrons are uncharged particles and for this reason they are highly penetrating. They are absorbed by different mechanisms than x-rays. They interact with the nuclei of the atoms of the absorbing material and set in motion fast recoil protons, alpha particles, and heavier nuclear fragments. Elastic scattering is the dominant absorption process at neutron energies of 100 KeV to 20 MeV. By this process, neutrons collide with the nuclei of the atoms of the absorber resulting in transfer of a portion of the kinetic energy of the neutron to the nucleus. In soft tissues interaction between neutrons and hydrogen nuclei, the most abundant atoms in tissue, is the dominant means of energy transfer. The hydrogen nuclei (recoil protons) are set in motion after interacting with the neutrons and as they pass through tissue they lose energy by excitation and ionization.

Inelastic scattering begins to occur at neutron energies above 6 MeV. By this process, the neutrons interact with carbon nuclei to produce three alpha particles or with oxygen nuclei to produce four alpha particles. These are called spallation products. Spallation products are densely ionizing and have an important effect on the biologic damage produced.

RADIATION UNITS USED IN RADIOLOGY

Exposure is the quantity which describes the output of an x-ray or gamma ray generator. It is the charge which results when a unit mass of air is exposed to ionizing radiation. An important milestone in radiology occurred in 1937 when the Fifth International Congress of Radiology accepted the roentgen as an international dosage unit for x-ray or gamma exposure. The roentgen (R) is equivalent to one electrostatic unit of electricity liberated from 1 cc of air at standard temperature and pressure (0 degrees C, 760 mm Hg) upon exposure to ionizing radiation. More recently, it has been recommended that exposure be expressed in SI units as coulombs per kilogram (C/kg) where $1R = 2.58 \times 10^{-4}$ Ckg^{-1}.

In 1953, the Seventh International Congress of Radiology adopted the rad as the unit of absorbed dose of any ionizing radiation equal to 100 ergs of energy absorbed per gram of any absorber. The energy absorbed per gram of air exposed to one roentgen = 0.869 rad. Recently, a special SI unit called the gray (Gy) has been introduced to replace the rad as the unit of absorbed dose. One Gy is equivalent to one Joule per kilogram (J/kg). The Gy is related to the rad and 1 Gy= 100 rad.

REFERENCES

1. Johns HE, Cunningham JR. The Physics of Radiology, Fourth Edition. Charles C. Thomas, Springfield Illinois, 1983.

2. Khan FM. The Physics of Radiation Therapy. Williams & Wilkins, Baltimore 1984.

Chapter 7

BASIC RADIATION CHEMISTRY
AND BIOLOGY

DIRECT VS INDIRECT IONIZATION

Ionizing radiation may be classified as directly or indirectly ionizing.[1] Charged particles are directly ionizing because they are capable of directly disrupting the atomic structure through which they pass to produce chemical and biological changes. Electromagnetic radiations such as x-rays and gamma rays are indirectly ionizing because they do not themselves produce chemical or biologic damage. When passing through tissue they interact with electrons in the atoms of the tissue and give up some of their energy to the electrons. These fast moving electrons are capable of producing ionization in the tissue resulting in chemical and biological injury.

COMPARISON BETWEEN PHOTONS AND PARTICLES

When ionizing radiations deposit energy in tissue, ionizing events tend to be localized along the tracks of the ionizing particles in a pattern which depends on the type of radiation involved. The tracks of fast electrons produced by the absorption of photons are marked by ionizing events which are spatially well-separated. Therefore, x- and gamma rays are sparsely ionizing. On the other hand, alpha particles give rise to ionizing events which are close together resulting in well-defined columns of ionization. Alpha particles, therefore, are densely ionizing. Neutrons give rise to tracks of intermediate ionizing density. Linear energy transfer (LET) is a term which refers to the energy transferred per unit of length of the track. X- and gamma rays are low LET radiations whereas alpha particles and neutrons are high LET radiations.

EFFECTS OF IONIZING RADIATION ON MOLECULES

In general, all types of ionizing radiations produce similar chemical effects, but it is important to distinguish between molecules which have been ionized directly by the incident radiation and those which have received the energy by transfer from another molecule. [2] The two processes are referred to as the direct and indirect effects of radiation. These direct and indirect effects should not be confused with the direct and indirect effects of ionization previously discussed. The indirect effect of radiation is important in materials such as tissue in which water is the most abundant molecule. In tissue, a water molecule may be ionized and then transfer its acquired energy to another molecule. The change in the second molecule is indirect.

FORMATION OF ION PAIRS

When an electron is ejected from a molecule a positive ion and a negative electron result, both of which contain energy:

$$A \rightarrow A^+ + e^-$$

The electron is rapidly captured by another molecule to yield a negative ion:

$$e^- + B \rightarrow B^-$$

The result of these events is the formation of two ions:

$$A + B \rightarrow A^+ + B^-$$

The positive and negative ions are referred to as the ion pair.

FORMATION OF FREE RADICALS

Ion pairs have a very short life ($<10^{-10}$ second). They then undergo further reactions to form free radicals. For example: $CD^- \rightarrow C^- + D^0$ where C^- is an ion having little energy and D^0 is a free radical with considerable energy. Free radicals are intermediaries between ion pairs and final chemical products. They are extremely reactive because they possess an unpaired electron in one of their outer orbits.

RADIATION EFFECTS ON WATER

Most biological systems are composed of about 80% water. The reaction for the radiation breakdown or radiolysis of water is:[3]

$$H_2O \rightarrow H_2O^{+0} + e^- \qquad (1)$$
$$e^- \rightarrow e_{aq}^- \qquad (2)$$
$$H_2O^+ + H_2O \rightarrow OH^0 + H_3O \qquad (3)$$

REACTIONS IN AQUEOUS (WATER) SOLUTIONS

When ionizing radiation interacts with a system such as tissue, the largest or most numerous molecules will be most often ionized because they occupy the greatest proportion of the volume. In a diluted aqueous solution, since most of the molecules are H_2O, most of the ionizations will occur in water molecules and the effect on the solute (dissolved substance) will be primarily indirect. The H_2O^{+0}, e_{aq}^-, or OH^0 radicals can have a variety of effects on the other molecules in the system. However, when an aqueous organic (carbon-containing molecule) solution is irradiated, the usual indirect reaction on the organic molecule is the removal of either the H atom or an entire radical group (such as the -CH3 "methyl" group) from the molecule. The general reaction for removal of a hydrogen atom is:

$$RH + OH^0 \rightarrow R^0 + H^2O.$$

Although breaks between carbon and hydrogen atoms are most common, carbon-carbon (C-C), carbon-oxygen (C-O), carbon-nitrogen (C-N), and carbon-sulfur (C-S) cleavages also occur.

MACROMOLECULAR REACTIONS

As a result of these chemical changes, very large molecules may undergo structural changes resulting in altered function. Degradation of large molecules into smaller ones and cross-linkings are structural changes which have been demonstrated. In cross-linking, a long molecule with a flexible structure can undergo intramolecular cross-linking resulting in its becoming attached to itself or to other molecules.

RADIATION EFFECTS ON PROTEINS

Proteins are intimately involved in all cellular functions. They make up many structural elements of the cell, the enzymes which catalyze the essential chemical reactions, the hormones which regulate metabolic processes, and the antibodies which defend against harmful foreign elements. All enzymes can be inactivated when irradiated in solution. However, if the substrate (the substances upon which an enzyme acts) of a specific enzyme is present in cells it is unlikely that enzymes are inactivated to a great degree by in vivo radiation. Furthermore, the radiation required to inactivate enzymes is high.

RADIATION EFFECTS ON NUCLEIC ACIDS

Nucleic acids, the carriers of genetic information, are made up of nitrogen containing bases called purines and pyrimidines. The bases are linked to 5 carbon sugars to make nucelosides which are linked by phosphate groups to form nucleic acid chains. There are two general types of nucleic acids. Ribonucleic acid (RNA) has D-ribose as its sugar and adenine, quanine, cytosine and uracil as its bases. Deoxyribonucleic acid (DNA) has 2-deoxy-D-ribose as its sugar and adenine, quanine, cytosine and thyme as its bases. DNA is a major constituent of chromosomes. DNA exists as a double-stranded helix consisting of two base-sugar-phosphate strands linked by hydrogen-bonding between bases with the entire structure coiled into a helical configuration.

A number of different kinds of radiation damage to the DNA molecule are known to occur:

1.   Change of a base

2. Loss of a base
3. Hydrogen bond breakage
4. Single strand fracture
5. Double strand fracture
6. Cross-linking within the helix
7. Cross-linking to the DNA molecules
8. Cross-linking to protein

RADIATION EFFECTS ON LIPIDS

Lipids are fats, waxes, and other substances which are soluble in organic solvents such as alcohol, acetone, and ether. Saturated and unsaturated fatty acids are simple lipids. Examples of other lipids are phospholipids and lipoproteins. Lipids are used in cells as nutrients and structural components. Radiation-induced alterations in lipids have been demonstrated in vitro but measurement of these in vivo has been difficult. Therefore, the importance of radiation-induced changes in lipids in biological systems is unknown.

RADIATION EFFECTS ON CARBOHYDRATES

Carbohydrates are compounds composed of carbon, hydrogen and oxygen. The simplest carbohydrates are 5 and 6 carbon sugars called monosaccharides. Some of these are constituents of nucleic acids and some are used in cellular respiration. Monosaccharides are joined together to form disaccharides, trisaccharides or polysaccharides. Polysaccharides such as glycogen are used by the body as energy reserves. Irradiation of polysaccharides in vitro causes chain breaking or depolymerization. In vivo, however this effect is probably not important because of the high radiation dose required to induce depolymerization.

RADIATION EFFECTS ON MEMBRANES

Large single radiation exposures (30-50 Gy) produce rupture of plasma membranes and dilation of endoplasmic reticulum. Mitochondria become swollen and their internal membranes become disorganized resulting in release of enzymes with further intracellular destruction. In addition, more subtle changes occur in the permeability of cells due to changes in the lipoprotein structure of the membranes. However, there is not conclusive evidence that permeability changes or enzyme release occurs with exposure to lower radiation doses.

RADIATION EFFECTS ON ENERGY METABOLISM

ATP production is reduced in some cells following moderate radiation exposure. This decrease appears to result from an uncoupling of the phosphorylation mechanisms from those of oxidation. Some investigators believe that uncoupling of phosphorylations is one of the primary mechanisms of radiation-induced cell death.

RADIATION EFFECTS ON SYNTHETIC PROCESSES

A decrease in the rate of DNA synthesis following radiation has been demonstrated. RNA synthesis is also reduced or delayed and, with large exposures, protein synthesis may be slowed. It is thought that radiation makes DNA molecules incapable of serving as a template for messenger RNA. The end result is that important enzymes and other proteins cannot be made and the cells can no longer maintain their ability to undergo cell division.

RADIATION EFFECTS ON CHROMOSOMES

Structural changes in chromosomes can be produced by irradiation of cells at any stage of their mitotic cycle. These structural changes, called aberrations, can be seen microscopically when the cells are in mitosis. When breaks in chromosomes are produced by radiation the broken ends may rejoin to give their original configuration. In this case, mitosis will precede normally. However, if the broken ends, fail to rejoin an aberration results. If the broken ends rejoin with other broken ends, distorted appearing chromosomes are formed. It is apparent that these effects are potentially lethal to the cell. Less obvious alterations in chromosomes can lead to alterations in cell function or synthetic activity.

RADIATION EFFECTS ON CELL DIVISION

Radiation causes delay in cell division and the length of the delay depends on the radiation dose and the phase of the cell cycle (Figure 7.1). Cells that are in mitosis at the time of irradiation complete the division; those about to enter mitosis are stopped in G_2 and those in S may be inhibited; those in G_2 are prevented from entering S. When the cells recover, more cells enter mitosis than normal.

Techniques have been developed by which it is possible to produce populations of cells in which all of the cells in the culture divide synchronously. If these synchronized cell populations are irradiated at various times following synchronization, survival curves for cells at G_1, S, G_2 and M can be produced (Figure 7.2). A number of investigators have studied different cell lines in this way and the main characteristics of the variation of radiosensitivity with cell age in the mitotic cycle are (a) that cells are most sensitive at or close to mitosis, (b) resistance is usually greatest in the latter part of the S phase and (c) G_2 is usually nearly as sensitive as M.

PRIMARY SITE OF RADIATION DAMAGE

Current evidence is overwhelming that the cell nucleus is the major site of

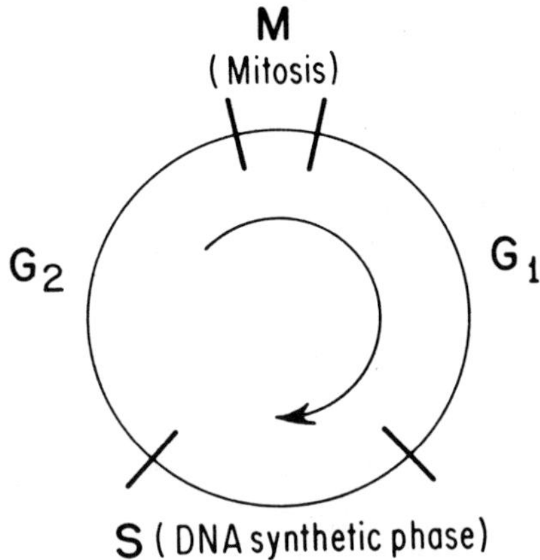

Figure 7.1 These are the phases of the cell cycle.

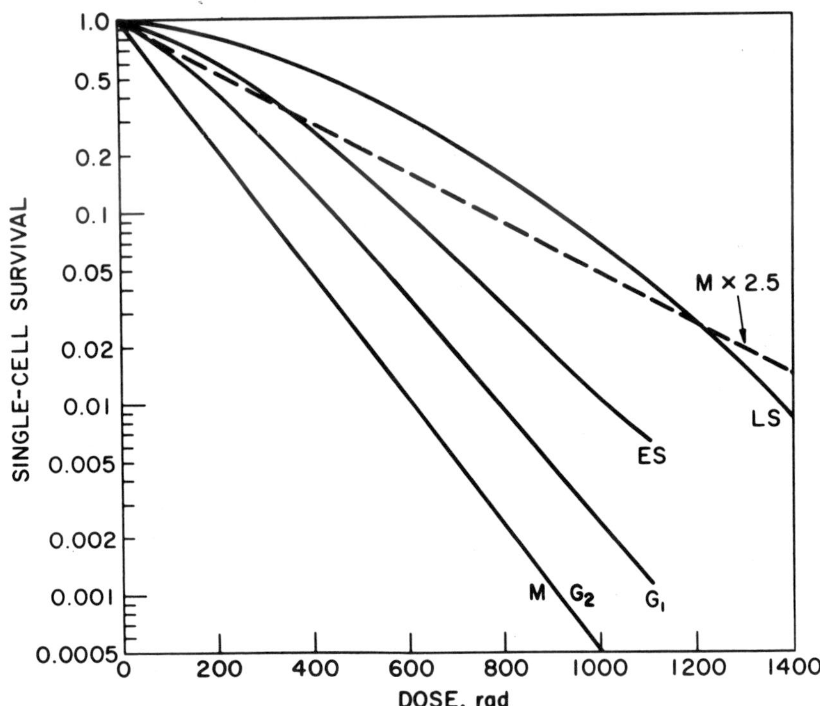

Figure 7.2 These survival curves for hamster cells synchronized and irradiated at the various phases of the cell cycle were produced by Dr.Warren Sinclair.

radiation damage leading to cell death. High-dose radiation exposures are required to inactivate enzyme systems or injure cell membranes, whereas low-dose exposures can cause chromosome alterations and mutations leading to cell death. However, alterations in membrane permeability and in other intracellular systems such as mitochondria cannot be disregarded and it is probable that cell death following radiation can result from any of several changes which could be lethal depending on the cell type, the cell activity at the time of exposure and the exposure conditions.

CELL SURVIVAL CURVES

A major advance in radiobiology occurred in 1956 when Puck and Marcus, using a strain of cells cultured from a cervix carcinoma called HeLa cells, produced a mammalian cell radiation survival curve.[4] A cell survival curve describes the relationship between the radiation dose and the proportion of cells which survive. A surviving cell is one which has retained its ability to proliferate indefinitely to produce a colony of cells. Such a cell is said to be clonogenic.

Survival curves are basic to an understanding of radiotherapy (Figure 7.3). To produce a survival curve, cells from a stock culture are placed in suspension. The number of cells per unit volume are counted by looking at the sample in a hemocytometer under low-power microscope. One hundred cells are placed on a Petri dish in growth medium and allowed to grow for 1-2 weeks. During this time, each cell will divide many times to form a colony which is easily visible. Not all of the original 100 cells will grow to form a colony and the term plating efficiency (PE) indicates the percentage of cells which grow into colonies. For example, if 70 colonies grow from an original seeding of 100 cells, the PE is 70%.

Another dish is seeded with cells and exposed to a radiation dose. The cells are allowed to grow for 1-2 weeks and the following observations are made: Some of the cells are single and have not divided; some of the cells have divided only a few times forming a small colony; some have grown into large colonies differing little from the irradiated controls. These cells in the third group are said to have survived. The surviving fraction is: Surviving fraction = colonies counted/cells seeded X (PE/100). The process is repeated so the surviving reactions are obtained for a range of doses.

Survival curves for mammalian cells are usually presented with dose plotted on a linear scale and surviving fraction on a logarithmic scale. For sparsely ionizing radiation, such as x- or gamma rays, the survival curve has a characteristic shape. At low doses, there is an initial shoulder followed by a portion which becomes straight or nearly straight. To define a curve of this shape two parameters must be specified. The first parameter is the slope of the final straight portion expressed as D_0. The D_0 is the dose required to reduce the number of surviving cells to 37% of their original number. The second parameter is the

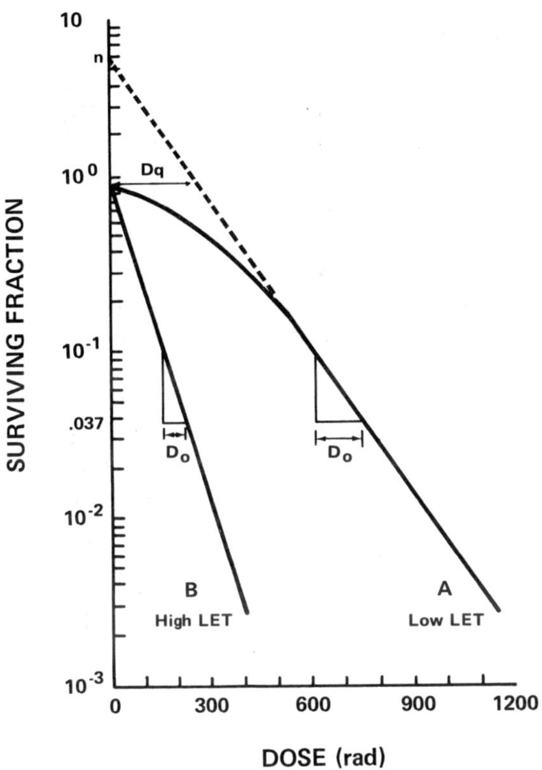

Figure 7.3 This is the shape of the survival curves for low LET (A) and high LET (B) radiation (produced by Dr. Eric Hall).

extrapolation number, n, which is found by extrapolating the straight portion of the curve to the point where it cuts the surviving fraction axis. The extrapolation number is a measure of the extent of the of the initial shoulder of the curve. If it is small the extrapolation number will be small and if it is large the extrapolation number will be large.

Another term used to describe the shoulder of the survival curve is the quasi-threshold dose (Dq). Dq is the dose at which the straight portion of the survival curve extrapolated backward intersects with the dose axis drawn through a surviving fraction of 1. All mammalian cells studied to date, regardless of their species of origin and whether they are normal or malignant, have similarly shaped survival curves. In most cases the D_0 values fall between 1-2 Gy and the n number falls in the range of 1.5-10.

FACTORS WHICH MODIFY SURVIVAL CURVES

Type of radiation For densely ionizing radiation such as alpha particles the survival curves do not have a shoulder and are described by a single parameter D_o. (Figure 7.3). Densely ionizing radiations differ from sparsely ionizing radiation in the magnitude of cell killing. In comparing different radiations it is customary to use 250 V x-rays as the standard. Relative biologic effectiveness (RBE) is a term used to compare the effectiveness of one type of radiation with 250 KV x-rays. For example, comparing fast neutrons with 250 KV x-rays, if the end-point chosen is a surviving fraction of 0.01 the dose of neutrons needed to reduce the surviving fraction to 0.01 might be 6.6 Gy and for 250 KV x-rays to 10 Gy. The RBE would be 1.5.

Dose rate For sparsely ionizing radiation, the rate at which the radiation is administered influences the severity of biological damage produced by a given radiation dose. If dose rate is reduced, the amount of injury is reduced because some of the injury is repaired during the exposure and if the dose rate is sufficiently low, cell division can continue during the exposure.

The oxygen effect The presence of oxygen sensitizes cells to the effect of radiation. The shape of the survival curves are the same for cells radiated in the presence of oxygen (aerated) and without oxygen (hypoxic), but the size of the dose needed to produce a given degree of biologic damage differs (Figure 7.4). The ratio of hypoxic to aerated doses needed to cause the same amount of damage is called the oxygen enhancement ratio (OER). The OER varies with the type of radiation used. For sparsely ionizing radiation the OER values range between 2.5-3.0, whereas for densely ionizing radiation OERs vary between 1-2. The mechanism of the oxygen effect is not completely understood, but it is thought that oxygen acts at the level of free radicals to produce more active radicals which increase the severity of chemical injury in the cell.

Other chemical modifiers These agents are classified as protectors or sensitizers depending on whether they diminish or increase the effect of a given dose.

Radioprotectors The sulfhydryl compounds including cysteine, cystamine, cysteamine, and WR2721 (a thiophosphate derivative of cysteamine), protect mammalian cells in tissue culture from radiation injury. The dose reduction factor (DRF) is the dose needed to produce a given biological effect in the presence of the radioprotector, divided by the dose producing the same effect without the drug. DRFs as high was 1.8 have been observed.

The mechanism of the radioprotecting affect of the sulfhydryl compound is

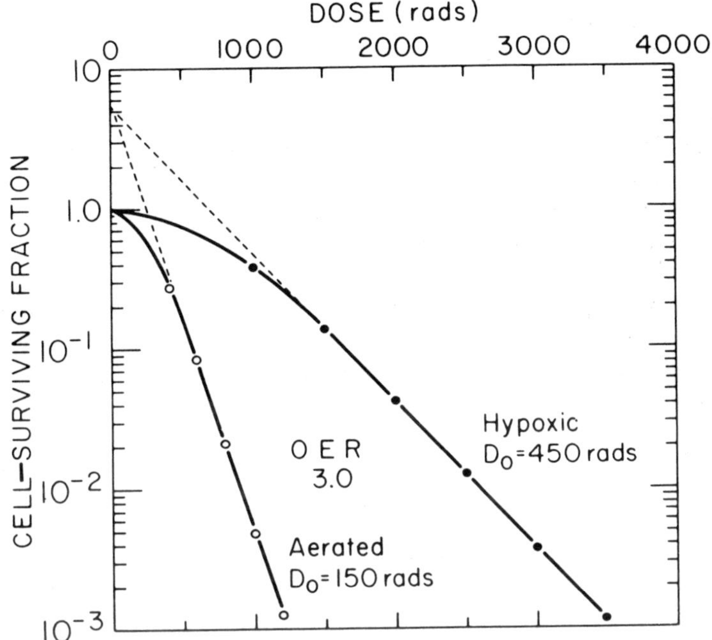

Figure 7.4 This is an illustration of the meaning of OER (Oxygen Enhancement Ratio) (Produced by Dr.Eric Hall).

not completely clear but it is thought that they act as free radical scavengers and, since they are electron affinic compounds like oxygen, they compete with oxygen for the unpaired electron on the free radicals.

Radiosensitizers True radiosensitizers are chemicals which have the capacity to increase the effect of radiation, but are non-toxic to cells when administered alone. Compounds classified as true radiosensitizers include 5-bromodeoxyuridine (BUdR) and 5-iododeoxyuridine (IUdR). These compounds are very similar to one of the normal constituents of DNA, thymidine, and can be incorporated in the DNA chain in the place of thymidine. The presence of the substances in the DNA chain makes it more susceptible to radiation damage.

Other compounds known to increase the killing effect of radiation are not true radiosensitizers because they are toxic to cells and part of their sensitizing ability may be simply additive toxicity rather than true radiosensitization. Compounds in this category include chemotherapy drugs such as actinomycin D, bleomycin and adriamycin.

RECOVERY FROM RADIATION INJURY

In cell survival experiments it has been demonstrated that cells can recover from radiation injury. A number of types of repairable injury have been described.

Sublethal injury Elkind was one of the first radiobiologists to demonstrate sublethal injury in irradiated cells.[5] He showed that a portion of the injury is repairable in split-dose experiments. In these experiments the effect of a single large radiation exposure to cells was compared to the effect of the same total dose divided into two equal fractions separated by varying time intervals (Figure 7.5). The data showed that when the time interval between the two doses was one-half hour the surviving fraction was greater than for a single dose. As the interval was further increased the surviving fraction increased until a plateau was reached at an interval of about 2 hours. This increase in the surviving fraction between the two fractions is believed to occur because a portion of the cellular injury is repaired following the initial fraction. The intracellular mechanisms responsible for repair are unknown. For alpha particles and other high LET radiations there is little repair of sublethal injury between fractions.

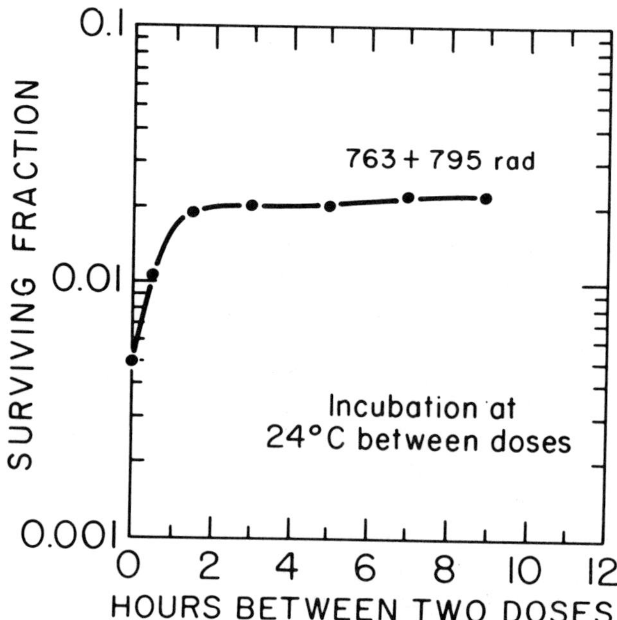

Figure 7.5 The classic work on recovery from sublethal injury was done by Dr. Mortimer Elkind. This illustrates the surviving fraction of hamster cells following two fractions with varying intervals between fractions.

Potentially lethal damage (PLD) This type of cellular injury is not well understood. PLD is injury which is usually lethal to the cell but under certain post-irradiation conditions can be repaired. Here are two examples of the PLD phenomenon: (1) Cells are usually incubated following irradiation in full growth medium but if they are incubated in balanced salt solution for several hours post-irradiation instead of full growth medium cell survival is increased; (2) cells are usually subcultured immediately following irradiation for assay of their colony forming ability, but if they are allowed to remain in crowded conditions in density-inhibited stationary-phase cultures for 6-12 hours post-irradiation, cell survival is increased. It appears, therefore, that repair of PLD is expressed following irradiation only if the conditions for cell proliferation are suboptimal. The releveance of PLD to clinical radiotherapy is unknown.

REFERENCES

1. Hall EJ. Radiobiology for the Radiologist, Third Edition, J.B. Lippincott Company, Philadelphia, 1988.

2. Casarett AP. Radiation Biology, Prentice-Hall, Englewood Cliffs, New Jersey, 1968.

3. Wardman P. Chapter 4, Principles of radiation chemistry, in The Biological Basis of Radiotherapy, Eds. Steel GG, Adams GE, Peckham JM, Elsevier Science Publishers B.V., Amsterdam, 1983, pp 51-59.

4. Puck TT, Marcus PI, Action of x-rays on mammalian cells, Journal of Experimental Medicine 103:653-666, 1956.

5. Elkind MM, Sutton, H. Radiation response of mammalian cells grown in tissue culture. 1. Repair of x-ray damage in surviving Chinese hamster cells, Radiation Research 12: 45556-592, 1962.

Chapter 8

EFFECTS OF RADIATION ON NORMAL TISSUES AND TUMORS

GENERAL FEATURES OF RADIATION INJURY

The changes seen by the pathologist in tissue following radiation injury are not unique.[1,2] Similar alterations are observed following injury due to heat, cold, infections, toxic substances, and ischemia. Radiation produces changes in tissues which can be classified as immediate, acute (within days or weeks following exposure), and late or delayed (months to years later). Immediate changes are rarely seen since they tend to be produced only by very large radiation exposures which are not used clinically.

Acute effects on tissues are seen only after doses above 0.5 Gy are delivered in a short time. The acute lesions consist mainly of cell necrosis but there are also vascular effects such as dilation of venous sinusoids and capillaries. In some tissues, such as skin and heart, there is also a cellular inflammatory infiltrate.

As the acute lesion resolves the necrotic cells are shed and the irradiated tissue is repopulated by new normal appearing cells and, for a time, no abnormalities are detectable to the naked eye or by light microscopy. However, residual lesions may be detected by electron microscopy.

Eventually, slowly progressive pathologic alterations develop. These delayed changes are usually limited to the stroma of the irradiated tissues but there may also be loss of functional cells. The changes in the stroma consist of edema followed by interstitial fibrinous exudate and progressive fibrosis. Capillaries and sinusoids are dilated and appear to be encased in collagen. Some of the most characteristic fibrotic lesions are seen in arterioles and small arteries. These late appearing lesions are usually apparent only after high radiation doses, but they are of great importance in clinical radiotherapy because they are irreversible and tend to progress with time.

RELATIVE RADIOSENSITIVITY OF THE NORMAL TISSUES

All mammalian tissues are susceptible to radiation injury and they can be classified according to their radiosensitivity (Table 8.1).[3] The term radiosensitivity refers to the dose level and rapidity following radiation at which lesions are clinically or pathologically detectable. The most radiosensitive tissues are those whose cells are constantly being replaced from a rapidly proliferating pool of stem cells such as bone marrow, intestinal epithelium, and gonadal epithelium. Tissues classified as highly radiosensitive also contain populations of rapidly

Table 8.1 Relative radiosensitivty of normal tissues

Radiosensitivity	Normal Tissue (Examples)
Very High	Lymphocytes Bone marrow Intestinal epithelium Testicular epithelium Ovarian epithelium
High	Hair follicles Epidermis Mucous membranes of oral cavity/oropharynx
Medium	Connective tissue Endothelium of small blood vessels Growing cartilage/bone
Fairly low	Mature cartilage/bone Pancreatic epithelium Thyroid epithelium
Low	Neuronal tissue Muscle

dividing cells, whereas those classified as medium and fairly low in radiosensitivity are composed of cells which repopulate slowly or only in response to injury. Those classified as low in radiosensitivity are composed of cells which do not replicate.

ACUTE EFFECTS ON INDIVIDUAL TISSUES

The following table lists the acute effects of irradiation which might be observed during a fractionated (administering multiple small dose over an extended time) course of irradiation to relatively small volumes of tissue such as occurs in clinical radiotherapy (Table 8.2). These effects occur only in the tissue irradiated.

FACTORS INFLUENCING THE SEVERITY OF THE RADIATION RESPONSE

The severity of the pathologic alterations seen in tissues following irradiation depend upon a number of factors:

1.   The type of tissue irradiated

Table 8.2 Doses for onset of acute effects (10 Gy/week/5 treatments)

Tissue	Acute Effect	Onset dose (Gy)
Skin	Epilation	15
	Erythema	20
	Dry desquamation	30
	Moist desquamation	40
Oral cavity	Patchy mucositis	30
	Confluent mucositis	40
Taste buds	Loss of taste	10
Esophagus	Esophagitis	25
Salivary Glands	Xerostomia	10
Stomach	Gastritis	20
Small intestine	Enteritis	25
Rectum	Proctitis	30
Urinary bladder	Cytitis	30
Testis	Oligospermia	0.25
Bone Marrow	Reduced cellularity	4
	Extensive hypoplasia	50
Lymphocytes	Lympopenia	0.25
Conjunctiva	Conjunctivitis	20

2. LET of the radiation -- the changes tend to be greater with high LET than low LET radiations
3. Dose -- the higher the dose the greater the effect
4. Dose-rate -- the changes are less severe at low dose-rates than high dose-rates for the same total dose
5. Fractionation -- fractionation tends to reduce the severity of the tissue reactions.
6. The volume of tissue irradiated -- the injury increases as the volume of tissue irradiated increases.

DELAYED EFFECTS OF FRACTIONATED IRRADIATION ON INDIVIDUAL TISSUES

The following table lists the delayed effect of irradiation which may be observed following a fractionated course of irradiation to relatively small volumes of tissues such as occurs in clinical radiotherapy (Table 8.3). The effects are seen only in the irradiated tissues

TOLERANCE DOSES FOR DELAYED EFFECTS

It is essential in radiotherapy that clinically significant delayed effects be avoided. Therefore, radiotherapists have attempted to establish dose thresholds for each effect (Table 8.3).The TD 5/5 is the dose in Gy which will produce injury in 1-5% of cases within 5 years post-irradiation. The doses listed are fractionated at 2 Gy per treatment, 5 treatments per week.

Table 8.3 Radiation tolerance doses (10 Gy/wk/5Rxs)

Organ	Injury at 5 years	Dose (Gy)/5%incidence
Skin	Ulceration/fibrosis	55
Oral mucosa	Ulceration	65
Esophagus	Stricture	60
Stomach	Ulcer, perforation	45
Intestine	Stricture	45
Colon	Stricture	45
Salivary	Xerostomia (permanent)	40
Liver	Liver failure	30
Kidneys	Renal failure	23
Bladder	Contracture	60
Ureters	Stricture	75
Testis	Sterility	5-15
Ovary	Sterility	2-3
Heart	Pericarditis/myocardopathy	35
Bone	Arrested growth in child	20
	Necrosis/fracture in adult	60
Brain	Necrosis	50
Spinal cord	Necrosis	45
Lens of eye	Cataract	5
Thyroid	Hypothyroidism	45
Pituitary	Hypopituitarism	60
Bone Marrow	Reduced cellularity	20
Lymph nodes	Atrophy	35

PATHOGENESIS OF DELAYED EFFECTS

The mechanism responsible for the development of the delayed effects is unknown but there are two theories.[7] The most commonly held theory is that the lesions develop primarily as a result of vascular injury. This theory holds that the delayed lesions develop as a result of occlusions to small arteries due to fibrosis, with secondary loss of tissue due to local tissue ischemia. The second theory suggests that the delayed lesions develop because of a primary effect on the irradiated tissue resulting in slow depletion of cells due to their progressive inability to divide and multiply. Both theories may be correct depending on the tissue irradiated, the dose administered and other factors.

Table 8.4 Important features of the acute radiation syndrome

Syndromes	Dose (Gy)	Period	Latent Pathology	Symptoms	Cause of Death	Time to Death
Hematopoietic	1	2-3 wks.	Depletion of marrow	Bleeding + infection	Infection	3 weeks
GI Syndrome	5	3-5 days	Depletion of small bowel epithelium	Diarrhea + electrolyte disturbances	Dehydration	10-14 days
Central Nervous Syndrome	20	15 min.- 30 hours	Edema of brain/death of neurons	Confusion + convulsions	Increased intracranial pressure	14-36 hours

THE ACUTE WHOLE BODY RADIATION SYNDROME

The signs and symptoms observed following intensive exposure of the whole body to penetrating radiation is known as the acute radiation syndrome.[3] This syndrome is characterized by three phases:

1. The prodromal phase develops within a few hours following an exposure of as little as 0.75-1 Gy. Symptoms experienced are apathy, loss of appetite, nausea and vomiting. This phase usually lasts less than 24 hours.

2. A latent period follows the prodromal phase during which the exposed individual feels well. The length of the latent period depends upon the dose received and is short following large exposures.

3. This is the principal phase of the illness. The clinical features of the acute radiation syndrome can be divided into three categories depending on the radiation dose received (Table 8.4).

The gastrointestinal and hematopoietic syndromes develop because the rapidly dividing stem cells in the crypts of the epithelium of the gastrointestinal tract and the bone marrow are killed or injured causing a delay in cell division. Since the epithelial cells on the villi in the intestine and the circulating blood cells are short lived, they must be replaced at a rapid rate by cell division in the stem cell population. Injury to the stem cells therefore, results in depletion of the lining cells of the intestine and the cellular elements of the blood. The severity of the acute radiation syndrome depends on the number of stem cells that survive.

The mechanism of the CNS syndrome is unknown, but it is thought that injury to small blood vessels in the brain is the initial event. This leads to increased permeability of vessels resulting in cerebral edema and increased intracranial pressure. At extremely high brain doses (100 Gy) rapid death can occur from direct injury to neurons.

Recovery following whole body irradiation occurs by two mechanisms: (1) Surviving cells repair non-lethal injury; (2) Surviving stem cells proliferate to repopulate depleted tissues. The latter is of prime importance in the bone marrow and gastrointestinal tract. Stem cell proliferation begins 24-48 hours after exposure and within 2-3 weeks there are more stem cells in the bone marrow than prior to irradiation. After an additional few weeks the normal steady state is again reached.

The $LD_{50(60)}$ is the dose of penetrating x- or gamma rays delivered to the whole body over a period of less than 24 hours that would be lethal to 50% of indivdiuals within 60 days. In a man the $LD_{50(60)}$ is believed to be between 3 and 4 Gy. The $LD_{50(60)}$ can be modified upward by treatments such as antibiotics, fluid and electrolyte replacement and bone marrow transplantation in severe cases.

ABNORMALITIES OF GROWTH AND DEVELOPMENT

The developing fetus and the preadolescent child are susceptible to radiation-induced disorders of growth and development.[6] The effects of radiation on the fetus are: (1) growth retardation; (2) prenatal or neonatal death; (3) congenital malformations. The radiation-induced defects are most severe in tissues undergoing their most rapid growth and differentiation at the time of exposure.

The type of abnormality seen depends on the stage of fetal development at the time of exposure.

1.   The pre-implantation stage extends from fertilization to the time of attachment of the fertilized ovum to the uterine wall. An exposure of 0.05-0.15 Gy may be sufficient to kill the fertilized ovum at this stage.

2.   The period of organogenesis extends from the time of implantation on day 8 or 9 through week six of gestation. An exposure of only 25 Gy may be sufficient to induce congenital abnormalities at this time.

3.   The fetal period extends from the sixth week of gestation to the time of birth. Since organ differentiation is complete, congenital anomalies would not be expected following a radiation exposure, but functional disabilities such as mental retardation would be expected following exposure in this period.

4.   The post-natal period extends from birth to the time of completion of growth and development. Impairment of bone growth is the primary abnormality expected following radiation exposure during this time.

RADIATION CARCINOGENESIS

Mortality data from atomic bomb survivors in Hiroshima and Nagasaki indicates that the rates of leukemia, lung, breast, urinary tract and colon cancer, and multiple myeloma were increased in the years following whole body exposures.

NON-SPECIFIC LIFE SHORTENING

Exposure to ionizing radiation appears to shorten the life span of small animals. This effect is observed even after corrections have been made for early deaths due to the acute radiation syndrome and radiation carcinogenesis. There is little evidence that a similar life shortening effect occurs in humans.

GENETIC ABNORMALITIES

Radiation can cause permanent change in the structure of DNA in germ cells called mutations. The consequences of mutations are experienced by the irradiated individual's subsequent generations. Since man has always been exposed to natural background radiation, exposure to radiation will not produce genetic defects that are new or characteristic. Rather, increases in the frequency of defects that occur spontaneously in the population are expected. However, evidence that radiation causes genetic defects on man is lacking. The largest group of humans exposed to man-made sources of radiation are the Japanese A-bomb survivors and, up to the present time, no increase in the frequency of prenatal or neonatal deaths or congenital malformations has been observed.

KINETICS OF TUMOR GROWTH

There are three factors that determine the growth rate of a tumor: (1) the cell cycle time of the proliferating cells in the tumor; (2) the fraction of cells that are proliferating called the growth fraction; (3) the rate of cell loss from the tumor.[5]

Tumors consists of a number of different subpopulations of cells (Figure 8.1). Some of the cells are proliferating and are distributed through the various phases of the cell cycle. The time required for a cell to progress through these phases is the cell cycle time, T_c. The cell cycle time is further subdivided into the time required for passage through the phases of the cell cycle and T_{G1}, T_s, T_{G2} and T_M can be measured with special techniques used to count cells labeled with radioactive thymidine.

The growth fraction (GF) is the ratio of the number of proliferation cells (P) to the total number of cells including those which are not proliferating (Q), GF+P/P+Q. Growth parameters have been measured for a number of human tumors and a few of these are shown in Table 8.5.

Cells in tumors can be lost through cell death from inadequate nutrition, damaged mitotic mechanisms and immunological attack. They can also be lost by metastasis and exfoliation or shedding from the surface of the tumor. The cell loss factor is a measure of the ratio of the rate of cell loss to the rate of new cell production. The cell loss factor ($\varnothing$) is defined as $\varnothing = 1 - T_p/T_d$ where T_p is the potential doubling time of a tumor (the time during which a tumor should be expected to double its volume) and T_d is the actual tumor volume doubling time. In experimental animal tumors, cell loss factors range from 0 to 90%. For human tumors the cell loss factor is usually about 7%. Therefore, cell loss from tumors is great and is an important factor in determining the rate of tumor growth.

THE EFFECT OF RADIATION ON
TUMOR GROWTH PARAMETERS

Changes in the growth parameters following radiation have been studied for a number of animal tumors. The results of these studies indicate that the effect of radiation on growth parameters varies from tumor to tumor. In one study, T_c was shortened following irradiation in two human tumors. Also, a number of studies have shown that radiation causes a prolongation in the volume doubling time. It has been postulated that the reason for this is, that radiation injures the endothelium of the capillaries supplying the tumor, rendering them incapable of

COMPONENTS OF A TUMOUR.

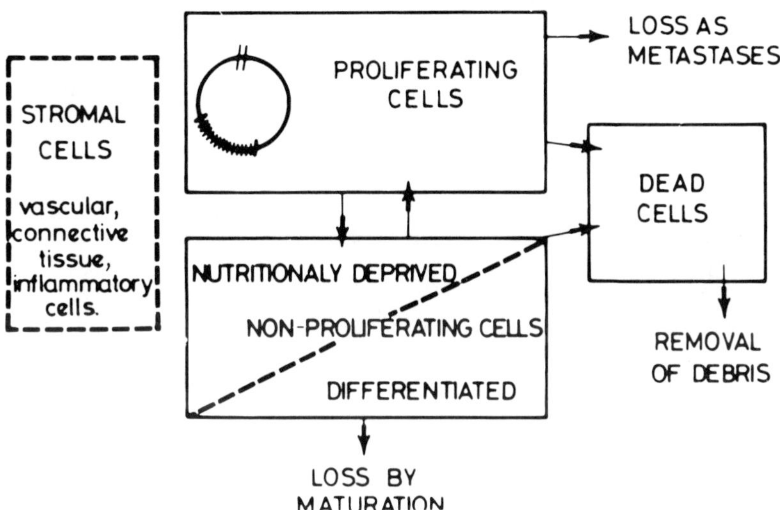

Figure 8.1 This is a schematic presentation of the components of a tumor which was produced by Dr. Julie Denekamp.

Table 8.5 Cell kinetic parameters for human carcinoma (from Denekamp)[5]

			Hours		
Tumor	T_c	G_1	S	G_2	%GF
Endometrial	113	50	48	7	25
Stomach	--	17	19	3	28
Breast	51	19	20	6	61
Squamous cell	52	22	18	7	36

continued growth. Therefore, the supporting stroma of the tumor is unable to support continued expansion of the tumor.

RADIOSENSITIVITY OF HUMAN TUMORS

Human tumors vary in their radioresponsiveness and can be classified as highly radiosensitive, intermediate or low in radiosensitivity (Table 8.6). Radiosensitivity in this context refers to the rate of regression and the dose at which the tumor is controlled in a high percentage of cases. In general, the radiosensitivity of the tumor corresponds to the radiosensitivity of the tissue of origin. In clinical radiotherapy, most of the tumors treated are intermediate in their radiosensitivity.

MORPHOLOGIC CHANGES IN IRRADIATED TUMORS

Histologic study of irradiated tumors in animals demonstrates reduced mitotic activity within a few hours. In human tumors, tumor necrosis has been observed early. Weeks to months after treatment there is a reduction in the number of nucleated tumor cells which are large irregular cells with giant nuclei. With time these large cells become surrounded by collagen and eventually, fibrosis. Eventually, if the treatment is successful, a dense fibrous scar is all that remains at the original tumor site.

RADIORESISTANCE IN HUMAN TUMORS

There are a number of factors which could cause a tumor to be radioresistant to the extent that it does not regress following treatment and is not controlled with doses usually tolerated by normal tissues:[8]

1. Intrinsic radioresistance of tumor cells -- The mechanisms responsible

Table 8.6 Relative radiosensitivity of selected human tumors

Radiosensitivity	Tumor	Tumor control dose (10 Gy/wk/5Rxs)
High	Leukemia	15
	Seminoma	20-25
	Wilms' tumor	20
	Lymphocytic lymphoma	30
Intermediate	Basal cell carcinoma	60
	Squamous carcinoma	65
	Adenocarcinomas of breast, prostate	65
Low	Astrocytoma of brain	80
	Renal cell carcinoma	80
	Malignant melanoma	80
	Osteosarcoma	100

for intrinsic radioresistance are unknown. However, radioresistant cells often have a large shoulder on their survival curve and are not killed with doses normally used in clinical radiotherapy.

2. Hypoxic tumor cells -- Most tumors contain hypoxic cells. These cells are hypoxic because they grow faster than their blood supply resulting in local

tissue ischemia. Hypoxic cells are 2.5-3.0 more radioresistant than fully oxygenated cells.

3.   Rapid repopulation of the tumor by surviving cells could occur during the course of treatment. The tumor could be composed of a large proportion of rapidly proliferating cells so that cell division is sufficient to balance the loss of cells due to cell killing.

4.   The size of the tumor -- Large tumors contain more tumor cells and require a larger dose for tumor control than small tumors.

5.   Redistribution of cells into resistant phases of the cell cycle could occur during a fractionated course of irradiation.

REFERENCES

1. Anderson RE. Chapter 6, Radiation injury, In Anderson's Pathology, Eight Edition, Eds. Kissane JM, The C.V. Mosby Company, St. Louis, 1985, pp 239-277.

2. Fajardo LF. Pathology of Radiation Injury, Masson, New York, 1982.

3. Rubin P, Casarett GW. Clinical Radiation Pathology, W.B. Saunders, Philadelphia, 1968.

4. Hall EJ. Radiobiology for the Radiologist, Third Edition, J. B. Lippincott Company, Philadelphia, 1988.

5. Denekamp J. Cell Kinetics and Cancer Therapy, Charles C. Thomas Springfield, Illinois, 1982.

6. Pizzarello DJ, Witkofski RL. Medical Radiation Biology, 2nd Ed. Lea and Febiger, Philadelphia, 1982.

7. Withers HR, et al, The pathobiology of late effects of irradiation,In Radiation Biology in Cancer Research, Eds., Meyn RE, Withers HR, Raven press, New York, 1980, pp 439-448.

8. Tubiana M. Chapter 2, The causes of clinical radioresistance, In The Biological Basis of Radiotherapy, Eds., Steel GG, Adams GE, Peckham MJ, Elsevier, Amsterdam, 1983, pp 13-33.

Chapter 9

THERAPY MACHINES AND EQUIPMENT

INTRODUCTION

Radiotherapy began late in the nineteenth century with the discovery of x-rays by Roentgen in 1895 and radium by Marie and Pierre Curie in 1898. Within months after each of these discoveries they were used for cancer treatment. Early x-ray machines were crude and unsafe, but with the introduction of the Coolidge tube in 1913, the development of transformers, and the placement of tubes in lead casings, improved performance and safety resulted. The era of deep x-ray therapy began in 1921 with the introduction of machines producing beams in the range of 200 KV.

The Curies were able to separate only 100 mg of radium from a ton of pitchblende. Therefore, it took a number of years to accumulate enough radium for use in clinical trials, but by 1920 it was known that implantation of radium into the uterus was a potentially curative treatment for cancer of the cervix. By the time of the Second World War radiotherapy had become an established medical specialty with steadily improving treatment results for a variety of neoplastic diseases.

ROENTGEN RAY MACHINES

Most radiotherapy departments have orthovoltage equipment which is used primarily in the treatment of skin cancer. Modern orthovoltage units are capable of treating at more than one energy level (Figure 9.1). Usually the unit can be used as a superficial x-ray machine operating in the range of 100-140 KV or as an orthovoltage machine operating in the range of 200-250 KV. The 100-140 KV beam is particularly useful for treatment of skin cancer.

The essential parts of an x-ray tube are shown in Figure 9.2. The envelope is constructed of tempered glass and the cavity of the tube is maintained at high vacuum. The filament is tungsten wire which is provided with a separate heating circuit. Targets are usually constructed of tungsten. When the target is bombarded with electrons, the phenomenon of secondary emission causes the production of high-energy secondary electrons, which can cause an electrostatic charge to be built up which interferes with focusing of the bombarding electrons on the target. To prevent this a hooded anode is used to absorb the secondary electrons produced in the target.

Heat production is a serious problem in x-ray tubes. The target is usually embedded in copper, an excellent heat conductor, and the tube is cooled by

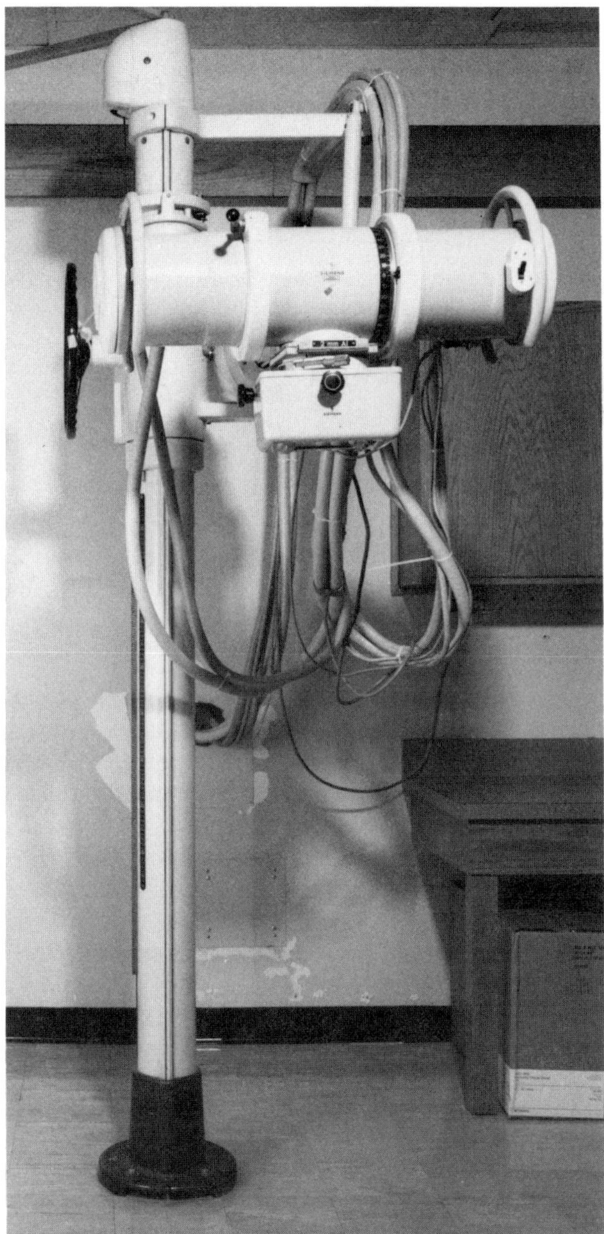

Figure 9.1 This orthovoltage unit generates 110 Kv x-rays used in the treatment of skin cancer. It can also produce 250 Kv x-rays.

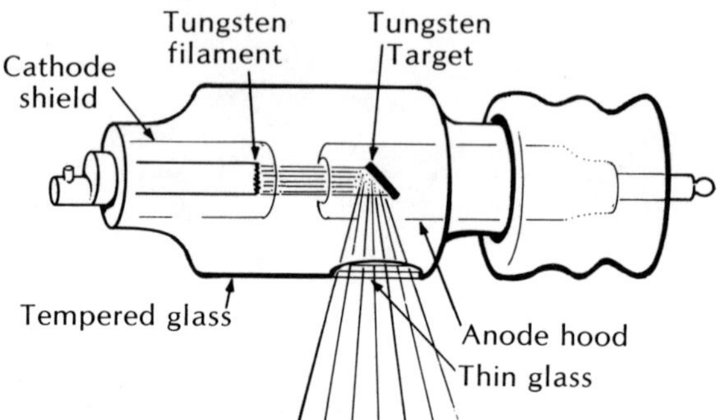

Figure 9.2 This is a diagrammatic illustration of an orthovoltage therapy tube.

circulating oil. The entire system is enclosed in a protective housing that absorbs x-rays in every direction except at the beam portal.

Special roentgen ray tubes designed for use in dermatology are available but these are primarily of historical interest. The grenz-ray tube produces 10-25 KV x-rays, the "contact" tube produces 45 KV x-rays and the Chaoul tube produces 60 KV x-rays. These x-rays have little penetrating power and they are used in the treatment of benign skin diseases.

COBALT-60

The era of megavoltage therapy began in 1951 with the installation of cobalt-60 units at two facilities in Canada. For 20 years cobalt-60 was the major source of radiation for cancer treatment throughout the world and these machines are still in use in hundreds of centers.

Cobalt-60 is produced by bombardment of cobalt-59 with neutrons in a nuclear reactor. Cobalt-60 decays to an isotope of nickel with the emission of two gamma rays with energies of 1.17 and 1.33 MV. The half-life of cobalt-60 is 5.20 years. Sources of very high activity, up to 20 curies per gram, are used in cobalt-60 units.

Cobalt-60 machines consist of a lead-filled steel container with the source placed near the center (Figure 9.3). Either a rotating wheel or sliding drawer mechanism is used to bring the source to the "on" position. Most units are mounted on a gantry so that the machine can be used for rotational therapy (Figure 9.4). The distance from the source to the center of rotation or isocenter is usually 80 cm.

LINEAR ACCELERATORS

The technology for linear accelerators was developed during the Second World War as a by-product of microwave radar research. The first linear

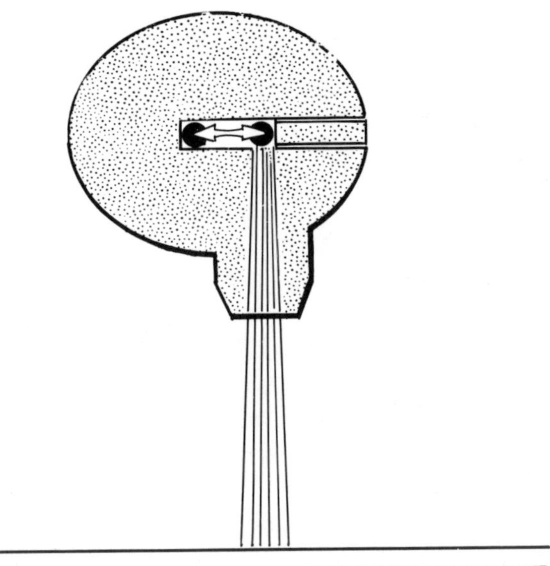

Figure 9.3 This is a diagrammatic illustration of a sliding-drawer on-off mechanism commonly used in cobalt-60 machines.

accelerator for medical use was installed at the Radiation Research Center of the Medical Research Council at the Hammersmith Hospital in London in 1952.[3] In the United States the first medical linear accelerator was installed at the Stanford University Hospital under the direction of Dr. Henry Kaplan.

To produce the radiation beam a power source produces high frequency electromagnetic waves which are transmitted down a wave guide tube (Figure 9.5). Electrons are injected into the wave guide and are carried along by the electromagnetic waves receiving increasing energy as they travel down the tube. At the end of the wave guide the electrons are used in one of two ways. If a tungsten target is placed into the electron beam, x-rays are produced, but if the target is not introduced the electron beam itself can be used.

Linear accelerators for medical use are available in varying sizes depending on the desired beam energy (Figure 9.6). Most are isocentrically mounted with the axis of rotation at 100 cm from the source. Very large linear accelerators have been built to produce high energy beams of nuclei. For example, at the University of California Lawrence Berkeley Laboratory, beams of helium, carbon, neon, or argon nuclei are being evaluated in clinical trials.[4]

BETATRONS

Betatrons are machines which accelerate electrons in a doughnut shaped

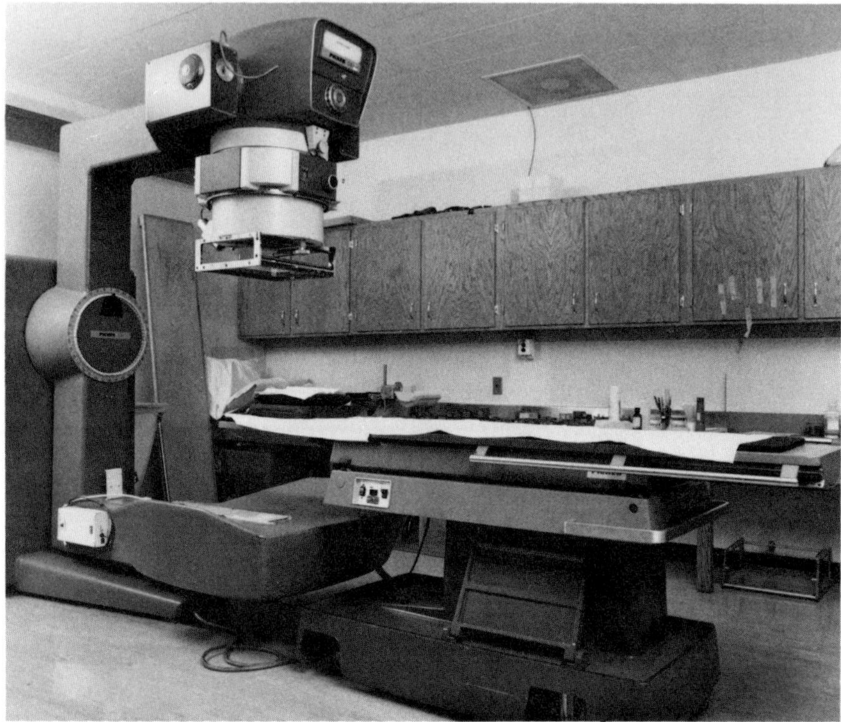

Figure 9.4 This is a rotational cobalt-60 unit. The treating distance is 80 cm SSD.

porcelain tube, operating at a high vacuum between the poles of a large magnet excited by an alternating electric field (Figure 9.7). The electrons are injected into the doughnut and drawn into a circular path by the magnetic field. As they circle around in the doughnut they are accelerated increasing their energy. The electrons themselves can be used for therapy or they may be accelerated into a target to produce an x-ray beam. Most betatrons manufactured in the U.S. produce 22-25 MV x-ray beams. Disadvantages of betatrons compared to linear accelerators are that they are not isocentrically mounted and the dose-rate is low.

CYCLOTRONS

Cyclotrons have been used in physics research for many years but they can also be used in radiotherapy to produce beams of protons or neutrons. The principle of the cyclotron is described simplistically. There are two hollow D shaped structures called Ds which face each other with a short gap between them. The Ds are placed between the poles of a large magnet and are connected to a high voltage oscillator which can rapidly change the electrical field between the Ds. Positively charged protons or deuterons are injected into the center of the system and are attracted into the negatively charged D where their trajectory becomes arced by the magnetic field. As they emerge from the D the electric field is suddenly changed so that the opposite D becomes negatively charged which draws the particles into the other D. As the particles circle from one D to the other their arc becomes progressively larger as they are accelerated. When they acquire sufficient energy to reach the periphery of the Ds the particles are removed. Neutrons are produced by accelerating deuterons into a beryllium target.

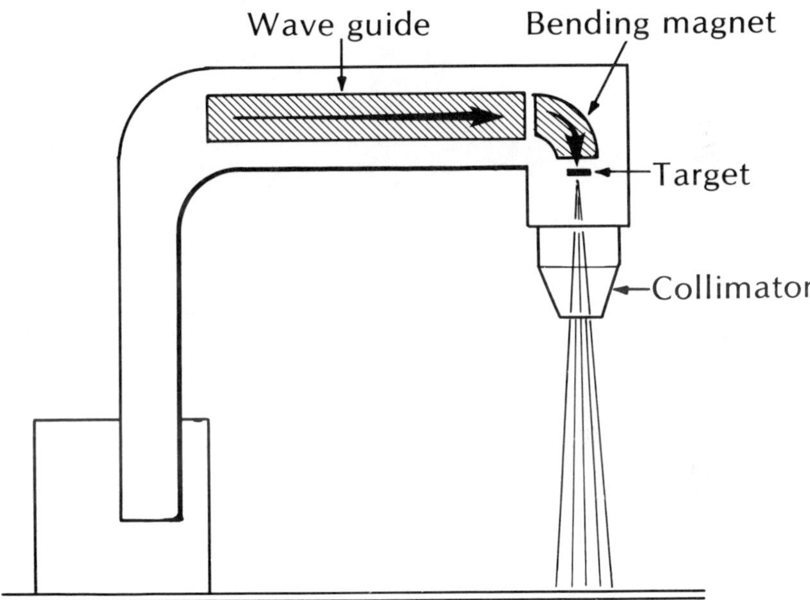

Figure 9.5 This is the configuration of the accelerating wave guide tube and bending magnet used for linear accelerators producing 10-20 MeV x-rays. Shorter tubes can be used for units producing x-rays in the range of 4-6 MeV and, for these, a bending magnet is not needed.

CHARACTERISTICS OF RADIOTHERAPY MACHINES

Depth dose The depth dose distribution in tissue from high energy beams differs from that seen with orthovoltage beams (Figure 9.8). High energy beams yield a low entrance dose with the maximum dose occurring beneath the skin surface, whereas the maximum dose occurs on the skin surface with orthovoltage beams. This depth dose pattern with high energy beams yields a skin sparing effect which has been largely responsible for improved treatment results. In the orthovoltage era, the tumor dose which could be delivered was limited because of severe skin reactions, but with modern machines, radiotherapists can give

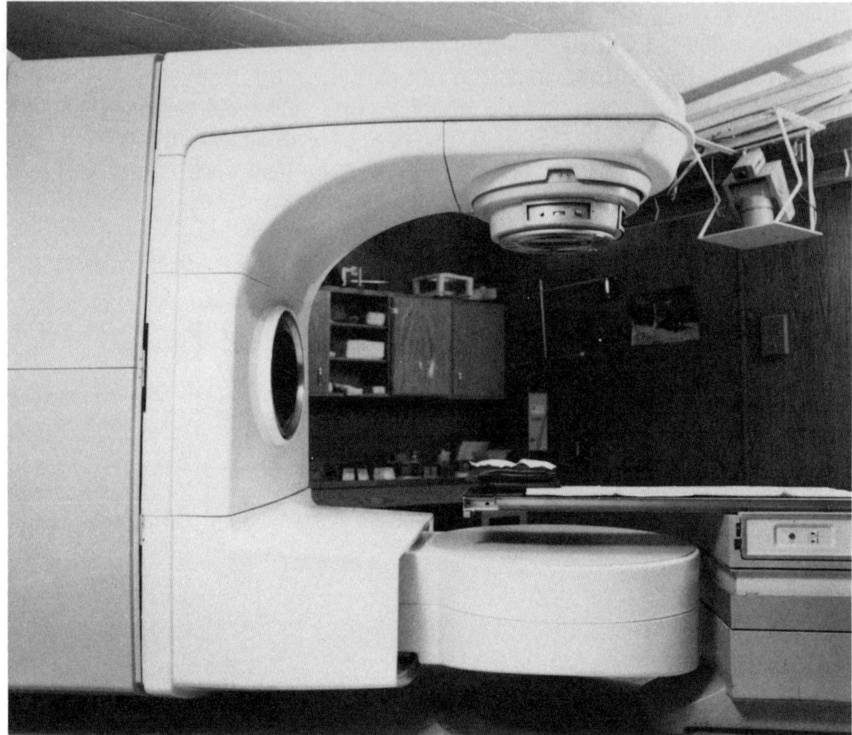

Figure 9.6 This linear accelerator produces 10 MeV x-rays and 6, 9, 12, 15, and 18 MeV electrons. The source-axis distance (SAD) is 100 cm.

higher tumor doses without severe skin reactions. In addition, the percent depth dose, deep in tissue, is higher with high energy beams which tends to spare superficial tissues allowing a higher tumor dose compared to orthovoltage. The depth dose distribution of electron beams is shown in Figure 9.9.

Collimator All radiotherapy machines have a collimating system which yields field sizes ranging from 4 x 4 cm to 40 x 40 cm.

Field Flatness The radiation beam should be uniform from the center to the edge. Cobalt-60 sources emit the same number of photons in all directions yielding a flat radiation field. Linear accelerators and betatrons require a special flattening filter to produce a flat field.

Penumbra All radiation sources yield radiation fields which are not sharply defined at the edges because the size of the source produces a penumbra (Figure 9.10). Early cobalt-60 sources were sometimes as large as 3 cm in diameter yielding radiation fields with a large penumbra, but modern cobalt-60 sources are only 1 cm in diameter and the size of the penumbra is no longer a problem.

Linear accelerators produce fields with a small penumbra because the source of the beam is small.

Light localizer A method is needed to allow the radiotherapy technologist to see the area which requires treatment so the radiation beam can be directed at the correct location. This is accomplished with a light localizer and skin markings. The light localizer consists of a light source and mirror located near the radiation source. When the light is "on" the skin surface is illuminated allowing the technologist to "fit" the light field to the skin markings. The radiation field will then approximate the light field.

Monitor Linear accelerators and betatrons have an uneven radiation output and therefore, sophisticated radiation monitors are needed to automatically turn the machine off after the pre-set dose has been given.

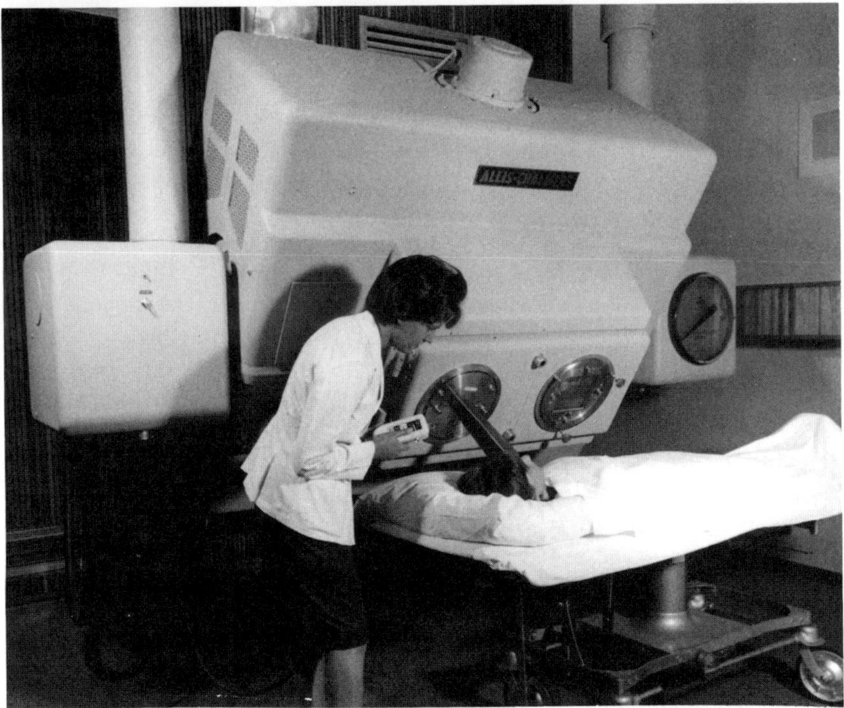

Figure 9.7 This is a photo of a betatron which produces 22 MeV x-rays.

PROTECTIVE BARRIERS

It is usually necessary to place barriers of lead, concrete or other materials between the radiation source and the position occupied by personnel, of sufficient thickness to reduce the exposure to a level which does not exceed the MPDE

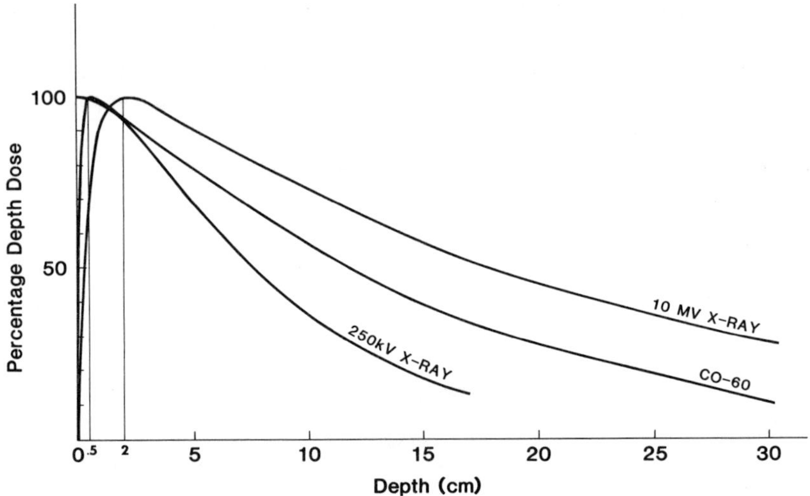

Figure 9.8 These are depth dose curves measured along the central ray in tissue equivalent material for 250 KV x-rays, cobalt-60 gamma rays and 10 MeV x-rays. A 10 X 10 cm field was used

(Maximum Permissible Dose Equivalent) recommendations. The areas surrounding the room where the source is contained are designated as controlled or noncontrolled depending on whether or not the area is under the supervision of the Radiation Protection Supervisor. For protection calculations the MPDE is 0.1 rem/week for controlled areas and 0.01 rem/week for noncontrolled areas.

In Figure 9.11 is the configuration of a high energy radiation therapy machine in a treatment room. Protection against three types of radiation is required, primary radiation, scattered radiation, and leakage radiation through the source housing. Primary radiation is radiation from the source that emerges through the collimating system. Scattered radiation results whenever a radiation beam strikes matter and, in a therapy room, the main source of scattered radiation is the patient. Leakage radiation is radiation that emerges from the head through its protective barrier.

The choice of barrier material depends on structural and spatial considerations. Concrete is relatively inexpensive and therefore, the walls and roof of the barrier are usually concrete. Lead or steel is used when there is too little space to accommodate thick slabs of concrete. A barrier designed for primary radiation provides adequate protection against leakage and scattered radiation.

The requirement for barrier protection from primary radiation is reduced when there is a beam stopper on the treatment unit. Since the beam stopper intercepts all of primary radiation, the main protection problem arises from leakage radiation.

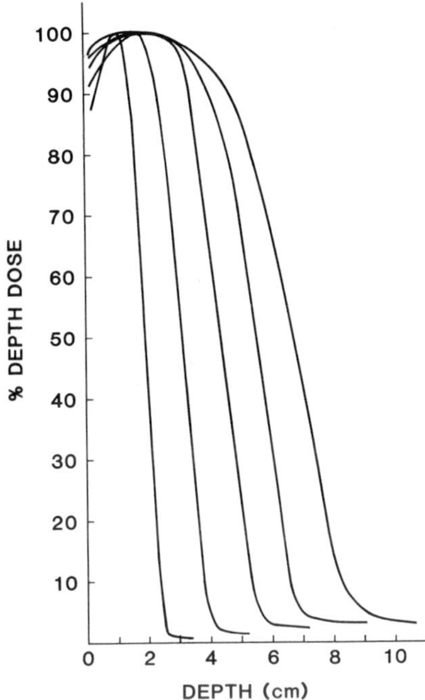

Figure 9.9 These are central axis depth dose curves for electrons. From left to right, the curves are for 6, 9, 12, 15, and 18 Mev electrons.

The requirement for door shielding is reduced by a maze entrance. If a maze arrangement is not used, the door must provide shielding equivalent to the wall surrounding the door. Therefore, for megavoltage units, an extremely heavy motor driven door is required. However, with a maze entrance of appropriate design, the radiation reaching the door has been multiply scattered, markedly reducing its energy.

High energy x-ray beams with energies above 10 MV are contaminated with neutrons produced by interaction of the photons and electrons with the materials in the target, flattening filter, collimators and beam stopper. Concrete barriers designed for x-ray shielding are usually sufficient for shielding against neutrons, but the door may require additional protective measures. The door shielding requirement for neutrons can be reduced by increasing the length of the maze. Also, hydrogenous material such as polyethylene can be added to the door to protect against penetration by neutrons.

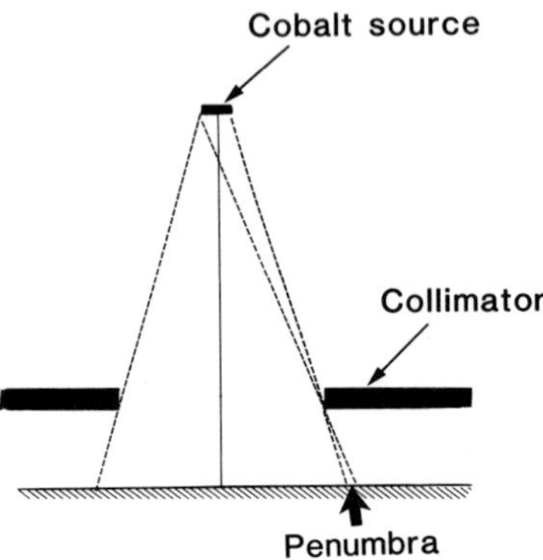

Figure 9.10 This illustrates the definition of penumbra. The penumbra is the distance on the edge of the beam between the point at which the radiation is at full intensity to the point where the intensity falls to 0.

Radiation protection guidelines for the design of structural shielding for radiation installations are discussed in several NCRP reports.

SIMULATORS IN RADIOTHERAPY

The development of treatment planning simulators has resulted in significant improvement in the accuracy of beam placement (Figure 9.12). Simulators allow the radiotherapist to use diagnostic x-rays to localize treatment volume with fields of the exact size and shape, treatment distance and beam angle that will be used on the treatment unit.

CT SCANNING IN RADIOTHERAPY

In recent years CT scanners have gained wide acceptance by radiotherapists as an aid to treatment planning. Clinical studies have shown that accuracy of simulated field placement can be increased by combining CT scanning with simulation in the treatment planning process.

COMPUTERS IN RADIOTHERAPY

Treatment planning computers are essential in modern clinical dosimetry to produce isodose curves for multiple field techniques (Figure 9.13). Newer

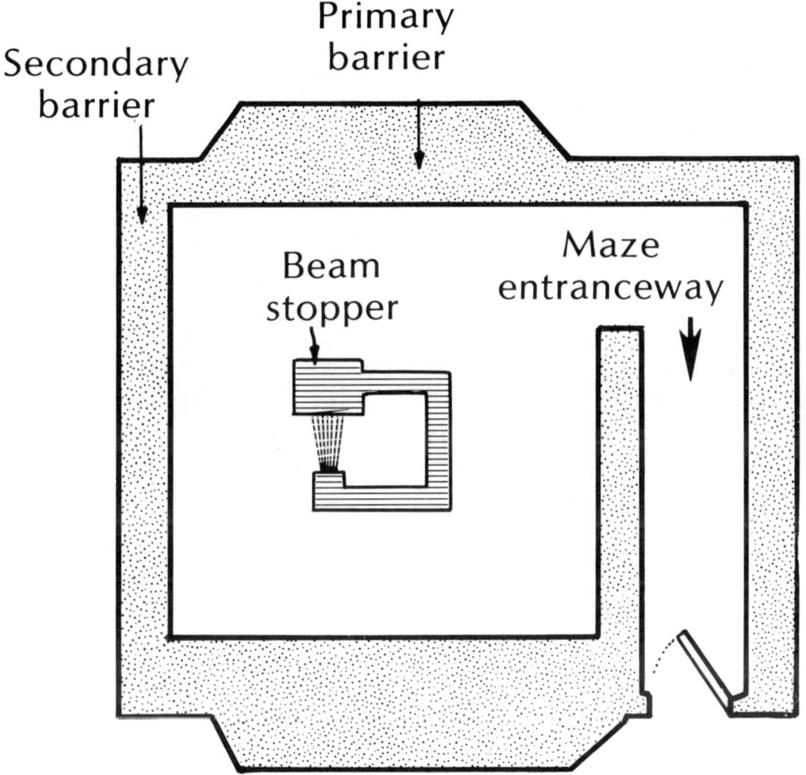

Figure 9.11 This is the configuration of a high energy treatment room. The beam stopper greatly reduces the requirements for primary barrier shielding. The maze entrance reduces the door shielding requirements.

computers are interfaced with CT scanners to yield accurate data about tumor location, patient contour and tissue inhomogeneities and they allow isodose distributions to be produced at a number of levels in the treatment volume. Computers are also used to produce accurate isodose curves around sources of interstitial and intracavitary brachytherapy implants. Finally, large computers are being used in several institutions to develop software for 3-dimensional treatment planning.

RADIUM AND RADIUM SUBSTITUTES

Brachytherapy (short distance therapy) is the placement of radioactive sources directly into tissues or body cavities. The former is called interstitial brachytherapy and the latter intracavitary brachytherapy. Cancer of the tongue

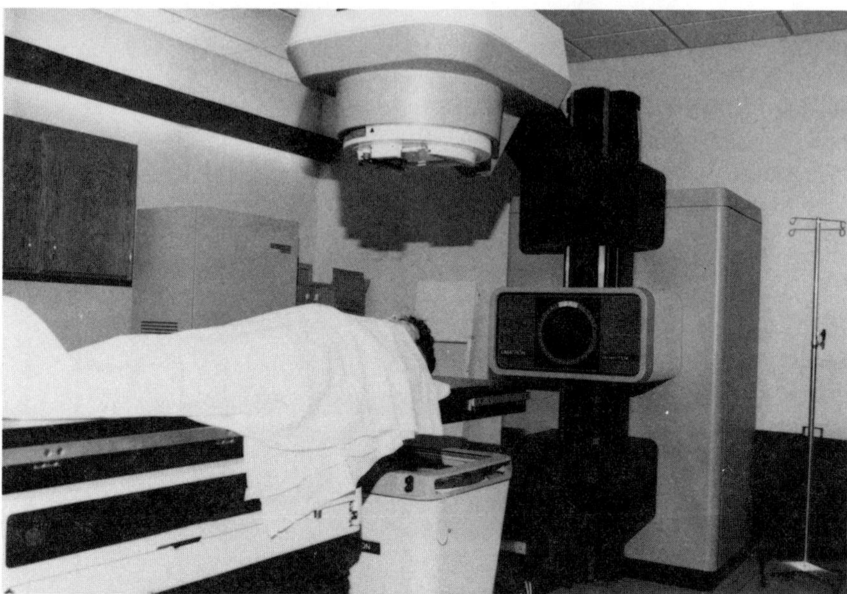

Figure 9.12 This is the treatment planning simulator in use at the Hershey Medical Center. It features computerized remote digital display of parameters, variable SSD from 60-135 cm and fluoroscopic capability.

or floor of the mouth and other accessible sites can be treated by removable implants in which radium or cesium-137 needles are implanted into the tumor and removed after the desired dose has been administered. Most departments own a stock of needles of various lengths and activity (Figure 9.14). They are inserted with a special forceps and held in position with sutures (Figure 9.15). However, iridium-192 had replaced needles in many departments for removable implants but because of the relatively short half-life of iridium-192 smaller departments must order the element for each case.

Permanent interstitial implants are used occasionally for prostate, head and neck, lung and pancreas tumors. In one popular technique, iodine-125 seeds are inserted directly into the tumor and left in place permanently. In another technique, gold-198 seeds are inserted with a special instrument (Figure 9.16).

Intracavitary therapy is used primarily for tumors of the uterus. Radium or cesium-137 tubes are placed into special applicators in the uterus and upper vagina and removed when the prescribed dose has been administered.

MEASUREMENT OF RADIATION

Ionization chambers A major advance in radiology occurred in 1924 when the free-air ionization chamber was introduced, making it possible to measure accurately, ionization in a well-defined mass of air. The most precise instrument

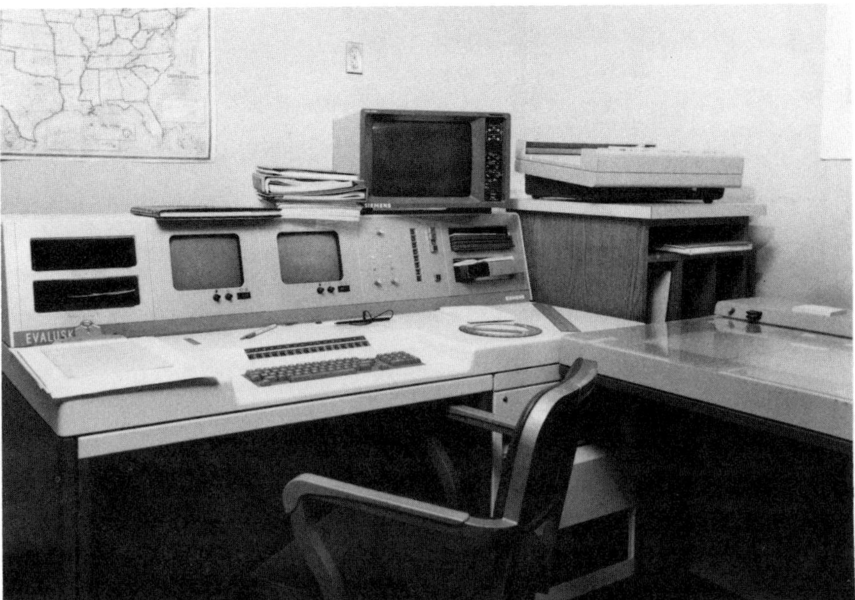

Figure 9.13 This is our treatment planing computer which interfaces with the CT scanner via floppy discs.

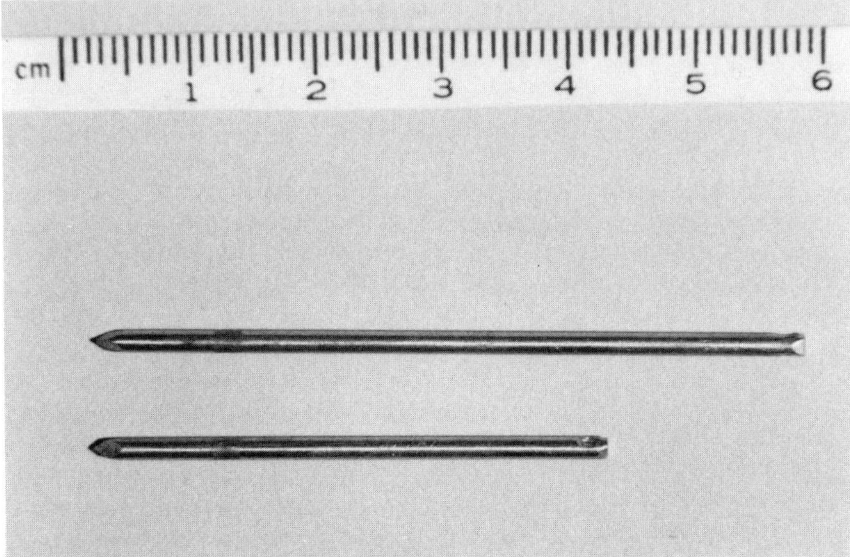

Figure 9.14 These are 2 lengths of cesium-137 needles. The active length of the upper needle is 4.5 cm and the lower 3.0 cm. The full strength needles contain 0.59 mg radium equivalents of Cs^{137} per cm and the half-strength needles contain 0.31 mg radium equivalents per cm.

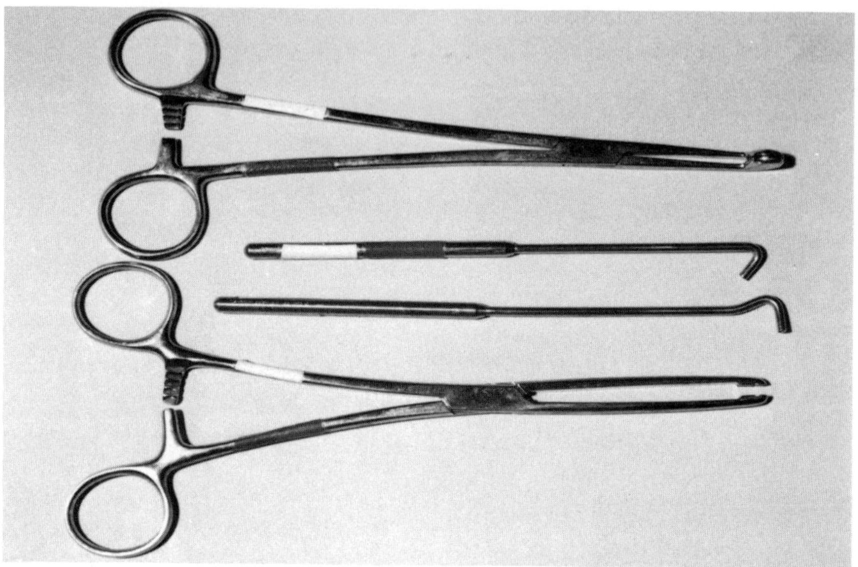

Figure 9.15 These instruments are used in the insertion of the cesium needles.

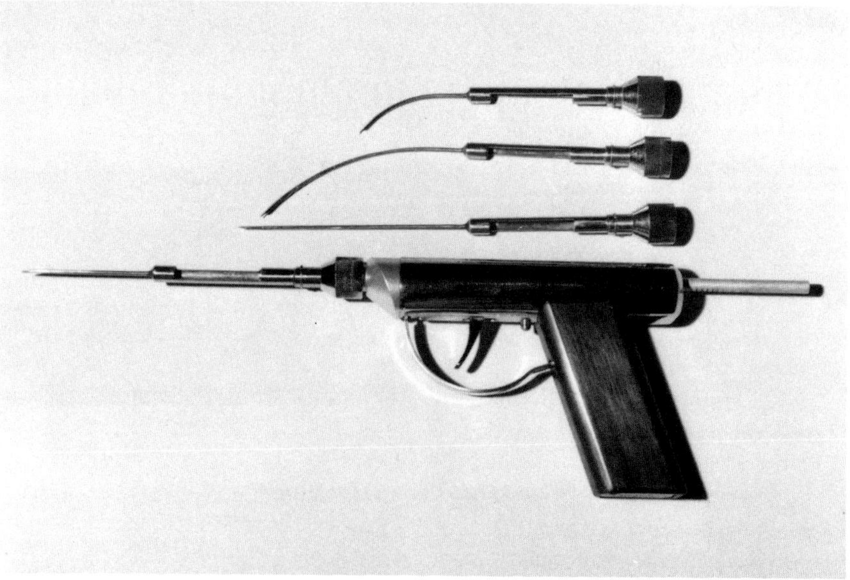

Figure 9.16 This is a Royal Marsden gun used to insert gold-198 seeds into tissue for permanent implants.

for measurement of radiation exposure is the Standard Air Chamber. This instrument is used by standardization laboratories such as the National Bureau of Standards in Washington, D.C., but it is too large to be practical for use in radiology departments.

Thimble chambers were introduced in 1925 and they are used in radiology for dosimetry of x- and gamma rays. Thimble chambers have a plastic outer wall which is lined with carbon. An aluminum electrode is located in the center surrounded by a small volume of air. The chamber is connected to an electrometer. The Farmer dosimeter is a thimble chamber which is widely used for energy therapy machines (Figure 9.17).

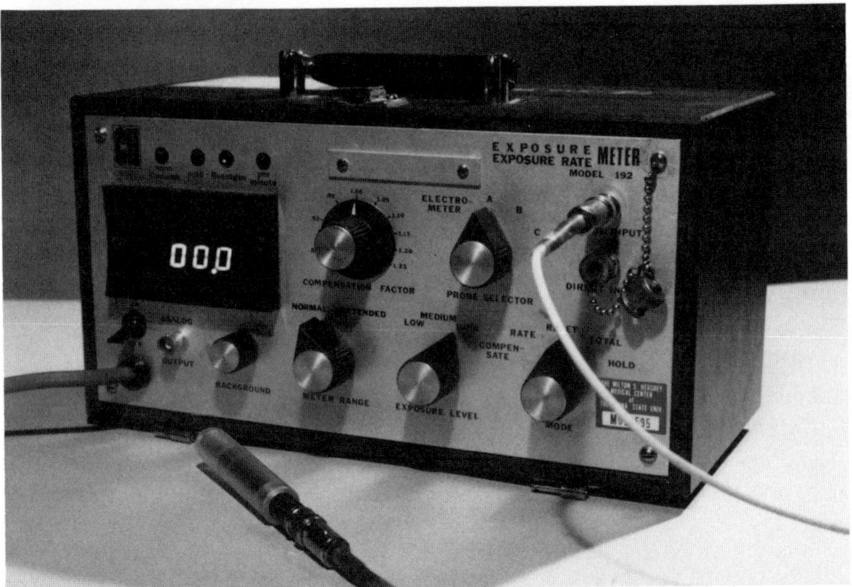

Figure 9.17 This is an electrometer attached by a long cable to a Farmer ion chamber. This system is used for routine dosimetry for cobalt-60 units and x-ray beams from linear accelerators.

Solid state detectors Solid state detectors measure the amount of ionization produced in a solid (diode). Diode detectors are being developed as detectors for diagnostic x-ray units.

Thermoluminescent dosimetry (TLD) Lithium fluoride (LiF) crystals are damaged when exposed to radiation and when heated they emit light in a quantity proportional to the radiation exposure. LiF rods can be placed into body cavities to measure exposure; they are used to calibrate high energy machines; they can be mailed to a group of centers to the dosimetry procedures between centers or used in personnel monitoring for radiation safety .

Film dosimetry Exposure of film to radiation makes silver bromide crystals in the film more sensitive to chemical change. When the film is developed the altered crystals are reduced to small grains of metallic silver. The film is then "fixed" which dissolves the silver bromide crystals, but does not affect the metallic silver. The film which was exposed to radiation appears dark and that which is unexposed appears light. The concentration of metallic silver is proportionate to the dose of radiation and can be measured in a densitometer. Film can be used for dosimetry for both diagnostic x-ray units and high energy therapy machines. Film is used in radiotherapy to determine the size, position of radiation fields, the position of shielding devices, the accuracy of light localizers, the size of the penumbra and for checking for leakage around collimators.

Film has also been used for many years in personnel monitors. Personnel monitoring must be used in areas for persons occupationally exposed to radiation. This is done with film badges which are worn on the chest or abdomen. The film badge is changed monthly and a cumulative record of life-time exposure is maintained for each worker.

Chemical dosimetry Various chemicals undergo chemical change following exposure to ionizing radiation. For example, ferrous sulfate is oxidized to ferric sulfate and this chemical reaction is used in the Fricke dosimeter. The Fricke dosimeter is useful in finding average radiation dose in a volume of complex shape. A ferrous sulfate solution is placed into a contact of the desired shape, exposed to radiation, agitated to mix the ferric ion throughout the volume and the average concentration of the ferric ion is measured.

Calorimetry Exposure of a substance to radiation results in a small elevation of its' temperature. This change in temperature can be measured. To date, however, calorimetry has not found wide application as a dosimeter in radiology.

HYPERTHERMIA EQUIPMENT

A recent addition to our therapeutic armamentarium is hyperthermia equipment. It has been shown that heating cells prior to or following radiation sensitizes them to cell killing by radiation. The mechanism of this effect is unknown, but it is thought that heating injures the metabolic functions of the cells making them more susceptible to radiation killing. Equipment has been developed for microwave heating of superficial tissues (Figure 9.18). This equipment has found widest application in the treatment of chest wall recurrences of breast cancer in combination with radiation.

REFERENCES

1. Goodwin PN, Quimby, EH, Morgan RH. Physical Foundations of Radiology, Fourth Edition, Harper and Row, 1970.

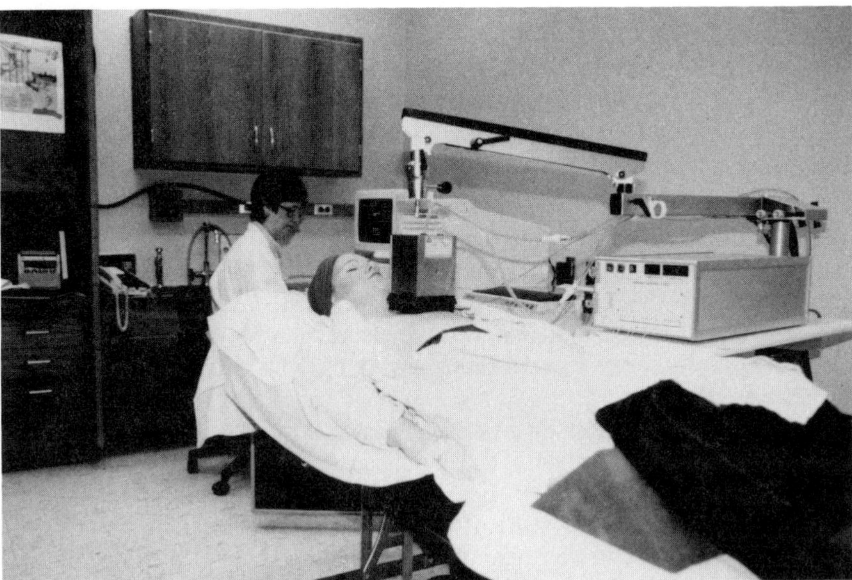

Figure 9.18 This hyperthermia unit generates 915 MHz microwaves. The applicator is water cooled. The temperature is computer monitored via gallium heat sensors.

2. Johns HE,Cunningham JE. The Physics of Radiology, Fourth Edition. Charles C. Thomas, 1983.

3. Schulz MD. The supervoltage story, Janeway Lecture, 1974, Am J Roentgenol 124:541-559, 1975.

4. Castro JR, et al. Treatment of cancer with heavy charged particles, Int J Radiation Oncol Biol Phys 8:2191-2198, 1982.

5. Khan FM. The Physics of Radiation Therapy, Williams & Wilkins, Baltimore, 1984.

6. NCRP Report No. 33: Medical X-ray and Gamma-ray Protection for Energies up to 10 MeV, Equipment Design and Use. National Council of Radiation Protection and Measurements, Washington, D.C., 1968.

7. NCRP Report No. 34: Medical X-ray and Gamma-ray Protection for Energies up to 10 MeV, Structural Shielding Design and Evaluation, National Council on Radiation Protection and Measurements, Washington, D.C., 1970.

8. NCRP Report No. 51: Radiation Protection Design Guidelines for 0.1-100 MeV Particle Accelerator Facilities, National Council on Radiation Protection and Measurements, Washington, D.C., 1977.

Chapter 10

PRINCIPLES OF RADIOTHERAPY
INITIAL PATIENT ASSESSMENT

Radiotherapy is a consultative speciality and patients are referred to the radiotherapist for an opinion as to whether radiotherapy may be of value in a particular situation. Usually the diagnosis of cancer has already been established and the clinical work-up is nearing completion when the consultation is requested. The radiotherapist reviews the medical record, takes a medical history, performs a physical examination, reviews the diagnostic radiographs and reviews the pathology reports concerning any biopsies or surgical resections that have been performed.

After evaluation of all of the clinical data, the radiotherapist must decide whether radiotherapy is indicated and, if indicated, whether the goal of treatment is cure or palliation. The radiotherapist reviews his findings and recommendations with the patient. The stage of disease, the prognosis and the proposed treatment plan are reviewed. If radiotherapy is recommended the patient is informed what area of the body is to be treated, the number of treatments to be given, and what the patient can expect from the proposed treatment, including possible beneficial effects, side effects and late effects.

INDICATIONS FOR CURATIVE RADIOTHERAPY

Radiotherapy alone Radiotherapy alone is indicated for curative treatment for a small number of tumors such as early vocal cord cancer, cancer of the cervix, and early Hodgkin's disease. However, in many patients, as in the case of locally advanced lung cancer, high radiation doses are given even though the chance of cure is not good.

Radiation combined with surgery Radiotherapy is used in combination with surgery for curative treatment in many patients. Patients with breast, endometrial, rectal, and head and neck cancer are often treated with surgery combined with pre-or post-operative radiation.

Radiation combined with chemotherapy Radiation is used in combination with chemotherapy for a growing number of patients, i.e., advanced head and neck cancer.

Radiation combined with surgery and chemotherapy In certain diseases all three modalities are used in planned combination.

It must be emphasized that communication among members of a multi-disciplinary treatment team is essential. Ideally, the discussion would take place at a multi-disciplinary tumor board meeting.

INDICATIONS FOR PALLIATIVE RADIOTHERAPY

Many patients are given radiotherapy for the purpose of providing tempo-rary relief of symptoms caused by advanced cancer. Painful metastasis to bone and symptomatic brain metastasis are the most common indications for palliative treatment.

SITUATIONS IN WHICH RADIOTHERAPY
MAY NOT BE INDICATED

1. The general medical condition of the patient may be such that a course of radiation would not be tolerated.
2. The stage of disease may be so advanced that radiotherapy would not be of benefit to the patient.
3. The disease might be more appropriately treated by another modality.
4. The patient may have previously received a high radiation dose to the site under consideration for re-treatment.
5. The tumor may be located so close to a radiosensitive organ that treatment would be life-threatening.

THE RADIOTHERAPY TREATMENT PLAN

Treatment planning is the most important task of the radiotherapist. Partici-pants in the process, in addition to the patient and radiotherapist, are the treatment planning technologist, the radiation dosimetrist, and the radiation physicist. It is important that special equipment be available including a simulator, a treatment planning computer, and a CT scanner.

The development of an appropriate treatment plan for any individual patient requires a knowledge of:
1. The location and extent of the tumor
2. The natural history of the tumor
3. The radiosensitivity of the tumor
4. The radiation tolerance of the structures to be included in the treatment volume
5. The physical characteristics of the radiation beam
6. The treatment technique to be used
7. The dose-time-fractionation regimen to be used

STEPS IN TREATMENT PLANNING

The treatment planning session should be well organized with each member of the team knowing his role in the process. The steps in treatment planning are as follows:

1. Make a precise description of the tumor volume
2. Select the beam energy
3. Select the treatment technique
4. Select the dose-time-fractionation regimen
5. Apply treatment fields and take simulator films
6. Check films for accuracy and make changes if indicated
7. Apply skin markings
8. Record field sizes, patient dimensions and special instructions for technologists on treatment unit
9. Order individualized shielding blocks when indicated
10. Take patient contour when indicated
12. Obtain computer plan if indicated
13. Calculate treatment plan

DESCRIPTION OF EXTENT OF DISEASE

It is important that the radiotherapy record contain a description of the extent of disease. This will include a detailed description of the location of the tumor, its dimensions, and whether neighboring structures are involved. Also, the presence, location and size of any metastases should be recorded. A supply of anatomical diagrams should be available so that a drawing of the tumor with its dimensions can be made.

SELECTING THE RADIATION BEAM

The ideal treatment technique will allow a high dose to be delivered to the tumor, while at the same time, keeping the dose to the surrounding normal tissue to a minimum. Here it is appropriate to introduce several concepts which are essential to an understanding of treatment planning.

The tumor volume The tumor volume is the volume of the actual tumor mass as detected on physical examination or imaging studies.

The target volume The target volume contains the tumor, but since the tumor usually has microscopic extensions beyond the tumor mass, a margin of at least 1 to 2 cm around the tumor mass is required and this is called the target volume. For some techniques, however, the target volume is much larger than merely 1 to 2 cm around the mass because the regional lymph nodes must be covered to treat possible microscopic deposits which may be present.

There are standard techniques for each tumor site and these will be reviewed in subsequent chapters. However, most of them are simple variations of or combination of one or more of the following treatment techniques.

The single direct portal technique The radiation beam is applied in a single portal perpendicular to the skin surface. This technique is used for other superficial tumors. It is also useful for palliative treatment of spinal metastasis.

The main disadvantage of this technique is that the subcutaneous dose is substantial, and therefore, it is not used for curative high-dose treatments.

The parallel opposing portals technique. This is the most commonly used technique because of its simplicity and accuracy. In it the tumor is treated between an opposing pair of portals. Tumors of the thorax and abdomen are treated with an anterior and posterior opposing pair (Figure 10.1), whereas, head and neck and tumors are treated with opposing lateral portals. The main disadvantage of this technique is that when high doses are required, the dose to superficial tissues such as subcutaneous tissue is high. This disadvantage can be minimized by using a high energy radiation beam.

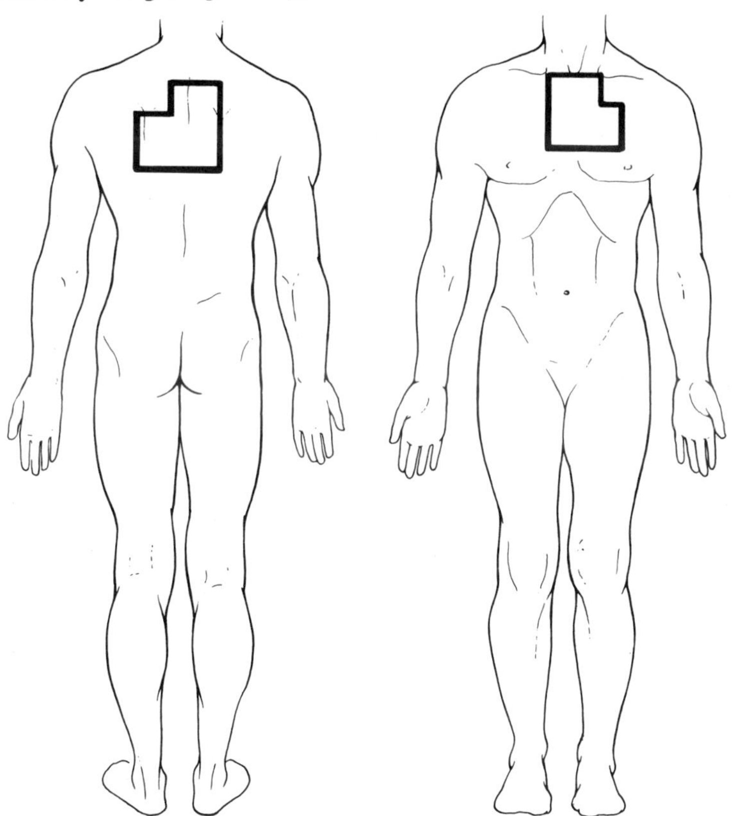

Figure 10.1 Opposing anterior and posterior portals are commonly used to treat the primary and mediastinum of patients with lung cancer.

Multiple portals technique In this technique the tumor is treated with three or more portals (Figure 10.2). This technique is used when high doses are

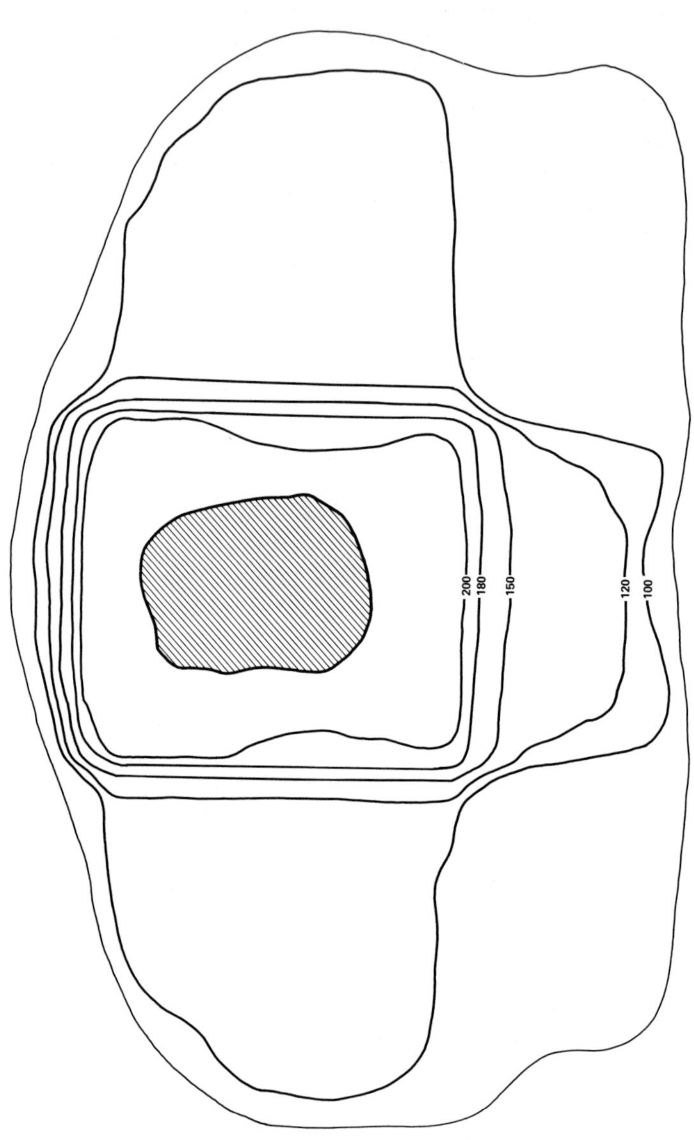

Figure 10.2 This is a typical set of isodose curves for a patient with bladder cancer treated with the four field "box" technique which employs AP-PA and right and left lateral portals.

required for curative treatment of deep seated tumors when radiosensitive structures must be included in the target volume. The main disadvantage is that since multiple portal techniques are more complicated, they are more susceptible to technical error. Also, set-up and treatment times are long compared to simpler techniques.

The wedge filter technique Occasionally, a technique is required in which radiation beams must be applied at right angles to each other. In this situation a method is needed to prevent a "hot-spot" in the target volume. This is accomplished with wedge filters. Wedge filters are wedge shaped pieces of lead or other metal which are attached to the treatment unit (Figure 10.3). The effect of wedge

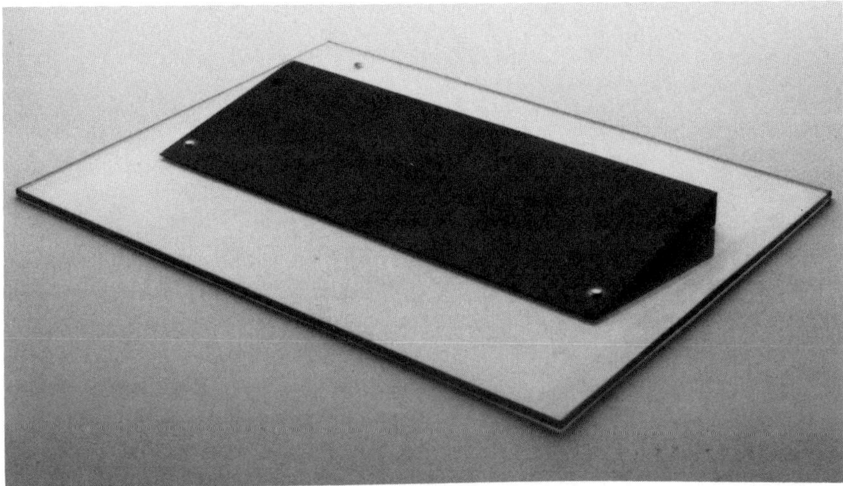

Figure 10.3 This is a wedge filter with a 30 degree wedge angle.

filters in the distribution of radiation in the target volume is shown in Figure 10.4. Different sized wedges are available and these are named according to the angle at which the isodose line is titled, i.e., 15°, 30°, 45°, and 60°.

The shrinking field technique This technique is used when a high dose must be given to a moderately radiosensitive tumor. In this technique the size of the treatment portal is reduced when enough radiation has been given to control microscopic extensions beyond the main tumor mass. Following field size reduction, treatment to the main tumor mass is continued. In this way the central portion of the tumor, which is relatively radioresistant and contains the greatest number of malignant cells, receives the highest dose. The shrinking field technique can be combined with any of the above techniques.

CHOOSING A DOSE-TIME-FRACTIONATION REGIMEN

Standard dose-time-fractionation regimens are used for each clinical situation and these will be covered in subsequent chapters. These regimens have

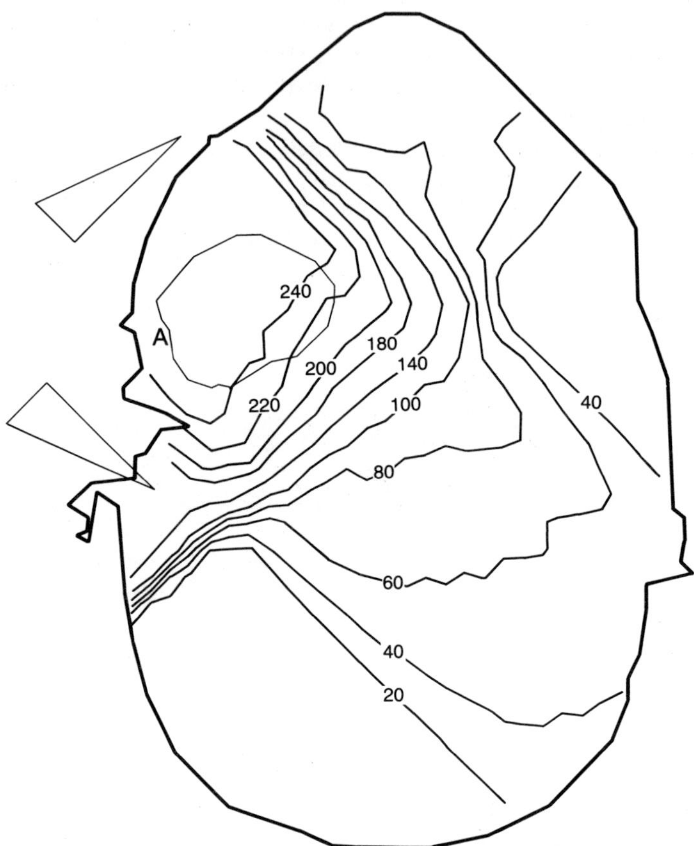

Figure 10.4 Here is a computer plan for a patient with a recurrent parotid gland tumor demonstrating the effect of wedges in the isodose distribution. The tumor dose each day was given to the 200 cGy line.

been arrived at through trial and error observations over many years. In general, however, the regimen selected will depend upon the treatment objective (cure vs. palliation), the radiosensitivity of the tumor, the size of the tumor, the volume of tissue to be irradiated and the age and general condition of the patient

The dose-time-fractionation regimens in current use are as follows:

Conventional fractionation Conventional fractionation is 2 Gy/fraction/ 5 fractions per week. For radiosensitive tumors, such as lymphocytic lymphoma, the treatment time is 3 weeks, whereas for tumors of intermediate sensitivity the treatment time is 6 1/2 to 7 weeks.

Protracted fractionation In this regimen the treatment time is extended and the dose per fraction is reduced to diminish the severity of the acute reaction. The dose per fraction is 1.7-1.8 Gy, 5 fractions/week (8.5-9.0 Gy). If protracted fractionation is used the total tumor dose is increased by 10%.

Split course-regimen In this regimen two courses of treatment areeach separated by a rest interval to allow normal tissues to recover from acute reactions. This method of fractionation may be better tolerated by elderly and debilitated patients. For example, for lung cancer, the patient receives 30 Gy/2 weeks-2 weeks rest-30Gy/2 weeks. This regimen should be used with caution since some studies suggest that treatment results are inferior with the split-course regimen because tumor cells are allowed to proliferate between courses.

Two or three days-a-week fraction This method is also occasionally used for elderly and debilitated patients because it reduces the number of trips to the treatment center. Caution is advised in using this method for curative high-dose regimens, however, since there is evidence that late tissue injury is greater with a smaller number of large fractions than is seen with conventional fractionation. If it is used, the total dose must be reduced by 10%.

High dose per fraction, few fractions This method is used exclusively for palliative treatments. Eight hundred to 1000 cGy in a single treatment, 20 Gy in 5 treatments and 30 Gy in 10 treatments are examples of regimens used for palliative treatment.

Multiple daily fractions In recent years, due to improved understanding of the radiobiology of fractionation, interest has arisen in the use of multiple treatments per day. Two methods are under investigation:

Accelerated fractionation In accelerated fractionation, 2 or 3 daily treatments are given with 4 or 5 hours between fractions, but the fraction size and total dose are similar to conventional fractionation. This results in a shorter overall treatment time. The rationale for this approach is that a tumor with a rapidly proliferating cell population may have significant cell proliferation between fractions with conventional fractionation. Therefore, with accelerated fractionation there is less time for cell proliferation between fractions. However, since the treatment time is shorter, more severe acute tissue reactions are expected with accelerated fractionation than are seen with conventional fractionation.

Hyperfractionation In hyperfractionation, 2 or 3 treatments are given daily in smaller than conventional fractions, i.e., 1.2 to 1.5 Gy/fraction. The overall treatment time is the same as with conventional fractionation but the total tumor dose is greater. Such a regimen may result in improved tumor control because an increase in the total tumor dose by 15% to 25% might be possible without increasing the severity of late effects. Early results suggest that improved local tumor control is seen following hyperfractionated treatment for advanced head and neck cancer.

APPLYING TREATMENT FIELDS AND
TAKING SIMULATOR FILMS

The desired treatment fields or portals are drawn on the skin with a "magic marker". The technologist sets the treatment field and takes a simulator film using the skin lines. The radiotherapist checks the film and, if changes are required in the treatment field, draws the changes on the simulator film. The technologist makes the alterations in the field and repeats the simulator film.

APPLYING SKIN MARKINGS

The final fields are marked on the skin with carbol fuchsin (Castaderm). In the event that the patient is reluctant to have red marks on the skin, the fields can be marked with tattoos. In this method the corners and central axis points of the fields are tattooed in India ink applied intra-dermally with a 22 gauge needle.

RECORDING FIELD SIZES, PATIENT DIMENSIONS
AND SPECIAL INSTRUCTIONS

The collimator settings for each field, the SSD (Source skin distance) and the treatment field sizes (the collimator field size corrected for blocking) are recorded on the treatment chart. A diagram is made of the anatomical location of each treatment field. Each treatment field is designated by a letter of the alphabet. In addition, any necessary patient measurements such as the thickness or diameter of the part to be treated opposite the SSD points, are recorded in the chart.

PREPARING INDIVIDUALIZED SHIELDING BLOCKS

Many treatment techniques require shielding of normal structures which do not require treatment but are located in the volume covered by a square or rectangular field. These structures can often be shielded with lead blocks placed on a lucite tray attached to the treatment unit (Figure 10.5). In many situations, however, the shape of the field is complex requiring individualized shielding devices. These are made with a low melting point lead alloy called cerrobend. The details of construction of cerrobend shields are shown in Chapter 24.

MAKING A PATIENT CONTOUR

Complex treatment techniques require computer generated isodose curves showing the radiation distribution in the target volume. In preparation for the computer plan a contour of the circumference of the body part to be treated is required. The contour is made with solderwire and transferred to paper. The contour is performed by the radiation dosimetrist or the treatment planning technologist.

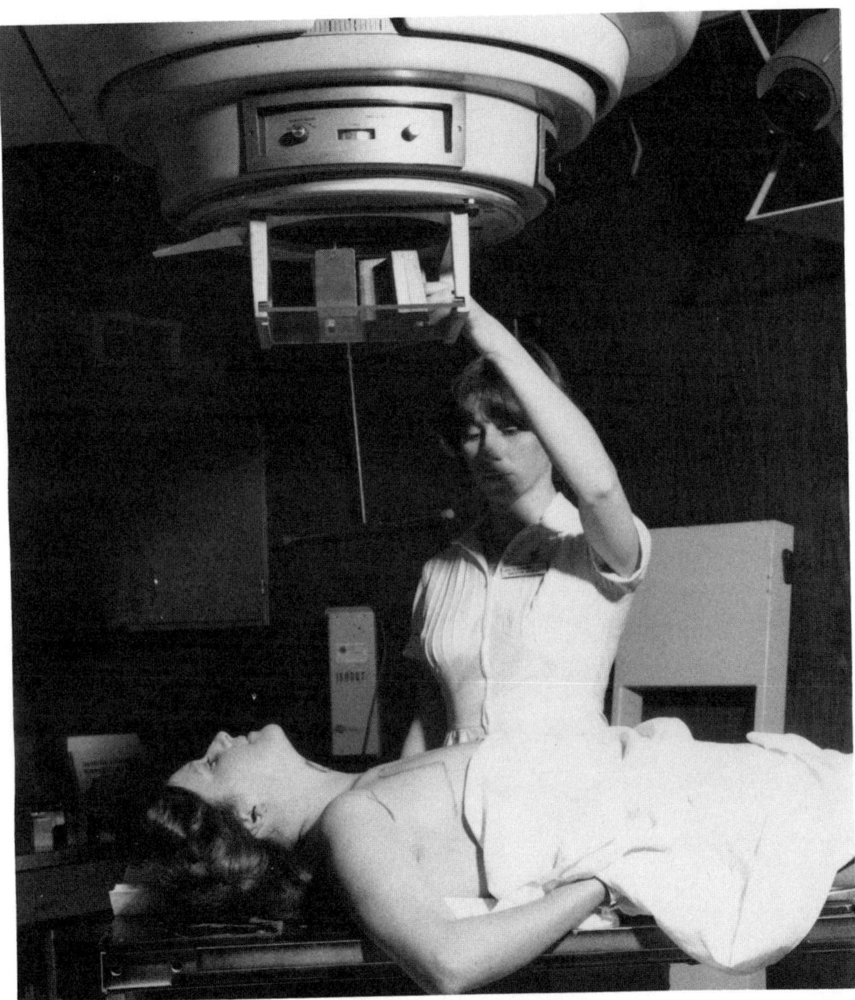

Figure 10.5 Shielding blocks are placed on a "shadow tray."

COMPUTER GENERATED ISODOSE CURVES

Computer generated isodose curves are obtained in the following situations:

1. For the parallel opposing portal technique when a precise knowledge of the radiation distribution in the target volume is required.
2. For most cases where multiple portal techniques are required.
3. Whenever angled beams are used.
4. Whenever wedge filters are needed.

The computer generated isodose curves are usually prepared by the physicist or the dosimetrist.

CT SCANNING FOR TREATMENT PLANNING

The addition of CT scanning has resulted in an improvement in the accuracy of treatment planning. CT scans are performed following completion of the simulation in the following situations:

1. When there is doubt about the true extent of the tumor in the target volume.
2. When multiple portal techniques are used to treat a deeply situated tumor.
3. When there is a need to know the exact position of a radiosensitive organ.

The steps in CT scanning for treatment planning are as follows:

1. The treatment planning technologist and the physicist accompany the patient to the CT scanner. The treatment planning technologist positions the patient on the CT scanner couch in the exact treatment position.
2. The skin markings are outlined with angiocatheters taped to the skin.
3. The CT scan is obtained.
4. The tumor volume is located on the scan and the coverage of the tumor in relation to the angiocatheters is assessed (Figure 10.6).

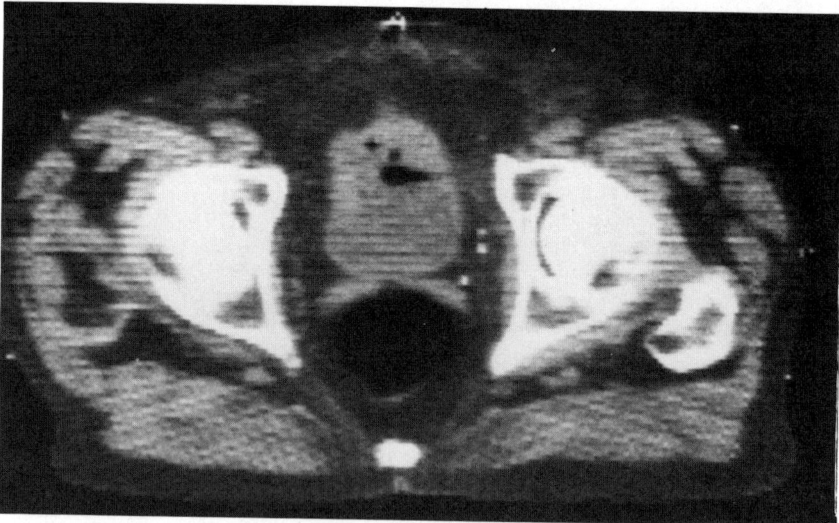

Figure 10.6 This is the treatment planning CT scan for a patient with locally advanced prostate cancer treated with the "box" technique. The white spots on the right and left lateral skin surfaces are radio-opaque angiocatheters which designate the anterior and posterior margins and SSD points for the lateral portals.

5. If changes in the plan are needed to cover the tumor, the computer generated isodose curves are made with the appropriate changes.
6. The changes in the skin markings on the patient are made.

CAUSES OF TREATMENT FAILURE

Treatment failure is defined as regrowth of tumor in a treated area or the occurrence of a significant treatment complication. The causes are:

Technical errors *Causes of recurrence:* 1) Geographical miss--part of the tumor was not irradiated and/or 2) "cold spots" (areas of underdosage)--a portion of the tumor received an insufficient dose. *Causes of complications:* 1) "Hot spots" (areas of overdosage) -- a portion of the tumor received an excessive dose and/or 2) excessive dose to radiosensitive organ in target volume.

Tumor dose excessive A cause of complications.

Tumor dose insufficient A cause of recurrence.

Radioresistant primary A cause of recurrence.

Large primary Local recurrence is more common with large tumors which contain many hypoxic cells.

New primary In some patients local failure occurs because a second primary tumor develops in the treatment area.

No obvious cause In many patients no cause can be identified to explain local treatment recurrence or complications.

Distant metastasis In many patients treatment failure occurs because of the development of distant metastases even though the local tumor has been controlled. This is less important than other causes in judging the success or failure of a local treatment method such as radiation.

EVALUATING TREATMENT RESULTS

Survival rate For most tumors the five-year survival rate is the standard for evaluating and comparing treatment results. The five-year survival rate is the percentage of the total number of patients treated who are surviving five years after treatment. For some tumors having a long natural history, such as breast cancer and prostate cancer, the survival rate at ten years is more appropriate. However, for rapidly growing tumors such as lung cancer, the two-year survival rate is an adequate end-point.

Local tumor control The rate of tumor control in the target volume is an important end-point in radiotherapy. The tumor control rate is the percentage of the total number treated in whom the disease is controlled in the treatment area at a specific time post-treatment i.e., 2 years or 5 years. Successful radiotherapy techniques have tumor control rates in excess of 80%.

Complication rate The complication rate is the percentage of the total number of patients treated who develop significant treatment complications within a specific time post-treatment. A successful radiotherapy technique must have a low complication rate (<5-10%).

THE THERAPEUTIC RATIO IN RADIOTHERAPY

The therapeutic ratio is the ratio between the incidence of tumor control and incidence of treatment complications (Figure 10.7). As can be seen from the figure, the rates of tumor control and complications can be plotted as sigmoid or S-shaped response curves. The goal of radiotherapy is to increase the therapeutic

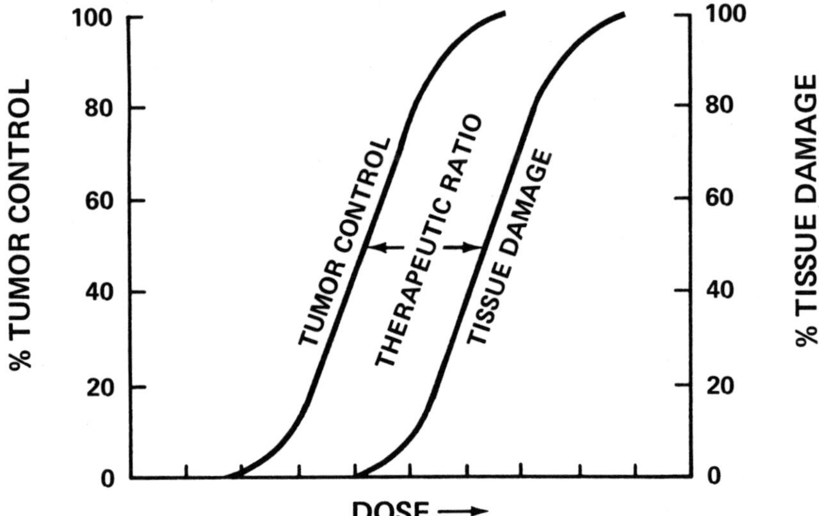

Figure 10.7 This is an illustration of the concept of therapeutic ratio in radiotherapy.

ratio by increasing the rate of tumor control without increasing the complication rates. A few examples of methods used to increase the therapeutic ratio are as follows:

Fractionation Fractionation spares normal tissue and increases the rate of tumor control.

Combining surgery and radiation A moderate dose of radiation is used to eliminate microscopic deposits of cancer which are beyond the surgical field, whereas the surgery eliminates the radioresistant central tumor mass.

Radiosensitizing drugs Research studies are underway to find a drug which can be used clinically to increase radiosensitivity of tumor cells without increasing the radiosensitivity of normal tissues. Several drugs of the class of drugs called nitromidazoles are capable of sensitizing hypoxic cells but not oxygenated cells. An example of one of these is called metronidazole. These drugs have promise because sensitization to the hypoxic cells of a tumor would result in increased tumor controls without an increase in complications.

Hyperbaric oxygen An early example of an attempt to increase the therapeutic ratio by reducing the fraction of hypoxic cells was to place the patient in a hyperbaric oxygen chamber during radiotherapy. The patients were treated at oxygen pressures of three to four atmospheres. One clinical trial from England suggested that control and survival rates for patients with advanced head and neck cancer were increased with hyperbaric oxygen plus radiation, compared to radiation alone.

Hyperthermia and radiation It has been demonstrated, that the addition of heat increases the damage produced by radiation in tumors and normal tissues. Clinical studies are underway investigating whether hyperthermia combined with radiation increases the therapeutic ratio. Various techniques are being investigated to provide local tissue heating including microwaves, ultrasound, hot water baths, short wave diathermy and radio-frequency induced current. These methods are designed to heat the tumor to 43 degrees centigrade for approximately one hour. The heating is effective if administered prior to, during, or following radiation.

Chemotherapy and radiation Studies are underway to evaluate the combined effect of chemotherapy drugs and radiation on tumors and normal tissue. Unfortunately, many drugs increase the severity of normal tissue reactions when combined with radiation. A drug is needed that acts synergistically with radiation to produce greater cell killing than the sum of both agents.

Charged particles and fast neutrons Clinical trials are proceeding in a number of centers evaluating the role of beams of charged particles, such as protons, which may increase the therapeutic ratio by improving the radiation dose distribution in tissue compared to conventional radiations. Fast neutrons may increase the therapeutic ratio by reducing the OER for hypoxic cells compared to conventional radiation.

REFERENCE

1. Fletcher GH. Chapter 2, Basic principles of radiotherapy, in Textbook of Radiotherapy, Lea and Febiger, Philadelphia, 1980, pp. 103-228.

2. Phillips TL. Clinical and experimental alteration in the radiation therapeutic ratio caused by cytotoxic chemotherapy, in Radiation Biology and Cancer Research, Eds. Meyn RE, Withers HR, Raven Press, New York, 1980, pp. 567-588.

3. Suit HD, Goitein M. Rationale for use of charged-particle and fast neutron beams in radiation therapy, in Radiation Biology in Cancer Research, Eds Meyn RE, Withers HR, Raven Press, New York, 1980, pp. 547-565.

Chapter 11

QUALITY ASSURANCE IN RADIOTHERAPY

Quality assurance is the continuing process by which human errors are detected and evaluated, and corrective and preventive measures instituted in all phases of radiotherapy. In curative radiotherapy high radiation doses must be delivered to the tumor to ensure a high rate of tumor control. Data from clinical studies suggest that if the tumor receives 5-10% less that the prescribed tumor dose a significant decrease in local tumor control will be observed. Likewise, if the actual tumor dose exceeds the prescribed tumor dose by 5-10% a significant increase in tissue injuries will be observed. Therefore, it is essential that all phases of radiotherapy are carried out for each patient as precisely as possible to ensure optimum treatment results. A comprehensive program of quality assurance is required in all activities in a radiation oncology department.

PERSONNEL

The most important requirement in any quality assurance program is that a sufficient number of qualified people be available in each personnel category to adequately process the work load. The Committee for Radiation Oncology Studies has published guidelines for optimal radiation therapy staffing and these are listed in Table 11.1.

Other personnel required for the effective operation of the radiotherapy service include social worker, dietician, administrative assistant, secretary, medical transcriptionist, medical record clerk, radiotherapy aid, transportation coordinator, electronics technician, machinist, statistician and data manager. These individuals may be shared with other hospital services.

QUALITY ASSURANCE IN DOCUMENTATION

An essential feature of any quality assurance program is the maintenance of adequate records. Each patient who undergoes treatment should have a radiotherapy chart that is separate from the hospital chart. The radiotherapy chart should contain the following: consultation reports, history and physical examination reports, anatomic drawings of the extent of the tumor, operative and pathology reports, diagnostic radiology reports, evaluations during the course of treatment and long-term follow-up data. In addition, all technical details of the treatment plan, dosimetry calculations and daily treatment documentation are recorded in the radiotherapy chart.

Table 11.1 Guidelines for optimal radiation therapy staffing

Personnel Category	Number per facility
Radiation oncologist director	1
Radiation oncologist	1 per 200-250 patients
Radiation physicist	1 per 400 patients
Treatment planning staff (physicist, dosimetrist, or treatment planning technologist)	1 per 300 patients
Radiation therapy technologist	
Supervisor	1
Staff	2 per megavoltage unit
Simulator	1-2 per unit
Nursing staff	1 per 300 patients

QUALITY ASSURANCE IN PATIENT EVALUATIONS

A list of important procedures to assure quality in initial assessment of the patient is as follows:

History and physical examination

Laboratory and radiographic studies

Pathology review

Staging classification

Treatment decision

Discussion with patient

New patient conference

QUALITY ASSURANCE IN TREATMENT PLANNING

Measures which can be used to assure quality in treatment planing are use of a simulator, checking simulations with CT scanning, using individualized immobilization devises, using accurate methods for obtaining patient contours, using a treatment planning computer to correct for tissue inhomogeneities and requiring all dosimetry calculations to be checked by a second person. Finally, the simulator films, CT scans, isodose curves and dose calculations should be reviewed at a treatment planning conference attended by members of the clinical, physics, and technical staff.

QUALITY ASSURANCE IN TREATMENT DELIVERY

The most common errors in treatment delivery are: 1. Errors in setting machine parameters and; 2. errors in field (portal) placement. Field placement errors are defined as deviations in the daily placement of the treatment field such that the treatment volume is different from the originally planned treatment volume. Several categories of field placement errors can occur including malposition of the cephalo-caudad and/or transverse dimension, rotation of the field, malposition of the patient and malposition of a beam shaping device or wedge filter.

Methods which can be used to reduce errors in treatment delivery include:

1. Requiring technologists to check each other in field placement and setting of machine parameters
2. Installing a record and verify system
3. Outline fields with skin markings
4. Measure distances of field margins from bony landmarks
5. Take photos of treatment fields and set-ups
6. Use easily reproducible techniques for patient positioning
7. Use isocentric treatment techniques which require little patient movement between set-ups
8. Use laser beam side lights for patient positioning
9. Take initial and weekly portal films
10. Daily portal film review sessions
11. Weekly clinical examination and evaluation of the patient
12. Weekly chart review
13. Regular quality assurance conferences attended by clinicians, physicists and technologists

PHYSICS QUALITY ASSURANCE

A list of procedures to be carried out by the physicist to assure proper equipment function is shown in Table 11.2. The list includes the maximum error that can be tolerated and the frequency that each factor should be checked.

QUALITY ASSURANCE IN BRACHYTHERAPY

Brachytherapy sources also require quality assurance procedures. All sealed sources must be leak tested every 6 months and an inventory log listing source locations must be maintained. The application and removal of all sources from patients should be the responsibility of the radiation oncology department. Quality is assured by strict adherence to established routines for handling radioactive sources. One or two trained individuals should have the responsibil-

Table 11.2   Quality assurance of external beam equipment

Parameter	Tolerance	Frequency
Central axis dose calibration	2%	Annually
Dose rate along central axis	3%	Daily
Depth dose	2%	Monthly
Beam uniformity	3%	Weekly
Dose monitor		
Timer accuracy		
Light field and radiation field agreement	3mm	Weekly
SSD lights and lasers	2mm	Monthly
Scale readouts		Monthly
Focal spot position		Annually
Jaw symmetry	2mm	Annually
Coincidence of collimator and gantry axis with isocenter	2mm	Annually
Stability of gantry arm and bearing under rotation		Annually
Couch motion and table top sag		Annually

ity for preparation of the sources for placement into the patient, for returning the sources to the safe and for maintaining the log. Orthogonal radiographs should be taken of each application to document the position of each source and computer generated isodose curves should be prepared. Experience has shown that the quality of brachytherapy is best in institutions where a large number of brachytherapy procedures are carried out.

Radiation safety   Any institution using radioactive materials must employ a Radiation Protection Supervisor who has the responsibility for establishing procedures and making recommendations regarding safe handling of radionuclides. He must determine exposure to anyone caring for or associating with radioactive patients.

Lead-lined safes for storing radioactive sources are commercially available (Figure 11.1). A source preparation bench should be located close to the safe and the preparation of the sources should be carried out behind a shield. Radioactive sources should be handled with long forceps. The operator should maximize the distance between himself and the sources and minimize the time that he works with the sources. The sources should be transported by long handled cart in a lead container (Figure 11.2).

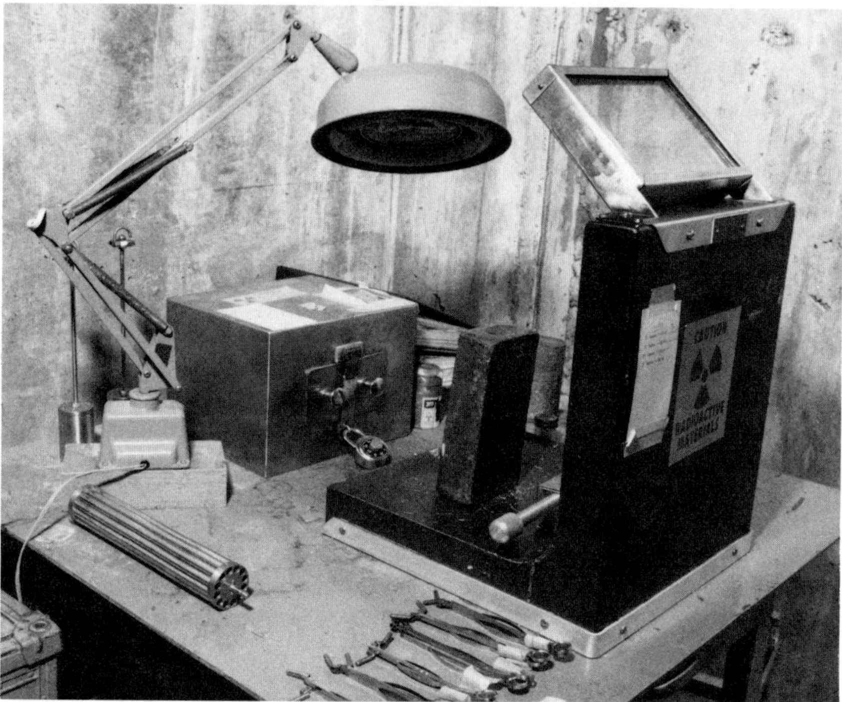

Figure 11.1 This safe is used for storage of cesium-137 needles and tubes. The dosimetrist works behind the shield.

Hospital routines for radioactive patients For all patients who have received radioactive material, an entry must be made in the patient's medical record which states the identity of the radionuclide and the date and time of administration.

The maximum exposure rate at a specified distance from the patient is determined immediately after administration of the material. The exposure rate is measured with an ionization chamber or survey meter (Figure 11.3). The exposure rate at a distance of 1 meter from the approximate center of the implant is recorded in the patient's chart. In most institutions, the exposure rate at 6 feet from the patient, at the door of the room and in the adjoining room is also measured and recorded.

A "Radioactivity Precautions" tag is placed on the medical record and on the patient, the bed and the door of the room. The tag specifies:

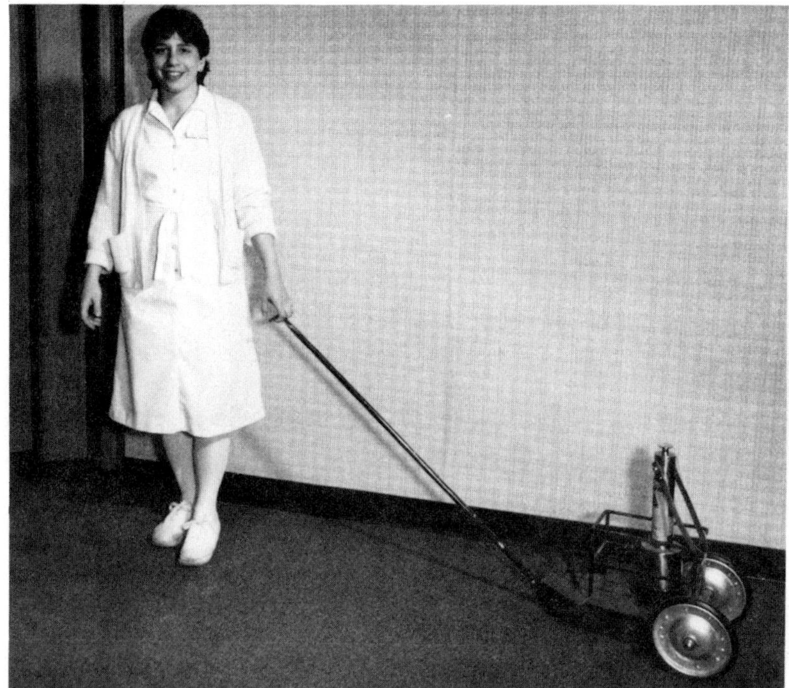

Figure 11.2 Radioactive materaials are transported in a lead container with a long-handled cart.

1. The radionuclide, activity of the sources and time of administration
2. The exposure rate at 1 meter, the time the determination was made and by whom
3. The date on which precautions cease to be required

The nurses caring for radioactive patients should be classified and instructed as radiation workers. Pregnant nurses should not be responsible for the care of radioactive patients. To minimize exposure to hospital personnel, radioactive patients should not be kept in one area but should be dispersed.

During interstitial and intracavitary therapy with sealed sources there is no danger of radioactive contamination except by damage or loss of a source. Therefore, no special precautions need be taken with regard to food, bedding, or excreta, except to be certain that no source is lost via these routes. Surgical dressings should be changed only by the physician and for gynecological implants perineal care is not given during the implant. However, care must be taken to ensure that the sources are not loosened or disturbed.

If a source should become dislodged, the nurse should pick it up with a forceps and place it in a lead container which is kept in the patient's room during

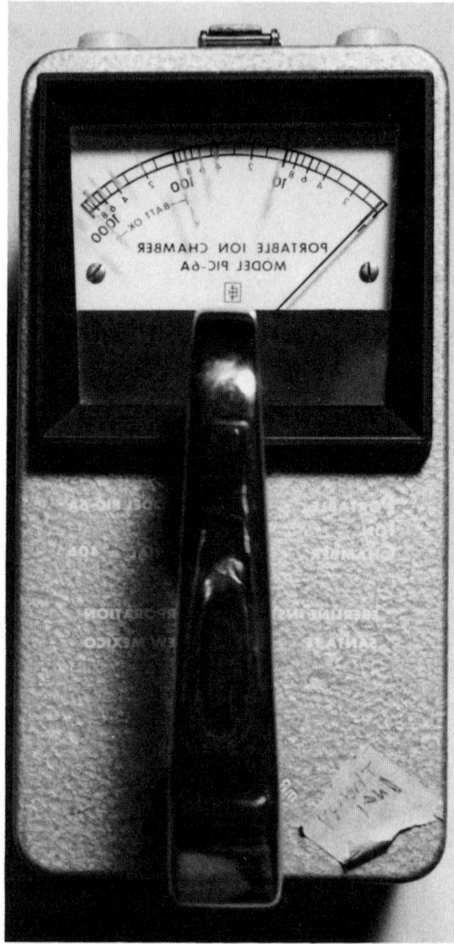

Figure 11.3 Room surveys are carried out with the aid of a small hand-held ionization chamber.

the implant. The physician and Radiation Protection Supervisor are both notified.

Persons visiting patients with radioactive implants should remain 6 feet from the patient. Pregnant women and children should not visit. Patients who are not receiving treatment with a radioactive implant and who are present in the same room or an adjoining room should not receive a dose of more that 100 mrem during any one hospital admission. The NCRP recommends that patients containing radioactive nuclides with half-lives greater than 125 days (radium-226, cobalt-60, cesium-137) be hospitalized for the duration of the treatment. For these patients, therefore, all sources must be removed prior to discharge.

Patients who have short-lived radionuclides such as iodine-125, gold-198, and radon may be discharged if the activity remaining in the patient will result in an exposure of less than 5 rem in one year at one meter from the patient. However, there are specific recommendations for contact with other individuals following discharge which vary according to the age of the other individuals in the household. The reader should consult NCRP Report No.37 for the recommendations.

REFERENCES

1. Criteria for Radiation Oncology in Multidisciplinary Cancer Management, Report to the Director of the National Cancer Institute National Institutes of Health by the Committee for Radiation Oncology Studies, Grant CA 25792, February, 1981.

2. Chaffey JT, Quality assurance in radiation therapy; Clinical considerations, Int J Radiat Oncol Biol Phys 10:Suppl 1, pp.115-117, 1984.

3. Kartha PKI, et al, Accuracy in clinical dosimetry, Brit J. Radiol 46:1083-1084, 1975.

4. Kartha PKI, et al, Accuracy in patient set up and its consequence in dosimetry, Medical Physics 2:331-332, 1975.

5. Byhardt RW, et al, Weekly localization films and detection of field placement errors, Int J Radiat Oncol Biol Phys 41:881-887, 1978.

6. Suntharalingam N, Teletherapy equipment and simulators, Int J Radiat Oncol Biol Phys 10: Suppl 1, 137-138, 1984.

7. NCRP Report No. 37; Precautions in the Management of Patients Who Have Received Therapeutic Amounts of Radionuclides, National Council on Radiation Protection and Measurements, Washington, D.C., 1970.

8. NCRP Report No. 40: Protection Against Radiation from Brachytherapy Sources, National Council on Radiation Protection, Washington, D.C., 1972.

Chapter 12

BASIC PRINCIPLES
OF CHEMOTHERAPY

MEDICAL ONCOLOGY

The administration of anticancer drugs should be carried out only by physicians trained in their use. Since these drugs may affect the function of many organs, the physicians must have knowledge of the pharmacology of the drugs and methods of evaluating the function of the various organs that might be injured. Physicians trained in the administration of chemotherapeutic agents are called medical oncologists. Medical oncologists are specialists in internal medicine who have taken additional training in oncology and cancer chemotherapy. They are trained to work closely with surgeons, radiotherapists and other members of the multidisciplinary team. Pediatric oncologists are physicians trained in pediatrics and cancer chemotherapy who are responsible for the overall care of children with cancer.

GENERAL PRINCIPLES

1.   A single malignant cell can give rise to sufficient progeny to kill the host. Therefore, it is essential that the entire population of malignant cells be eradicated.

2.   In contrast to antimicrobial chemotherapy where there are major contributions by the immune system, in malignancy immune mechanisms appear to contribute little to cure unless there are only a small number of malignant cells present.

3.   The cell killing caused by chemotherapeutic drugs is similar to that of radiation and follows first order kinetics. This means that a constant percentage, rather than a constant number of cells, is killed by a chemotherapeutic agent. For example, a patient with advanced acute lymphocytic leukemia might have a tumor burden of 10^{12} cells. A drug capable of killing 99.99% of the cells would reduce the tumor burden to 10^8 cells. This fact has led to chemotherapy regimens utilizing several drugs concurrently, or in sequence, in an attempt to obtain total cell kill.

4.   In general, chemotherapeutic agents are more effective against small tumor burdens than against large tumor burdens.

5.   Chemotherapeutic agents usually act at specific phases of the cell cycle, and therefore, are active only against cells that are in the process of cell division. For this reason, tumors that are most susceptible to chemotherapy are those with a large growth fraction (a high percentage of cells in the process of cell division).

6.   All chemotherapeutic agents affect normal as well as neoplastic cells. Normal cells which divide rapidly, such as hair follicle epithelium, bone marrow cell and gastrointestinal epithelium are usually most sensitive. The toxic effects of each agent are known and supportive care programs are available. Blood component therapy with transfusion of red cells and platelets, and antibiotic therapy are frequently necessary to control the problems of anemia, bleeding, and infection which are common side effects of chemotherapy.

CLASSIFICATION OF CHEMOTHERAPEUTIC AGENTS

A classification scheme for the major classes of chemotherapeutic agents and a list of several examples of diseases that each agent is active against is shown in Table 12.1.

Table 12.1 Classification of chemotherapeutic agents			
Class	**Type of agent**	**Drug**	**Diseases**
Alkylating agents	Nitrogen mustards	Mechlorethamine	Hodgkin's disease
		Cyclophosphamide	Acute leukemia, breast, lung
	Nitrosoureas	Carmustine (BCNU)	Primary brain tumors
		Lomustine (CCNU)	Primary brain tumors
Antimetabolites	Folic acid analogs	Methotrexate	Acute leukemia, head & neck, bone
	Pyrimidine analogs	Fluorouracil (5FU)	Breast, GI, head & neck
	Purine analogs	Mercaptopurine	Acute leukemia
Natural products	Vinca alkaloids	Vincristine	Acute leukemia, lymphomas
	Epipodophyllotoxins	Etoposide	Testis, lung
	Antibiotics	Doxorubicin	Soft tissue, bone, breast, lymphomas
		Bleomycin	Lymphomas, lung, head & neck
Miscellaneous agents	Platinum coordination complexes	Cisplatin	Testis, head & neck, bladder

MECHANISMS AND SITES OF ACTION OF CHEMOTHERAPEUTIC AGENTS

Most chemotherapeutic agents act specifically on processes such as DNA synthesis, transcription or the function of the mitotic spindle and are called cell cycle specific. Examples of the sites of action of selected agents are shown in Table 12.2.

COMBINATION CHEMOTHERAPY

It has been found for a number of tumors that the response rate and duration is improved if multiple agents are administered in combination. Successful multi-drug regimens have the following criteria: 1. Each drug in a combination should be active against the tumor when used alone; 2. The drugs should have

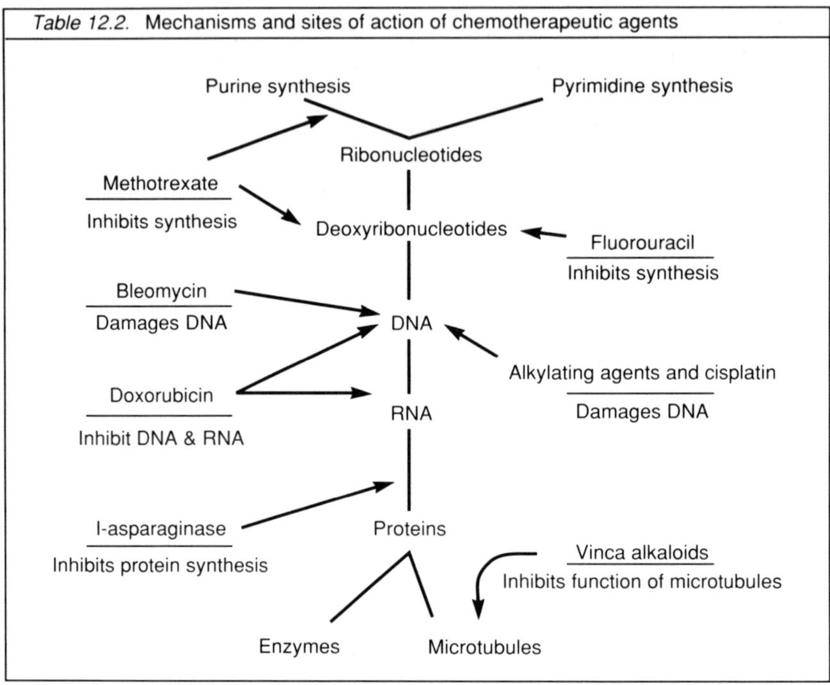

different mechanisms of action; 3. The toxic effects of the drugs should not overlap. Combination chemotherapy has yielded improved treatment results for Hodgkin's disease, some non-Hodgkin's lymphomas, acute leukemias, disseminated breast cancer and testicular cancer.

ADJUVANT CHEMOTHERAPY

Clinical studies have shown that even after operations thought to be curative, local recurrences and distant metastases may occur. The reason for these failures is that micro-metastases occurred prior to the operation. Chemotherapy administered immediately following surgery, called adjuvant chemotherapy, may eradicate these microscopic foci yielding improved cure rates. Clinical studies evaluating adjuvant chemotherapy are underway for breast, colon, head and neck and lung cancer as well as various pediatric neoplasms.

CRITERIA FOR EVALUATING RESPONSE TO CHEMOTHERAPEUTIC AGENTS

Objective response A patient undergoing chemotherapy is said to have had an objective response if the following criteria are met:

1. There must be a reduction in the product of the longest perpendicular diameters of the most easily measurable tumor mass by at least 50%.
2. There must be no increase in the size of other masses.
3. No new areas of disease appear.
4. This result must be maintained for at least 2 months.

Performance status Response to chemotherapy is also evaluated by the change in the patient's performance status. An improvement in performance status suggests a beneficial effect of the treatment on the tumor. A commonly used system for quantifying performance was described by Karnofsky:

Karnofsky Performance Status Scale

Index	Definition
100	Asymptomatic
80-90	Symptomatic but fully ambulatory
60-70	In bed less than 50% of each day
40-50	In bed more than 50% of each day
20-30	Completely bedridden

Survival The ultimate proof of the effectiveness of a drug is its ability to produce improved survival. This is usually demonstrated in a randomized clinical trial in which patients with a malignant disease are randomly assigned to receive the test drug or drug combination versus no treatment or another standard treatment. The objective response rate and the survival time in days, months or years for the two treatments are compared.

THE IMPACT OF CANCER CHEMOTHERAPY

Chemotherapy was not introduced into medical practice until the late 1950s and was not widely and consistently used until the specialty of medical oncology was established in the late 1950s. Since this time there has been an overall 30% improvement in survival rates which can be attributed to improvements in radiation therapy and the increased use of chemotherapy alone or in combination with surgery and radiation.

A partial list of diseases, curable by chemotherapy alone or in combination with surgery, in the adjuvant setting is shown in Table 12.3. Also listed are some diseases which are responsive to chemotherapy, but not curable, and some that are poorly responsive to currently available drugs and drug combinations.

RATIONALE FOR COMBINING RADIATION AND CHEMOTHERAPY

In a relatively high percentage of patients treated for a locally advanced tumor by radiation alone failure occurs because of local recurrence or distant

Table 12.3 Tumors responsive to chemotherapy

Tumors curable in advanced stages by chemotherapy

Choriocarcinoma	Wilms' tumor	Hodgkin's disease
Acute lymphocytic leukemia	Diffuse large cell lymphoma	Testicular cancer Burkitt's lymphoma
Ewing's sarcoma	Embryonal rhabdomyosarcoma	
Small cell lung cancer		

Tumors curable by adjuvant chemotherapy combined with surgery

Breast cancer	Osteogenic sarcoma	Soft tissue sarcoma
Colorectal cancer		

Tumors responsive in advanced stages, but not curable

Bladder cancer	Head & Neck cancer	Gastric carcinoma
Chronic mylogenous leukemia	Cervical cancer	Breast cancer Prostate cancer
Multiple myeloma	Hairy cell leukemia	Chronic lymphocytic leukemia
Soft tissue sarcoma		

Tumors unresponsive in advanced stages to chemotherapy

Pancreatic cancer	Renal cancer	Colorectal cancer
Melanoma	Non-small cell lung cancer	

metastases. For this reason, there is great interest in developing methods of combining radiation and chemotherapy for the purpose of reducing the incidence of local and distant failure. This field is in its developmental stages and much more research is needed before combined modality therapy with irradiation and chemotherapy becomes widely used.

REFERENCES

1. Calabresi P, Chabner BA. Section XII, Chemotherapy of neoplastic diseases, in Goodman and Gilman's The Pharmacologic Basis of Therapeutics, Eight Edition, Eds. Gilman AG, Rall TW, Nies AS, Taylor P, Pergamon Press, 1990, pp 1202-1263.

2. DeVita VT. Chapter 16, Principles of chemotherapy, in Cancer Principles and Practice of Oncology, 3rd Edition, Eds. DeVita VT, Hellman S, Rosenberg SA, J. B. Lippincott Company, Philadelphia, 1989, pp. 276-300.

Chapter 13

PRINCIPLES OF
ENDOCRINE THERAPY

Endocrine therapy is a valuable treatment method for cancers derived from hormone-sensitive tissues such as breast and prostate gland. At the present time, endocrine therapy is not curative for any neoplasm, but useful palliation for a large number of patients is possible with endocrine therapy.

Hormones influence cell function and growth by penetrating the susceptible cells to become bound to specific hormone receptors. The hormone receptor complex is then transported to the nucleus of the cell where it attaches to the responsive cell genome. The stimulated genome induces increased protein synthesis resulting in changes in cell growth, division and function. These steps in the transport and incorporation of the hormone molecule can be blocked or altered at a number of points. Endocrine therapy is unique in cancer therapy because hormones do not cause cell death by destruction of DNA as in radiation and chemotherapy. Hormones exert their effect on cell growth division and function through physiologic mechanisms. Therefore, hormone responses occur more gradually and one to three months of therapy may be necessary before improvement is seen.

An important improvement in endocrine therapy occurred when it became possible to measure hormone receptor levels in tissue samples. For example, breast cancer tissue can be assayed for estrogen receptors and this has made therapy more rational because only those tumors which have estrogen receptors would be expected to respond to endocrine therapy.

The mechanism of action of the majority of hormonal agents is unknown. In many cases, the removal of a hormone or the administration of the same hormone will lead to tumor regression.

METHODS OF ENDOCRINE THERAPY

Surgical ablation One of the earliest methods of endocrine therapy was surgical removal of endocrine organs. Bilateral oophorectomy (removal of ovaries), to eliminate the major source of estrogen production is an important technique for management of advanced breast cancer in patients having estrogen receptor (ER) positive (+) tumors. Other surgical techniques which have been successful in management of advanced breast cancer include bilateral adrenalectomy and hypophysectomy (pituitary ablation). Bilateral orchiectomy (removal of testes), to eliminate the main source of testosterone is an important treatment for advanced prostate cancer.

Estrogens Estrogens are responsible for the stimulation and maintenance of secondary female sex characteristics. Estrogens are also used as treatment for advanced prostate and breast cancer. Diethylstilbestrol (DES) is the most widely used estrogen in cancer treatment. The mechanism of action in prostate DES causes a reduction in testosterone levels.

Antiestrogens Antiestrogens are useful in the treatment of advanced breast cancer. Tamoxifen is the most widely used antiestrogen. Tamoxifen binds to estrogen receptors which depletes the receptor pool and thus interferes with normal estrogen action. Tamoxifen is also effective in the adjuvant treatment of breast cancer. Postmenopausal patients withStage II (+ nodes) breast cancer who have an ER (+) tumor experience a longer disease-free survival when placed on tamoxifen compared to those treated with surgery alone.

Aromatase inhibitors Aminoglutethamide, an inhibitor of steroidogenesis, is effective in the treatment of metastatic breast cancer. This drug is used in postmenopausal women who have already had an oophorectomy. Aminoglutethamide acts on the adrenal gland and on the peripheral cells to inhibit estrogen production so that the net effect is a further reduction in the already low levels of estrogens.

Androgens Androgens are responsible for secondary male sex characteristics, promotion of spermatogenesis and anabolic effects such increasing muscle mass and promoting general body growth. Androgens are secreted primarily by the testes but also by the ovaries and adrenal glands. Androgens are effective in the treatment of advanced breast cancer but the response rate is lower than with other endocrine agents. The mechanism of action is unknown. The most commonly used agent is fluoxymesterone (Halotestin).

Antiandrogens Antiandrogens compete with testosterone for receptor sites in cells. Several of these have activity in prostate cancer. Flutamide is an orally administered antiandrogen which is under investigation in prostate cancer.

Gonadotropin-releasing hormone antagonists Gonadotropin-releasing hormone (GnRH) is secreted by the hypothalamus and causes the pituitary gland to secrete LH and FSH. Several analogues of GnRH have been synthesized. One of these agents, leuprolide, is active in treatment of advanced prostate cancer. Long-term administration causes LH and testosterone levels to reach very low levels. In addition to suppressing testosterone production by the testes, the drug suppresses androgen production by the adrenal glands.

Progestins Progesterone is secreted primarily by the ovaries but also by the testes and adrenal glands. Tissues that are influenced by progestins contain PR receptors. Progesterone causes development and maintenance of a secretory endometrium, changes in the vaginal epithelium and secretions, proliferation of glands in the breasts and an elevation of basal body temperature. Progestins are used in the treatment of endometrial and breast cancer. In endometrial cancer the mechanism of action is thought to be through blocking of PR receptors. The most widely used agent is megestrol acetate (Megase).

REFERENCE

1. Allegra JC, Hamm JT. Chapter 23, Hormonal therapy for cancer, in Manual of Oncologic Therapeutics, Ed. Wittes RE, J. B. Lippincott Company, Philadelphia, 1989, pp. 170-176.

Chapter 14

BIOLOGIC RESPONSE MODIFIERS

A biologic response modifier (BRM) is an agent or treatment that modifies the host response to tumor cells. Traditional treatments for cancer employ methods designed to destroy tumor cells directly. BRMS, on the other hand, do not directly destroy cancer cells but effect tumor cells by indirect means through the action of natural host defense mechanisms or administration of natural substances. The term immunotherapy was in the past synonymous with BRM therapy, but in recent years the term BRM has also been applied to non-immunologic treatments.

TYPES OF HOST RESISTANCE TO CANCER

Animal studies have shown that tumor cells contain antigens which are not found on normal cells of the host. These are called tumor-associated antigens. Furthermore, there are natural processes which recognize these antigens as foreign leading to the destruction of the tumor cells. This process is called immune surveillance system. It is not known how tumor cells escape immune destruction to become clinical cancer. The following is a partial list of possible ways that the immune system can defend against cancer:

Antibody Antibodies are large protein molecules called immunoglobulins which are secreted by plasma cells. Plasma cells arise by differentiation from a subpopulation of small lymphocytes called B cells. Each B lymphocyte that undergoes this differentiation develops antigen-binding molecules on its surface which have the ability to recognize specific foreign molecules called antigens. When B cells come in contact with the specific antigen they become activated and migrate to lymph tissue where they proliferate. As they proliferate they differentiate into plasma cells which secrete antibodies against the antigens which originally activated them. The secreted antibodies are not themselves capable of killing tumor cells but they become attached to the surface of the tumor cells to assist in their killing by a number of mechanisms: (1) phagocytosis by macrophages; (2) destruction by killer cells; (3) lysis of cell membranes by activation of the blood enzyme system called complement. Antibodies are not strong enough to eradicate gross tumor masses once they have developed.

T lymphocytes T lymphocytes are a population of cells that have undergone differentiation in the thymus gland. In the thymus gland these cells develop the capacity to recognize antigens. They enter the circulation to be distributed to the lymphatic tissues of the body. There are a number of subpopulations of T cells which have different functions: Helper T cells assist B cells in antibody synthesis, suppressor T cells which act to suppress the immune response, and killer T cells which can recognize and destroy tumor cells.

Macrophages Macrophages are phagocytes which can ingest bacteria, foreign particles or other cells. They have numerous roles in the normal function of the immune system. They are widely dispersed in the body and may be fixed in specific tissues or wandering in the circulation. Macrophages can be activated by products of T lymphocytes called lymphokines, to kill tumor cells or inhibit their proliferation. Macrophages are responsible for digestion of cellular debris and are one of the means of tumor cell destruction after recognition of their antigens by T and B lymphocytes.

Natural killer cells Natural killer (NK) cells constitute a distinct subpopulation of cells within the immune system. They lack the characteristics of B or T cells but are thought to be lymphocytes. NK cells are found in the circulation and in lymph tissue. They have the capacity to destroy tumor cells without previous exposure to their antigens. NK cell activity is increased following treatment with bacterial vaccines such as Bacillus-Calmette-Guerin (BCG) and Corynebacterium parvum (C. parvum).

Lympokine-activated killer cells (LAK) LAK cells are lymphocytes that can destroy an array of normal and malignant cells following activation by interleukin-2 (IL-2).

Cytokines Cytokines are a class of proteins, produced in small amounts by immune cells, that act as hormones to mediate cell destruction at a distance from their sites of secretion. Examples of cytokines include IL-2, interferons (IFN), and tumor necrosis factor (TNF).

IMMUNOTHERAPY

Immunotherapy is the process by which therapeutic measures induce the immune defense mechanisms of the body to eradicate cancer. The following is a short list of approaches that have been used:

Active non-specific immunotherapy Bacterial vaccines, toxins or products, or other biological substances are injected into the patient in an attempt to induce an immune response. Examples of non-specific immunostimulants include BCG, C. parvum, levamisole and interferon. Since immunotherapy is effective only against small tumor burdens, most clinical trials have used the immunostiumlant as an adjuvant to surgery, radiation or chemotherapy in the hope that only a small amount of tumor will remain after treatment by the primary modality.

BCG BCG is an attenuated strain of Mycobacterium bovis. The possible mechanisms of BCG mediated tumor regression are complex and not fully characterized. Lymphocytes and macrophages may be stimulated by BCG to participate in tumor killing directly or by releasing cytokines. BCG has been administered by subcutaneous, intradermal, intravenous, and intrapleural injection, by instillation into the urinary bladder, and by injection into the tumor. For example, intralesional BCG injections have been used to induce regression of skin metastases from malignant melanoma.

Interferons Alpha-interferon is the only BMR which has received Food and Drug Administration (FDA) approval for use in the treatment of hairy-cell leukemia. Interferons (IFNs) are a group of proteins and glycoproteins subdivided according to differences in antigenic, biologic and chemical properties. There are three distinct types of IFNs, designated as alpha, beta and gamma. Alpha-IFN and beta-IFN can be induced in a wide range of cell types by various inducers and can activate cells by binding to a common receptor. Gamma-IFN is induced in T lymphocytes by mitogens or antigens and activates cells via a distinct receptor.

All classes of IFNs possess antiviral, immunomodulatory and antiproliferative activities that may play a role in tumor control. Their antiproliferative activities suggest that IFNs play a role directly in tumor control, but they may also act indirectly to enhance the cytotoxicity of NK cells, killer cells, T cells and macrophages. In addition to hairy-cell leukemia, other malignancies which have occasionally responded to IFN include chronic lymphocytic leukemia, chronic myelogenous leukemia, non-Hodgkin's lymphoma, renal cell carcinoma, Kaposi's sarcoma in patients with AIDS, mycosis fungoids, superficial bladder cancer, malignant glioma, malignant melanoma, breast cancer, osteosarcoma, carcinoid tumors and multiple myeloma.

Interleukin-2 Interleukin-2 (IL-2) is a lymphokine produced by T lymphocytes after antigen stimulation of NK cells. No consistent therapeutic responses have been observed and early clinical testing is underway for numerous malignancies. Several trials are evaluating combination therapy with two BMR agents such as IL-2 and IFN or IL-2 and LAK cells.

Tumor necrosis factor (TNF) TNF is a family of cytotoxic glycoproteins, induced in mice, pretreated with an immune stimulant such as BCG, and then given lipopolysaccharide. Serum from such animals contains factors that cause tumor necrosis in animal model tumor systems. TNF is produced in B lymphocytes and macrophages. TNF has cytotoxic activity against certain tumor cell lines and recombinant human TNF is now being studied in early clinical trials.

Active specific immunotherapy This is treatment utilizing a tumor antigen preparation. The objective is to increase the immune response to tumor-associated antigens which may already be active in the host. In active specific immunotherapy the patient is injected with a vaccine prepared from his own tumor cells or from other patients with a similar tumor. The cells are killed or modified with radiation or chemicals prior to vaccination. This form of treatment is also used primarily in conjunction with other modalities.

Adoptive immunotherapy Adoptive immunotherapy involves the sensitization in vitro of lymphoid cells such as peripheral lymphocytes to tumor-associated antigens. The sensitized lymphocytes are then returned to the host. An alternative method is to transfer lymphoid cell extracts rather than the cells themselves. This subcellular material, known as transfer factor, is thought to have the capacity to transfer immunological information.

LAK cells Rosenberg,et al, has used LAK cells, prepared by incubating human lymphocytes with IL-2, to treat human tumors. The LAK cells are usually administered concomitantly with IL-2. Results from clinical trials suggest that partial and complete responses in patients with advanced cancer are seen with IL-2 and LAK cells.

Monoclonal antibodies Monoclonal antibodies are products of immune B lymphocytes fused with an established myeloma cell line. Production of monoclonal antibodies involves immunizing mice with a source of antigen such as human tumor cells. Spleen cells from immunized animals containing immune B cells are fused with a mouse myeloma cells line. The resulting hybrid cells combine the immune B cell's ability to produce specific antibody and the myeloma cell's capacity to replicate indefinitely. These hybrid cells are isolated by cell cloning procedures that allow the hybrid clones, secreting the desired antibody, to be identified.

The mechanism of action of monoclonal antibodies in cancer treatment are complicated but probably involve immune mediated mechanisms such as compliment mediated and cell mediated (i.e., NK cells and macrophages) cytotoxicity as well as direct cytotoxicity. Preliminary clinical trials in which antitumor antibodies are injected into the patient have been reported with a number of tumor types, especially lymphomas and malignant melanoma, have produced mixed results. Future studies will employ larger quantities of antibodies administered alone or in combination with other BMR agents such as interferon or IL-2. There is also great interest in the use of monoclonal antibodies attached to radionuclide such as iodine-131 to deliver radiation therapy directly to the tumor site.

REFERENCES

1. Fundenberg, HH, Stites DP, Terr AI. Basic and Clinical Immunology, Seventh Edition, Appleton & Lange, Norwalk, Connecticut, 1991.

2. Krown SE,Chapter 24, Biologic response modifiers, in Manual of Oncologic Therapeutics, Ed. Wittes RE, J. B. Lippincott Company, Philadelphia, 1989, pp 177-185.

3. Rosenberg SA, Longo DL, Lotze MT. Chapter 17, Principles and applications of biologic therapy, in Cancer Principles and Practice of Oncology, 3rd Edition, Eds. DeVita VT, Hellman S, Rosenberg SA, J.B. Lippincott Company, Philadelphia, 1989, pp 301-347.

Chapter 15

SKIN CANCER

BASAL AND SQUAMOUS CELL CARCINOMA

Etiology and epidemiology Skin cancer is the most common neoplastic disease in man. Skin cancer is more common in men (2:1) and more than 95% are basal or squamous cell carcinomas. Many carcinogens are known to cause skin cancer including arsenic, ionizing radiation, ultraviolet light and polycyclic aromatic hydrocarbons such as coal and petroleum products. The risk of skin cancer is increased in geographic areas having the most days of sunlight per year, such as the southern U.S., Australia, South America, and South Africa. They are more common in white persons having light complexions.

Clinical presentation and behavior Basal cell carcinomas are slow growing and rarely metastasize. They most commonly develop in sun-exposed areas such as the face, ears and neck. They are usually seen as a small nodule with distinct margins having a pearly gray color and fine blood vessels. In larger lesions central ulceration is seen.

Squamous cell carcinomas are also slow growing but do occasionally metastasize to regional lymph nodes. The commonest sites are the cheek, ear, lower lip, preauricular area, neck, nose, and dorsum of the hands. Initially they are scaly, reddish in color and raised with an ill-defined border. Larger lesions become nodular and ulcerated.

Treatment methods Excellent cure rates and cosmetic results can be achieved for basal and squamous cell skin cancer by a number of modalities. Few patients die of basal or squamous cancer because recurrences can usually be salvaged.

Surgical excision Surgery is the standard treatment for skin cancers because it is quick and inexpensive. Modern techniques of plastic surgery yield excellent cosmetic results.

Superficial x-rays Radiation is used when surgery would cause excessive cosmetic defects. One of the commonly used modalities is 100-140 KV x-rays. The 5 year tumor control rate is 95% for basal cell carcinoma and 93% for squamous cell carcinoma.[1] The cosmetic result is excellent in most cases.

Electron beam Skin cancers of any size can be treated with electrons. Six MeV electrons are used for superficial lesions and 9 or 12 MeV for thick lesions. Electrons are particularly useful for tumors involving large areas of skin, i.e., diffuse cancer of the scalp or chest wall.

Brachytherapy Sealed sources such as radium-226, cesium-137, and iridium-

192 can be used for interstitial implants or surface applications.[2] This method is not often used and is primarily of historical interest.

Chemosurgery This method, known as Mohs' chemosurgery, is gaining wide acceptance as a primary treatment method for lesions.[3] In it, chemical destruction of the tumor is achieved through local application of zinc chloride. The tumor is then excised and frozen-section samples are taken of the tumor bed to locate areas still containing tumor. These are further excised until there is no evidence of tumor.

Topical chemotherapy 5-Fluorouracil cream is used in treating premalignant or in-situ carcinomas involving large skin areas.

Cryosurgery Intense cold in the form of liquid nitrogen can destroy basal cell carcinomas with cure rates that are comparable to those seen with standard methods.

Electroexcision Electrocoagulation or eletrodesiccation involves destruction of skin cancer by intense heat. Very satisfactory results have been reported with this method.

Laser Beam Satisfactory results have also been reported in patients treated with laser surgery.[4]

Technical considerations for external beam therapy

Dose The radiation dose-time-fractionation schedules used for various size tumors is shown in Table 15.1.

Table 15.1 Dose-time-fractionation schedules			
Size of tumor	**Dose (Gy)**	**No. Treatments**	**Time**
2 cm or less	40	10	12-14 days
2-3 cm over cartilage	45	15	3 weeks
Eyelids	50	20	4 weeks
3-5 cm	60	25	5 weeks
5-8 cm	65	33	6.5 wks
>8 cm	75	40	8 weeks

Technique The single direct portal technique is used for most skin tumors.

Margins A 2 mm margin of normal appearing skin around palpable tumor is adequate for small tumors, but for large tumors the margin should be 5 mm. The margins are defined with a lead sheet in which a hole has been cut (Figure 15.1). The thickness of lead required will vary according to the type of radiation used and its energy (Table 15.2).

Shielding (1) <u>Eyelids</u>-Shielding of the underlying eye is required during treatment of eyelid tumors (Figure 15.2). (2) <u>Lip</u>-Shielding of underlying teeth

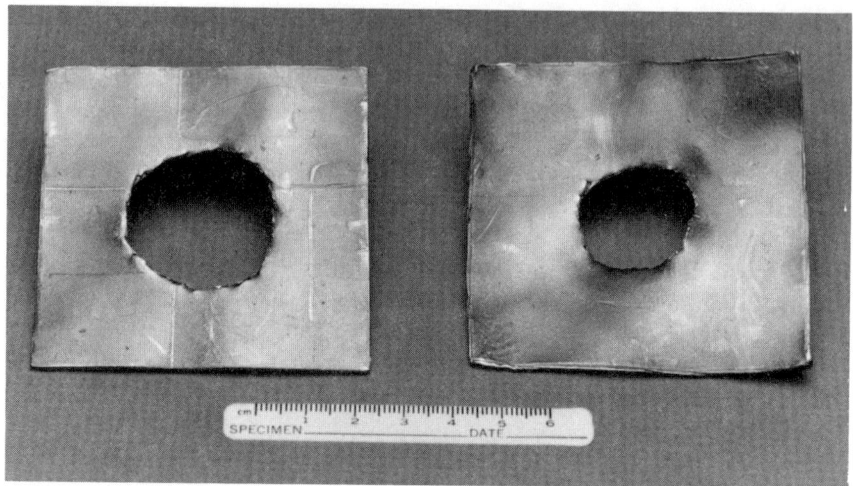

Figure 15.1 Lead cut-outs are placed on the skin over the tumor during treatment of small skin cancers to shield skin that does not require treatment.

and other oral structures is necessary during treatment of tumor of the lip. (3) <u>Nose</u>-The underlying nasal septum is shielded during treatment of tumors of skin of the nose.

MALIGNANT MELANOMA

Etiology and epidemiology Malignant melanoma is a cancer which originates in melanocytes. One-third of cases arise in a pre-existing nevus or mole but most arise de novo. The incidence of malignant melanoma is increasing due to increasing sunlight exposure among susceptible populations. Individuals with pale skin, blue eyes, blond or reddish hair and an intolerance to sun exposure are

Table 15.2 Thickness of shielding according to beam energy

Type of radiation	Energy	Shielding (mm lead)
X-rays	140 KV	1.5
X-rays	250 KV	3.0
Electrons	6 MeV	1.5
Electrons	9 MeV	3.0
Electrons	12 MeV	6.0

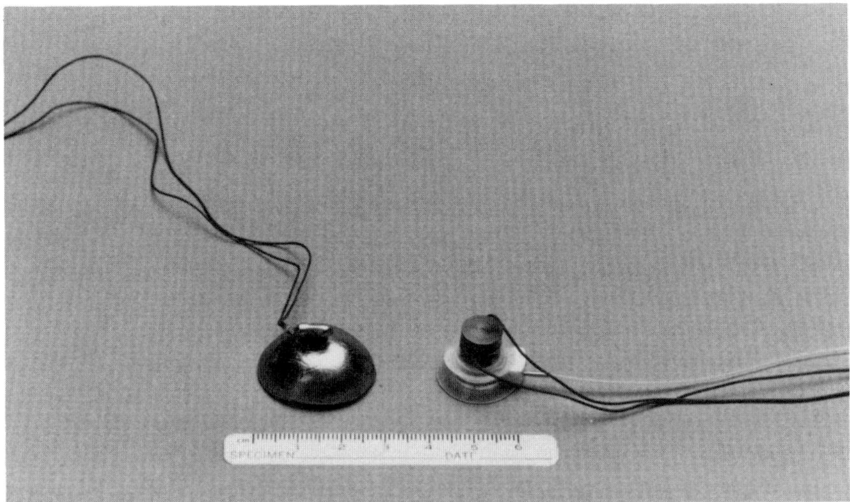

Figure 15.2 These are eye shields used during treatment of lesions near the eye. Local anesthesia with eye drops is essential since they must be inserted into the conjunctival sac. The shield on the left is used for tumors of the eyelid. The shield on the right is useful for treatment of lesions involving the conjunctiva, since it shields only the cornea and lens.

particularly susceptible. In addition to ultraviolet light exposure, genetic, hormonal and immunologic factors and chronic trauma may play a role.

Clinical presentation Malignant melanomas can arise in the skin in any part of the body. They may vary in color from brown to black. Much less commonly, they may originate in the mucosa of the head and neck region, anus, genitalia, choroid of the eye, central nervous system, bladder, and respiratory or GI tracts. There are three clinical types of skin melanomas: superficial spreading melanoma (60%), nodular melanoma (30%), and lentigo maligna melanoma (10%). Lentigo maligna melanomas occur on sun-exposed skin in the elderly, whereas superficial spreading and nodular melanomas occur on any part of the body in all age groups above age 15. Nodular melanomas tend to grow vertically, whereas superficial spreading and lentigo maligna lesions are flat and have large areas of horizontal growth until late in their course. Regional lymph node and distant metastases are common particularly with nodular melanomas.

Melanomas of the skin are classified by the pathologist according to the depth of invasion (Table 15.3). The overall 5 year survival rate of lentigo maligna melanoma is 75%, for superficial spreading melanoma, 60%, and for nodular melanoma, 50%. Involvement of regional lymph nodes adversely affects prognosis and cures are rare for patients with distant metastases.

Treatment *Surgery* Radical local excision is the appropriate treatment for

Table 15.3 Clark's pathologic staging classification		
Clark's Level	**Depth of involvement**	**5 year survival**
I	Confined to epidermis	100%
II	Invasion into papillary dermis	90%
III	Invasion to interface between papillary and reticular dermis	70%
IV	Invasion into reticular dermis	55%
V	Invasion into subdermal fat	10%

most melanomas. Regional lymph nodes are dissected if they are clinically involved. Elective dissection of uninvolved regional nodes does not improve survival. Surgery is used for local recurrence and some distant metastases.

Chemotherapy Chemotherapy is used for patients with disseminated disease. The overall response rate is less than 20%.

Immunotherapy BCG injection of skin metastasis has been used experimentally. Any immunotherapy approach is currently considered experimental and should be used only in research settings.

Radiotherapy Radiotherapy has never found a role in curative treatment because these tumors are usually radioresistant. Therefore, the role of radiotherapy has usually been limited to palliative treatment of distant metastases. However, radiobiological studies suggest that the shoulder on the survival curve is large in melanoma cells compared to other tumors. If this is the case, melanomas would not be expected to respond to conventionally sized fractions, i.e., 2 Gy per treatment. It is possible, therefore, that improved responses will be seen with larger fractions, i.e., 4-6 Gy per treatment.[5] Clinical studies are underway to evaluate this possibility. Other clinical studies suggest that the response rate to radiation can be increased by hyperthermia.[6]

MYCOSIS FUNGOIDES

Mycosis fungoides is an uncommon form of malignant lymphoma which originates in the skin and has a chronic prolonged course. The disease appears in the form of flat reddish lesions involving large areas of the body which progress over years to become tumor masses. Involvement of lymph nodes and deeper organs eventually develops. The tumor is very radiosensitive and one form of treatment involves the use of low energy electron beam treatment (2-4 MeV) to the entire skin surface. Special techniques have been developed for this purpose using linear accelerators.[7] Topical application of chemotherapeutic agents such as nitrogen mustard is the most commonly used current therapy for this disease.

Radiation is effective for palliation of local symptoms due to advanced skin lesions. Doses in the range of 6-8 Gy in a single fraction are effective for short-term palliation.[8] When long-term palliation is required, doses in the range of 30 Gy in 15 treatments are needed.

KAPOSI'S SARCOMA

Kaposi's sarcoma is a slow-growing malignancy of the skin which usually presents as purple colored nodules on the hands and/or feet. The disease originates in the skin at multicentric sites. Prior to the AIDS epidemic, the incidence of Kaposi's sarcoma was low and the tumor was seen primarily in Jewish or Italian men between age 50 and 70. However, in recent years, the incidence of the disease has increased dramatically and the disease is seen most commonly among young men who are victims of AIDS.

Radiotherapy is useful in palliation since the lesions are radiosensitive. Single fractions of 8 Gy are effective for small lesions.[9] For fractionated treatments, total doses of 20 to 30 Gy have been used. The response of Kaposi's sarcoma lesions in AIDS patients is similar to that seen with patients who do not have AIDS.

METASTASIS

Metastasis to the skin from carcinomas of breast and other sites are not rare and radiotherapy can provide useful palliation for painful or ulcerating lesions.

KELOID

A keloid is an excessive, but benign, healing response of the skin to trauma such as burns, incisions, insect bites or vaccinations resulting in large, nodular accumulations of scar tissue. Keloids may be a cosmetic problem or may be symptomatic due to pain or itching. The most effective therapy is surgical excision followed the same day by radiotherapy to the incision line.[10] Fifteen to 18 Gy in 3 Gy fractions given every other day for 12-14 days is effective in preventing further keloid formation.

HEMANGIOMA

Hemangiomas of the skin are benign blood vessel tumors which may be present at birth or appear in the first months of life. They can grow rapidly over a few months which is alarming to the parents. However, nearly all hemangiomas regress spontaneously and they rarely require treatment. Occasionally, however, as in the case of hemangioma of the larynx, they can cause life-threatening obstruction of the airway or other system and in these, a single treatment of 2 or 3 Gy may be helpful.

PLANTAR WARTS

Radiotherapy is effective treatment for plantar warts.[11] Ten Gy in a single treatment is usually successful, but a second 5 Gy treatment 3 weeks later may be needed.

RADIATION SKIN REACTIONS AND THEIR CARE

Treatment of skin cancers will usually be accompanied by a skin reaction in the surrounding irradiated normal skin. Radiation skin reactions occur in five degrees of severity depending on the radiation dose, the size of the area treated and the area of the body treated. The five stages are epilation, erythema, dry desquamation, moist desquamation and ulceration. The reaction begins in the third week of a fractionated course and is usually healed within the weeks following completion of treatment. Epilation is usually temporary but may be permanent with doses above 50 Gy. Erythema and dry desquamation can be pruritic and can be treated by local application of eucerin cream or topical steroids. Moist reactions should be cleaned frequently with hydrogen peroxide. Ulcerations should not occur with proper technique but chronic non-healing ulcers may require surgery.

REFERENCES

1. Fitzpatrick PJ, et al. Basal and squamous cell carcinoma of the eyelids and their treatment by radiotherapy, Int J Radiation Oncol Biol Phys 10:449-454, 1984.

2. Paterson R. Chapter 11, The skin, in Treatment of Malignant Disease by Radiotherapy, Second Edition, The Williams & Wilkins Company, Baltimore, 1963, pp. 174-195.

3. Swanson NA. Mohs' surgery: Technique, indications, applications and the future, Arch Dermatol 119:761-, 1983.

4. Kozlov AP, Moshalik KG. Pulsed laser radiation therapy of skin tumors, Cancer 46:2172-2178, 1980.

5. Katz HR. The results of different fractionation schemes in the palliative irradiation of metastatic melanoma, Int J.Radiation Oncol Biol Phys 7: 907-911, 1982.

6. Kim JH, et al. Combination hyperthermia and radiation therapy for malignant melanoma, Cancer, 49:2289-2294, 1982.

7. Tadros AAM, et al. Total skin electron irradiation for mycosis fungoides: Failure analysis and prognostic factors, IN J Radiation Oncol Biol Phys 9:1279-1287, 1983.

8. Cotter GW, et al. Palliative radiation treatment of cutaneous mycosis fungoides-a dose response, Int J Radiation Oncol Biol Phys 9:1477-1480, 1983.

9. L o TCM et al. Radiotherapy for Kaposi's sarcoma, Cancer 45:684-687, 1980.

10. Levy DS, Salter MM, Roth RE. Postoperative irradiation in the prevention of keloids, Am J Roentgenol 127:509-510, 1976.

11. Macht SH, Corderro JM. Superficial radiotherapy of warts: Results of treating 531 warts, Radiology 122:231-232, 1977.

Chapter 16

HEAD AND NECK CANCER

ETIOLOGY AND EPIDEMIOLOGY

Head and neck cancer occurs predominately in men over age 50. Alcohol and tobacco abuse are the leading etiologic factors suggesting that chemical carcinogenesis is the predominant cause of head and neck cancer. Head and neck cancer occurs with increased frequency among some occupation groups. For example, in some locations, workers in the furniture and textile industry have a high incidence of cancer of the nasal cavity and sinuses suggesting that chemical carcinogens may be involved in etiology.

Genetic factors may be involved in some cases. For example, the incidence of nasopharynx cancer is excessive among Chinese. However, viruses may also be involved in the etiology of nasopharynx cancer because patients with the disease may have elevated antibody levels to Epstein-Barr virus in their blood. Finally, nutritional factors may be involved in some cases since individuals with deficiency of the vitamin riboflavin are at increased risk for oral and larynx cancer.

SYMPTOMS OF HEAD AND NECK CANCER

Some of the common symptoms of head and neck cancer according to primary site are shown in Table 16.1.

Table 16.1 Symptoms of head and neck cancer

Site	Common Symptoms
Oral cavity	Sore which doesn't heal
Oropharynx	Pain on swallowing, lump in neck
Nasopharynx	Lump in neck, difficulty hearing, stuffy nose, headaches
Nasal cavity	Stuffy nose, bleeding from nose
Paranasal sinus	Stuffy nose, pain in face or teeth
Larynx	Hoarseness of voice, lump in neck
Hypopharynx	Pain on swallowing, hoarseness of voice, lump in neck

DIAGNOSIS

The diagnosis of head and neck cancer is usually the responsibility of the otorhinolaryngologist. Tumors of oral cavity and oropharynx can be visualized directly and biopsied in the clinic. Inaccessible tumors such as those originating in the nasopharynx, paranasal sinuses and larynx may require hospitalization for visualization and biopsy under general anesthesia. Specialized radiographic studies such as CT and MRI scans are used to assess tumor extent at the primary site and neck.

PATHOLOGY

Most head and neck cancers originate in the mucous membrane epithelium and are squamous cell carcinomas. However, adenocarcinomas can occur in the minor salivary glands of the epithelium and malignant melanomas can occur rarely in the mucous membranes of the head and neck. Major salivary gland tumors if they are malignant, are most common in the parotid gland and are usually glandular in origin. Malignant lymphomas and primary bone and soft tissue tumors occur rarely in the head and neck region.

ORAL CAVITY

Anatomy the oral cavity extends from the skin-vermilion junction of the lips to the junction of the hard and soft palate above and to the circumvallate papillae of the tongue below. The oral cavity is divided into the following areas:

Lip The lip begins at the skin-vermilion junction and includes only the portion of the lip which comes into contact with the opposing lip.

Buccal mucosa All mucosa lining the cheeks.

Lower alveolar ridge Mucosa of the lower gum or gingiva.

Upper alveolar ridge Mucosa of upper gingiva.

Floor of mouth Mucosa extending from the lower alveolar ridge to the undersurface of the tongue.

Anterior 2/3 of tongue The mobile portion of the tongue anterior to the circumvallate papillae. It is subdivided into the tip, dorsum, lateral borders and the undersurface. Most carcinomas develop on the lateral borders or undersurface.

Hard palate The mucosa covering the palatine bones.

Retromolar trigone A triangular area of mucosa covering the mandible posterior to the last molar tooth.

Distribution of cases according to primary site Table 16.2 shows the distribution of cases according to primary site in a large published series.

Incidence of lymph node metastasis from oral cavity primaries The predominant initial pattern of spread from tumors of the lip is to submental and submandibular lymph nodes; carcinomas of the tongue and floor of mouth

Table 16.2 Distribution of oral cavity cases according to site
(Memorial Hospital, New York)[1]

Site	Number of cases (%)
Oral tongue	312 (28%)
Floor of mouth	290 (26%)
Upper and lower gum	185 (16%)
Buccal mucosa	147 (13%)
Lip	118 (11%)
Hard palate	68 (6%)

metastasize most commonly to submandibular, subgastric and mid-jugular lymph nodes. Ten to 15% of lip and hard palate cancers present with clinically positive nodes; 30-40% of tongue, floor of mouth, buccal mucosa and alveolar ridge carcinomas present with clinically positive nodes.

Staging of lip and oral cavity tumors

Primary tumor (T)

T1 Tumor 2 cm or less in greatest dimension

T2 Tumor more than 2 cm but not more than 4 cm

T3 Tumor more than 4 cm in greatest dimension

T4 Tumor invades adjacent structure, i.e., bone

Regional lymph nodes (N)

N0 No regional lymph node metastasis

N1 Metastasis in a single ipsilateral lymph node 3 cm or less in greatest dimension

N2 Metastasis in a single ipsilateral lymph node more than 3 cm but not more than 6 cm in greatest dimension; or in multiple ipsilateral lymph nodes none more than 6 cm; or in bilateral or contralateral lymph nodes none more than 6 cm

N3 Metastasis in a lymph node more than 6 cm in greatest dimension

Distant metastasis (M)

M0 No distant metastasis

M1 Distant metastasis

STAGE GROUPING

Stage I T1 N0 M0

Stage II T2 N0 M0

Stage III T3 N0 M0, or T1-T3 N1 M0

Stage IV T4 N0 or N1 M0, any T N2 or N3 M0, any T any N M1

Treatment of oral cavity tumors Surgery and radiation are competing modalities for stage I and II oral cancer. However, the results of treatment in stage III and IV are unsatisfactory, and therefore, combined modalities are used in advanced disease.

Surgery Small cancers (1 cm or less) can be treated by local excision but more advanced lesions require extensive resection. For example, a 4 cm cancer on the lateral border of the tongue is treated by hemiglossectomy combined with radical neck dissection. The results of surgical treatment from a large cancer center for cancers of the oral cavity are shown in Table 16.3.

Table 16.3 Ten year cure rates following surgery for cancer of the oral cavity (Memorial Hospital, New York)[2]

Site	Number patients	% cured
Oral tongue	191	48%
Floor of mouth	147	54%
Upper and lower gum	75	56%
Buccal mucosa	66	58%
Hard palate	15	33%

Radiation Small cancers can be treated by local techniques such as interstitial implant, intra-oral cone, or smaller external beam portals. For larger lesions, because of the possible presence of occult lymph node metastasis, radiation of the neck is combined with local techniques. In general, for tumors of the oral tongue, floor of mouth and buccal mucosa, interstitial implants should be used for a portion of the treatment because local control is improved compared to external beam alone. The results of radiotherapy from a large cancer center for cancers of the oral cavity are shown in Table 16.4.

Table 16.4 Five year results following radiotherapy for cancers of the oralcavity (M.D. Anderson Hospital, Houston)[3]

Stage	Number of patients	%NED
T1	36	56
T2	115	60
T3	68	47
T4	35	17

NED-surviving without evidence of disease.

Combining surgery and radiation The rationale for combining radiation and surgery is that the surgery is effective for large tumor masses, whereas radiation is effective for microscopic deposits which may be present beyond the surgical field or spilled into the wound at the time of the operation.

Preoperative radiation Treatment is given preoperatively to the entire planned surgical area. The advantages of preoperative radiation compared to postoperative radiation are: 1) tumor cells escaping into the circulation are less likely to be viable cells; 2) the amount of viable tumor handled by the surgeon is less, resulting in a reduced likelihood of spillage of tumor cells into the wound. A number of preoperative regimens have been used:

1) <u>High-dose, conventional fractionation</u> (50 Gy/25 treatments/5 weeks) with surgery delayed for 4 to 6 weeks following radiation to allow the acute reaction to heal. This is the most commonly employed method.

2) <u>Low-dose conventional fractionation</u> (20-30 Gy/10-15 fractions/2-3 weeks) with minimal delay prior to surgery. This method has not found favor among radiotherapists because the radiation dose is not high enough but surgeons favor it because there are fewer wound healing problems compared to the high-dose regimen.

3) <u>Small number of large fractions</u>, i.e., 5-10 Gy in a single fraction, followed by surgery the same day. This regimen is favored by surgeons because there is no delay prior to surgery.

Postoperative radiation This is the most commonly employed method of combining radiation with surgery. Treatment is given postoperatively to the entire surgical area. Radiation is delayed following surgery for 10 to 14 days to allow for wound healing. The doses used for postoperative RT vary somewhat with the situation, but for head and neck cancer, 60 Gy/30 fractions/6 weeks is well-tolerated.

The advantages of postoperative RT compared to preoperative RT are: 1) the pathologist has the opportunity to study an unirradiated tumor, and therefore, the prognostic information is more accurate; 2) problems with wound healing are less likely.

Chemotherapy combined with radiation Since treatment results for advanced oral cavity cancers are unsatisfactory, there is great interest in combining the two modalities in hopes of improving survival. For example, experimental protocols in which radiation is combined with concurrently administered cisplatin and 5-fluorouracil intravenous infusions for patients with advanced head and neck cancer are being evaluated in a number of centers.

Radiotherapy techniques used for oral cavity tumors

Interstitial brachytherapy Interstitial implants are used for cancers of the oral tongue, floor of mouth and buccal mucosa. Radium or cesium-137 needles or iridium wires or ribbons are the most commonly used sources. The implants are performed in the operating room under general anesthesia. There are three types of implants:

1) <u>Single plane implants</u> are used for superficial cancers. The needles are inserted into the tissue immediately beneath the tumor (Figure 16.1). Following the procedure, AP and lateral orthogonal radiographs are obtained for computer dosimetry. Small tumors less than 2 cm in size can be treated with brachytherapy alone (65-70 Gy in 5-7 days.) However, most tumors are treated initially with external beam to ensure adequate treatment of the lymphatics of the upper neck. For example, 50 Gy/5 weeks is given with external beam followed by 30 Gy in 3 days from an implant.

2) <u>Double plane implants</u> are used for tumors that are too thick for a single plane implant (>1 cm). The tumor is sandwiched between 2 planes of needles.

3) <u>Volume implants</u> are used for massive tumors of the tongue or floor the mouth that are too large to be treated by single or double plane implants. The needles are placed in concentric circles to form a vertical cylinder. Each needle is placed 1 cm from it neighbor. Iridium-192 is ideal for volume implants because the ribbons or wires are longer than radium or cesium needles and the implants are less painful because the sources are thinner and more flexible.

External beam therapy for oral cavity tumors

Equipment Most cancers of the head and neck are adequately treated with cobalt-60 or 2-6 Mv x-rays. Electron beams of 6 to 18 MeV are useful for treating superficial tumors (i.e., lip or parotid gland) or boosting neck masses.

Technique The parallel opposing portals technique is used to treat the primary and upper neck (Figure 16.2). The patients are treated in the supine position with the head immobilized with the aid of a head holder (Figure 16.3). When there are clinically positive neck nodes the lower neck is also treated.

Doses Radiation doses used for external beam therapy in various situations are shown in Table 16.5.

Intra-oral cone therapy Small superficial cancers of the oral cavity can be treated with intra-oral cone therapy (Figure 16.4). This technique is usually feasible only in edentulous patients. It is usually combined with external beam in which treatment is initiated with opposing lateral fields (45-50 Gy/5 weeks), covering the primary and the upper neck lymphatics and completed with a boost to the primary with an intra oral cone (27-30 Gy/9-10 fractions).

OROPHARYNX

Anatomy The oropharynx extends from the level of the hard palate superiorly to the hyoid bone inferiorly. The oropharynx is subdivided into the following areas.

Faucial arch Includes the mucosa of the soft palate, uvula and right and left

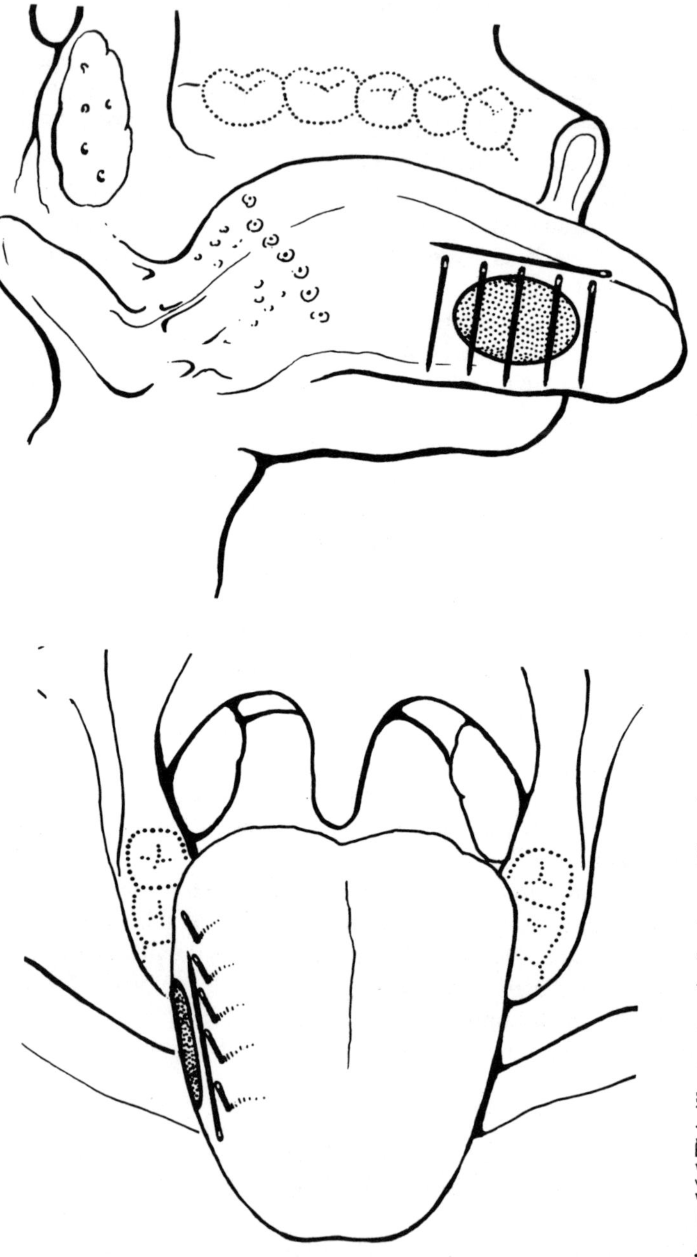

Figure 16.1 This illustrates a single plane radioactive needle implant for a squamous cell carcinoma of the lateral border of the tongue. The needles are held in place with sutures.

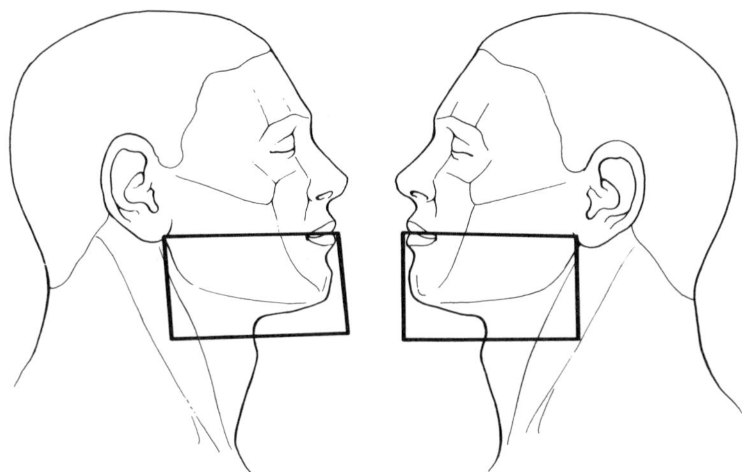

Figure 16.2 This diagram illustrates the treatment portals used for patients with carcinomas of the tongue or floor of mouth. The portals cover the primary site and the submental, submandibular and upper jugular lymph nodes.

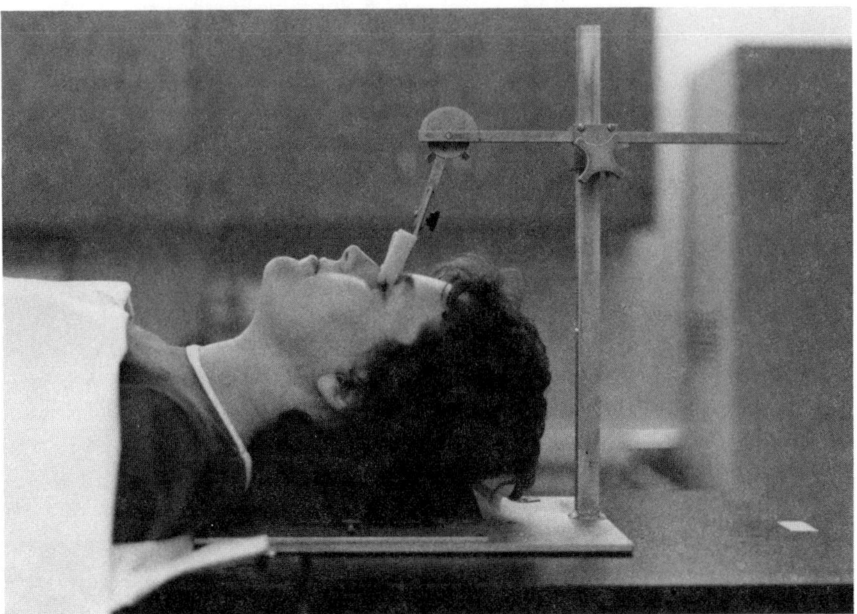

Figure 16.3 This is the immobilizing device that we use for many of our head and neck patients

Table 16.5 Doses for external beam therapy for oral cavity tumors
(1.8-2.0 Gy/treatment/5 treatments per week)

Total Dose (Gy)	Treatment Situation
45-50	Primary and upper neck prior to implant Preoperative RT to primary + neck Elective RT to neck
60	Postoperative treatment to primary area and upper neck
65-70	External beam to primary without surgery or implant

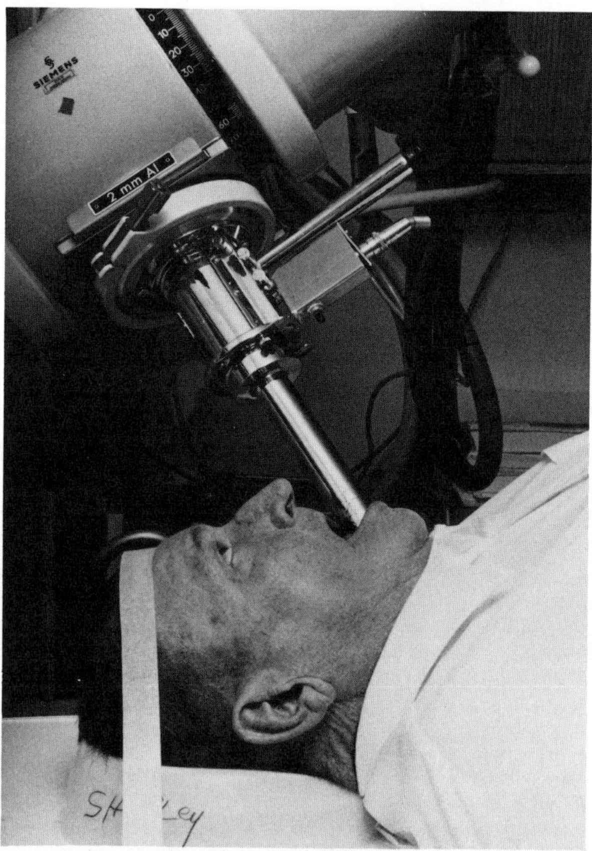

Figure 16.4 Intra-oral cone therapy for cancers of the anterior tongue or floor of mouth.

anterior tonsillar pillar.

Tonsillar fossae and tonsils Right and left.

Base of tongue Extends from the circumvallate papillae to the base of the epiglottis or vallecula.

Pharyngeal walls Includes the mucosa of the lateral and posterior walls.

Distribution of cases The distribution of cases according to primary site is shown in Table 16.6.

Table 16.6 Distribution of oropharynx carcinomas according to primary site (M.D. Anderson Hospital, Houston)[4]	
Site	**Number of Patients (%)**
Retromolar trigone/anterior tonsillar pillar	146 (24.5%)
Base of tongue	145 (24%)
Pharyngeal wall	145 (24%)
Tonsillar fossa	102 (17%)
Soft palate /uvula	59 (10%)

Incidence of lymph node metastasis The predominant pattern of lymphatic spread of tumors of the oropharynx is to the subdigastric nodes and mid-jugular lymph nodes. The incidence of positive lymph nodes on initial clinical examination according to primary site is as follows: soft palate 44%, retromolar trigone/anterior pillar 45%, base of tongue 78%, tonsillar fossae 76%, and pharyngeal walls 59%.

Staging The TNM classification and stage grouping is the same as for the oral cavity.

Treatment of carcinomas of the oropharynx Stage I and lesions can be treated by surgery or radiation. However, most patients present with advanced disease are treated with combined modality therapy. Surgical operations vary from local intra-oral excisions for small tumors to extensive resections of soft tissue and bone for large tumors.

Radiotherapy techniques utilize external beams primarily since interstitial implants are not easily adaptable for most oropharyngeal tumors. Chemotherapy combined with radiation and/or surgery is under evaluation for advanced disease. The results of surgical treatment for oropharyngeal tumors from a large cancer center are shown in Table 16.7 and the results of radiotherapy alone are shown in Table 16.8.

Radiotherapy techniques and doses The parallel oposing portals technique is used for the primary and upper neck (Figure 16.5). Small tumors are given 65 Gy in 6 1/2 weeks and larger tumors receive 70-80 Gy in 7-9 weeks. The shrinking field technique is used whenever feasible. The spinal cord dose should not exeeed 45 Gy.

Table 16.7 Ten year cure rates following surgery for cancers of oropharynx (Memorial Hospital, New York)[2]

Site	Number of Patients	%cured
Base of tongue	110	36%
Tonsil	89	54%
Soft palate	65	40%

Table 16.8 Results of radiotherapy alone for carcinoma of oropharynx (M.D. Anderson Hospital, Houston)[4]

Stage	Number of Patients	%NED
T1	98	56%
T2	90	47%
T3	86	38%
T4	63	18%

NED=surviving without evidence of cancer

The lower neck is treated for all patients with base of tongue and tonsil primaries even if the neck is clinically negative. For soft palate tumors, the lower neck is treated if there are clinically positive nodes. If lymph node metastases are to be treated with radiation alone, the dose to the nodal masses should be at least 65-70 Gy. Electron beam boosts are often used to bring the dose to this level.

Postoperative radiotherapy for oral cavity and oropharynx

Postoperative radiotherapy is indicated for patients with carcinomas of the oral cavity or oropharynx when there is histologic evidence of positive or close surgical margins or positive lymph nodes in the neck. The entire surgical area, including all wound extensions and both sides of the neck down to the clavicles are irradiated.

Fifty to 60 Gy in 5 to 6 weeks is given to the primary and upper neck with the opposing lateral portals techniques and 45 Gy in 5 weeks to the lower neck with an anterior portal. Sites of positive surgical margins can be boosted with an additional 10-15 Gy. Electron beam fields can be used to treat wound extensions, i.e., into the posterior neck area.

NASAL CAVITY AND PARANASAL SINUSES.

Anatomy The nasal cavity consists of three regions:

Vestibule The cavity which forms the inner aspect of the anterior portion of the nasal septum divides the vestibule in the midline.

Olfactory region The roof of the nasal cavity.

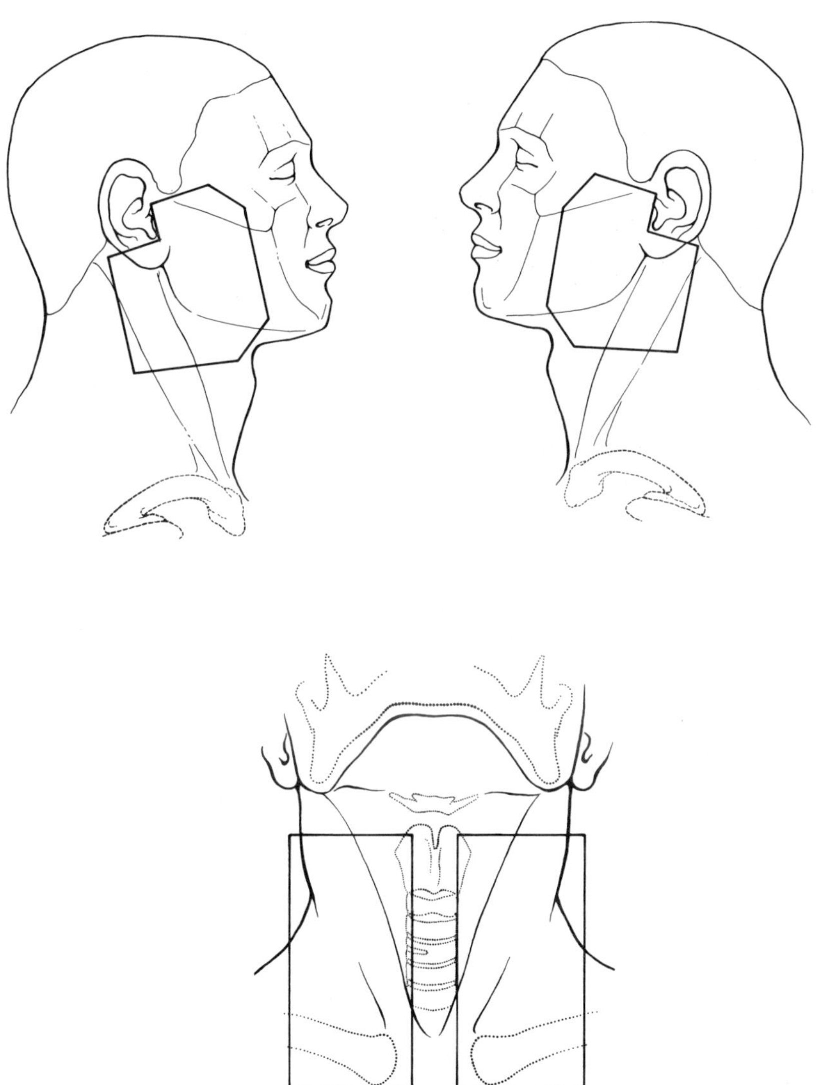

Figure 16.5 These diagrams illustrate the treatment portals used for patients with cancer of the tonsil. The upper portals cover the priamry site and upper jugular and posterior cervical lymph nodes. The portals must be reduced in size at 45 Gy to shield the spinal cord.

Respiratory region Consists of the lateral walls, the turbinates, most of the septum and the floor of the nasal cavity.

The paranasal sinuses consist of the maxillary, ethmoid, frontal and sphenoid sinuses.

Treatment *Maxillary sinus* There is not a standard treatment for carcinomas of the maxillary sinus. Patients are treated by a combination of surgery and radiation. T1 and T2 lesions are treated by radical maxillectomy combined with either pre- or postoperative irradiation; T 3 and T4 tumors usually receive preoperative irradiation followed in 4 to 6 weeks by exploratory surgery; inoperable cases are treated palliatively by radiation alone or combined with chemotherapy. Reported 5 year survival rates range from 30% to 45%.

Ethmoid sinuses Treatment is individualized. Some patients will be treated by radiation alone but most will need a combination of surgery and radiation. Tumors originating in the low ethmoids require radical maxillectomy, whereas tumors extending upward toward the brain require a craniofacial resection in which neurosurgeon and head and neck surgeon operate together to remove the tumor from above and below.

Frontal sinuses These are rare tumors that can be treated with surgery or radiation or a combination of the two. If surgery is used, most will require craniofacial resection involving a cooperative effort between neurosurgeon and head and neck surgeon.

Sphenoid sinus These are very rare tumors. Because of their location, surgical resection is usually not feasible and most are treated with radiation.

Nasal cavity Treatment is individualized. Small tumors can be treated by surgery or radiation alone, whereas large tumors usually require a combination of surgery and radiation. Survival rates, at 3 years post-treatment,of 75% have been reported following RT.

Nasal vestibule Excellent results are seen with surgery or radiation for small tumors of the nasal vestibule. Large tumors are often treated by radiation alone because the cosmetic result is superior. If extensive surgery is required a prosthesis or multiple surgical procedures will be required to cover the defect.

Radiotherapy techniques Nasal cavity and paranasal sinus tumors require techniques in which wedged filters are used. Tumors of the nasal vestibule can be treated by wedge filtered external portals (Figure 16.6). Electron beams and interstitial brachytherapy techniques can also be used for tumors of the nasal vestibule.

NASOPHARYNX

Anatomy The anterior limit of the nasopharynx is the nasal cavity. The roof is attached to the base of the skull and slopes downward to become continuous with the posterior pharyngeal wall. The lateral wall is composed of the torus tubarius, the eustachian tube orifice and the fossa of Rosenmuller. The inferior is the plane of the hard palate.

Incidence of lymph node metastasis Nasopharyngeal carcinomas metastasize initially to retropharyngeal, posterior cervical, superior deep jugular, and

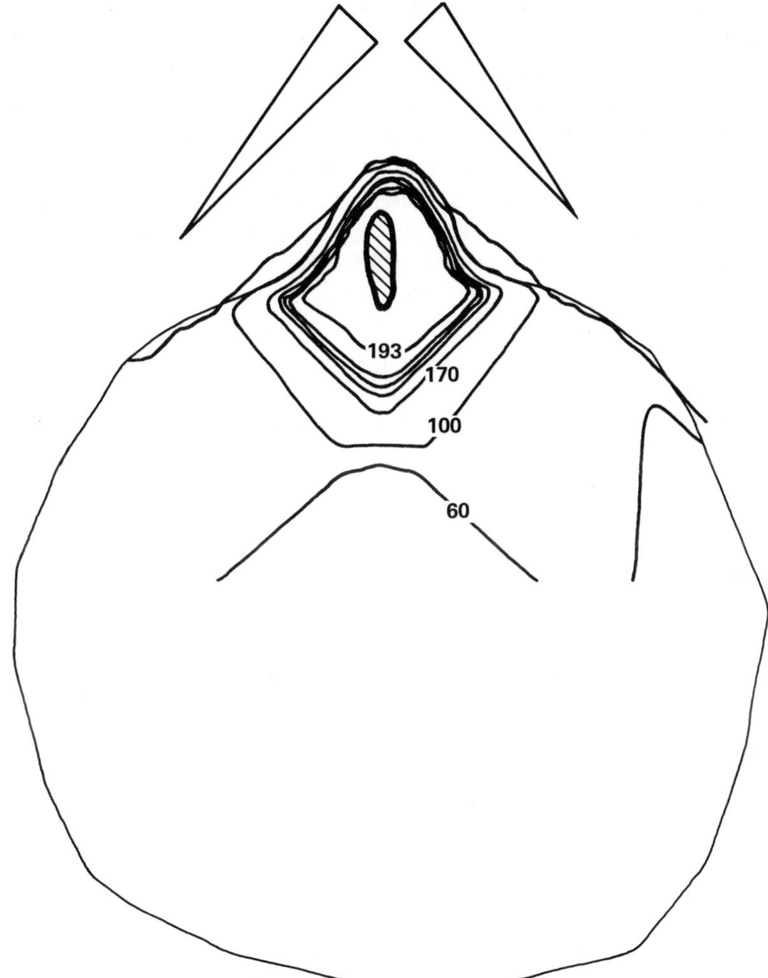

Figure 16.6 This is the computer plan for a patient with a small cancer on the anterior nasal septum.

subdigastric lymph nodes. Eighty-seven percent of patients have neck metastasis when first seen.

      Staging   T1 Tumor confined to one site in nasopharynx

                        T2 Tumor invades more than one subsite

                        T3 Extensions to nasal cavity and/or oropharynx

                        T4 Invasion of base of skull or cranial nerves.

                        N and M stages and stage grouping same as oral cavity.

Radiotherapy techniques and doses Radiation alone is the usual treatment for nasopharynx cancer. The nasopharynx and upper neck are treated with the parallel opposing portals technique and the lower neck is treated in every patient (Figure 16.7). Tumor dose to the primary site range from 65 to 75 Gy in 6 1/2 to 8 weeks with the higher doses reserved for T4 disease. Lymphoepithelioma is a histologic variant of squamous carcinoma which appears to be more radiosensitive and durable than squamous cell carcinomas. Tumor doses as low as 60 Gy may be effective for T1 and T2 lymphoepitheliomas.

The neck is usually treated with RT alone. Areas which do not contain clinically positive nodes receive 45 Gy, whereas areas which contain clinically positive nodes receive at least 60 Gy. Electron beams are useful for boosting large neck masses with doses ranging from 5 to 30 Gy depending on the size of the residual mass.

Intracavitary brachytherapy Recent reports suggest that improved local control rates result when external beam therapy is combined with intracavitary brachytherapy.[5] External beam therapy is given initially, followed by a boost with a radium or cesium tube applied to the nasopharynx.

Results Reported 5 year survival rates following external beam therapy alone range from 15% to 50%. [6,7]

Recurrent disease Local recurrence is a major problem for patients with nasopharyngeal carcinoma and the question of reirradiation frequently arises. Retreatment can result in an occasional long term cure and should be attempted in patients with localized disease. Complications following retreatment are frequent. A few patients with local recurrence are salvaged with radical surgery as practiced in a small number of centers in the U.S.

HYPOPHARYNX AND LARYNX

Anatomy *Hypopharynx* The hypopharynx extends from the plane of the hyoid bone to the lower border of the cricoid cartilage. It consists of three regions: pyriform sinus, posterior surface of the larynx or post-cricoid area and posterior pharyngeal wall.

Larynx The larynx consists of three regions: supraglottis, glottis and subglottis. The supraglottis is composed of the epiglottis and the right and left aryepiglottic folds, arytenoids and false vocal cords The glottis consists of the right and left true vocal cords. The subglottis is the region extending from the lower boundary of the glottis to the lower margin of the cricoid cartilage.

Distribution of cases *Hypopharynx* Pyriform sinus, 75% of cases, posterior pharyngeal wall, 20% of cases, post-cricoid, 5%.

Larynx Glottic, 65% of cases, supraglottic, 34% subglottic, 1%. In the supraglottic area the distribution is: epiglottis 44%, false vocal cords 30%, aryepiglottic folds 21%, arytenoids 5%.

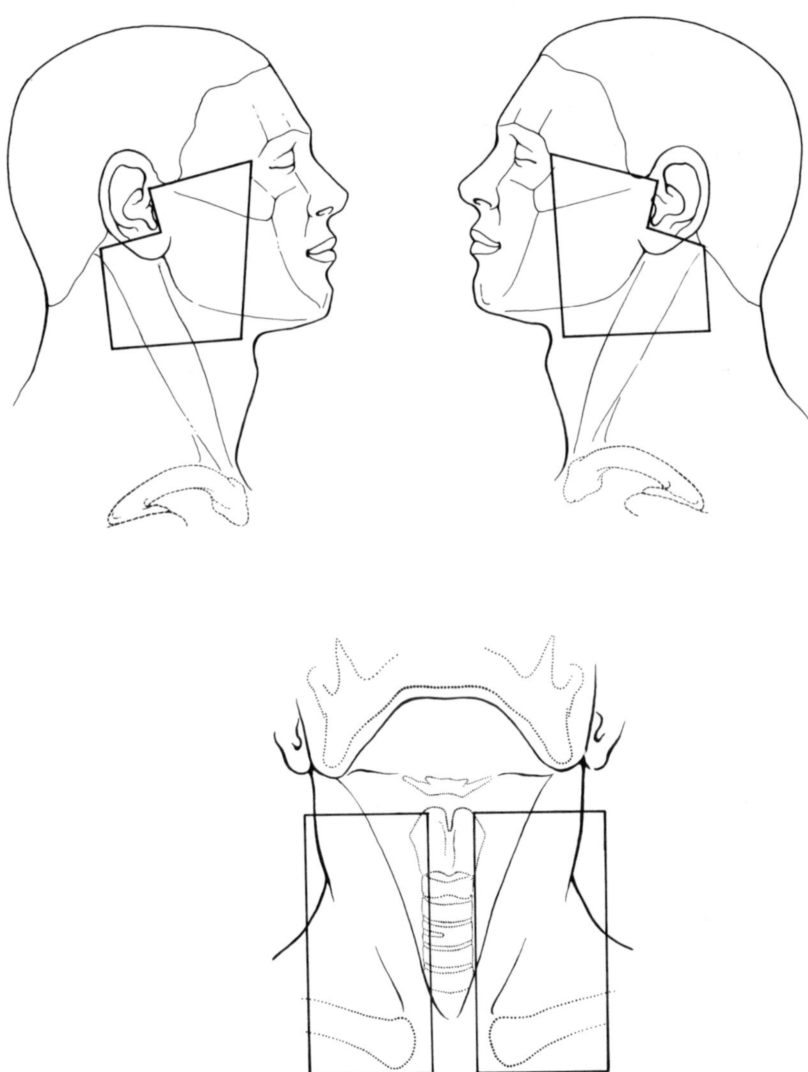

Figure 16.7 These diagrams illustrate the portals used for patients with cancer of the nasopharynx. The upper portals cover the primary site, the retropharyngeal, upper jugular and posterior cervical lymph nodes. The portals are reduced off the spinal cord at 45 Gy.

Incidence of lymph nodes metastasis *Hypopharynx* These tumors metastasize primarily to parapharyngeal, retropharyngeal, subdigastric and midjugular lymph nodes; 75% have clinical positive lymph nodes at presentation.

Larynx There are no lymphatic vessels in the vocal cord and for this reason, lymphatic metastasis does not occur from vocal cord tumors unless there is spread to supraglottic or subglottic structures. The lymph nodes most commonly involved with metastasis from tumors of the supraglottic larynx are the subdigastric and midjugular nodes. Less than 1% of early glottic tumors present with lymph node metastasis; 55% of supraglottic and 20% of subglottic carcinomas present with metastasis.

Staging

Hypopharynx

T1 Tumor confined to one site

T2 Tumor invades more than one subsite of hypopharynx or
adjacent site without fixation of hemilarynx

T3 Tumor invades more than one subsite of hypopharynx or adjacent site
with fixation of hemilarynx

T4 Tumor invades adjacent structures such as cartilage or soft tissue of
neck

Supraglottis

T1 Tumor limited to one subsite of supraglottis with normal
vocal cord mobility

T2 Tumor invades more than one subsite of supraglottis with normal cord
mobility

T3 Tumor limited to larynx with vocal cord fixation and/or invades
postcricoid area, pyriform sinus or pre-epiglottic tissues

T4 Tumor invades through the thyroid cartilage and/or extends to other
tissues beyond the larynx

Glottic

T1 Tumor confined to vocal cord(s) with normal mobility of vocal cord

T2 Supraglottic and/or subglottic extension with normal or impaired
mobility of vocal cords

T3 Tumor confined to larynx with cord fixation

T4 Massive tumor with destruction of thyroid cartilage and/or extension
beyond larynx

The N and M classification and stage groupings are the same as for the oral cavity. Fixation of the vocal cord means that the vocal cord does not move when the patient vocalizes, while the cords are being visualized by indirect examination with a laryngeal mirror. This is an indication that the tumor is extensively infiltrating the underlying muscle of the larynx.

Treatment *Glottic* The treatment options in early carcinoma of the vocal cord are: transoral removal, resection through a neck incision called cordectomy, hemilaryngectomy and external beam irradiation. Transoral removal is used for patients with very early tumors limited to the true cord(s). The techniques for transoral removal include electrocoagulation, laser surgery and cryosurgery.

Hemilaryngectomy, in which half of the larynx is removed, is used for large stage I and stage II tumors. However, most patients with T1 and T2 tumors are treated with radiation because the quality of the voice is superior following treatment. Surgery is used to salvage radiation failures.

Advanced vocal cord cancer (T3 and T4) is treated by removal of the larynx called total laryngectomy. Radiotherapy is given postoperatively if there are lymph node metastases or if there is cartilage invasion or extensive subglottic extension.

Supraglottic Early supraglottic cancers can be treated equally well by radiation and surgery. Partial laryngectomy, in which the upper portion of the larynx is removed with preservation of the vocal cords, is the operation used. Advanced supraglottic cancer requires total laryngectomy and radical neck dissection. Radiotherapy is used postoperatively for patients with lymph node metastases. Treatment results following radiotherapy for glottic and supraglottic cancer are shown in Table 16.9.

Table 16.9 Results of radiotherapy for squamous cell carcinoma of the larynx (M.D. Anderson Hospital, Houston)[3]

Site	Number of patients	%local control *	5 year NED (%)
Glottic			
T1	176	99%	84%
T2	84	93%	75%
Supraglottic			
T1	12	100%	50/%
T2	27	96%	70%
T3	17	94%	35%
T4	9	78%	33%
*Includes patients salvaged by surgery NED=surviving without evidence of disease			

Subglottic Radiotherapy and surgery can be used in early cases. Total laryngectomy is used for advanced cases. Postoperative radiation is used if there are node metastases.

Hypopharynx Early cancers can treated by surgery or radiation alone. Most patients, however, present with advanced disease and require a combination of surgery and radiation. When surgery is needed, the larynx can be saved in only a small number of cases and most patients require a total laryngectomy with partial pharyngectomy. Radiotherapy is usually given postoperatively.

Carcinoma of the pyriform sinus, the most common hypopharyngeal tumor, is one of the most aggressive of all head and neck carcinomas. Reported overall 5 year survival rates for this tumor are usually in the range of 15% to 20%. However, patients with advanced disease who are able to complete an aggressive combined treatment program have a somewhat better prognosis. Chemotherapy combined with surgery and/or radiation is under investigation as a means of improving treatment results.

Radiotherapy techniques and doses *Glottic* T1 and T2 carcinomas are treated with small parallel opposing portals (Figure 16.8). Small, superficial tumors receive 60 Gy; moderately large tumors receive 65 Gy; large tumors 70 Gy. The usual daily tumor dose is 2 Gy. When postoperative radiotherapy is indicated, the upper neck is treated with parallel opposing portals (60 Gy) and the lower neck is treated with an anterior portal (45 Gy). Postoperative treatment is started 4 to 6 weeks after surgery.

Supraglottic T1 and T2 tumors with no clinically positive lymph nodes can be treated with parallel opposing portals (Figure 16.9). The tumor dose for small tumors is 60 to 65 Gy and for larger tumors 70 Gy. The lower neck is usually treated electively.

Postoperative radiation is indicated for advanced disease and treatment must be given to the entire neck; opposing lateral portals are used to cover the upper neck and an anterior portal covers the lower neck and stoma. The dose to the upper neck is 60 Gy and to the lower neck 45 Gy. Care must be taken to avoid "hot spots" on the spinal cord with blocking of the lower corners of the lateral portals. The spinal cord dose should not exceed 45 Gy and therefore, field reduction is required. If surgical scars extend posteriorly over the cord, electron beams are used to boost the dose to these incision lines.

Hypopharynx When postoperative radiation is required for tumors of the pyriform sinus, the mid and upper jugular and parapharyngeal lymph nodes, up to the base of skull, are treated with opposing lateral portals to 60 Gy. When the surgical incision extends posteriorly over the spinal cord, field reduction is required at 45 Gy; a portion of the treatment to the posterior neck must then be given with electrons. The lower neck is treated with a separate anterior field.

CANCER OF THE EXTERNAL AUDITORY CANAL, MIDDLE EAR AND MASTOID

Cancers of the external auditory canal, middle ear and mastoid are rare. Most are squamous cell carcinomas. Tumors of this region are usually extensive and involve the temporal bone. Radiotherapy alone is not indicated because there is a high incidence of radionecrosis of the temporal bone and tumor control rates are poor. Therefore, resection of the temporal bone is the usual treatment. Postoperative radiotherapy is indicated in most cases because there is a high incidence of recurrence following surgery alone. Radiotherapy can be given with angled anterior and posterior or superior and inferior wedged portals or with a direct electron beam. Sixty Gy is the usual tumor dose. Reported 5 year survival rates range from 15 to 40%.

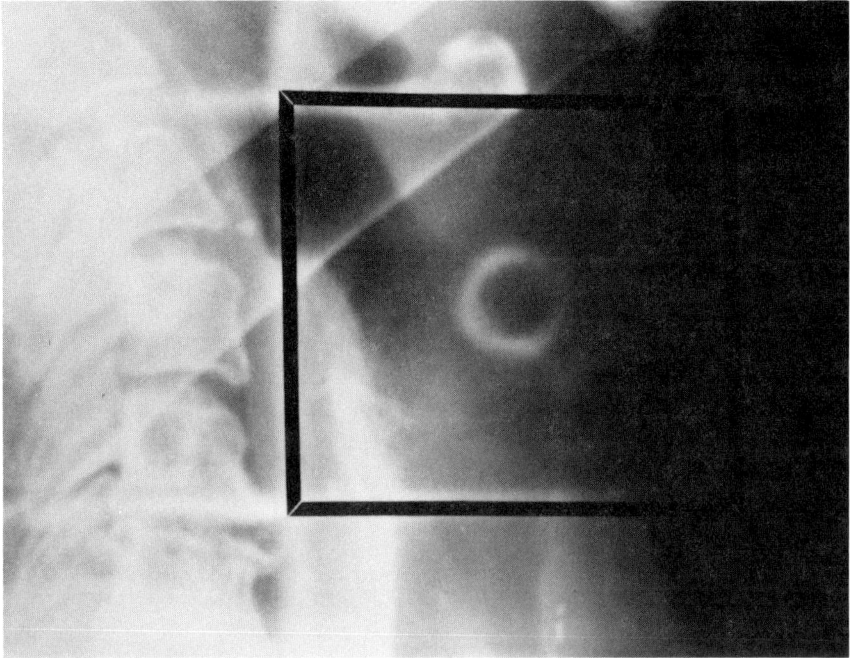

Figure 16.8 This is the simulator film for a patient with a T1 lesion of the vocal cord. Opposing lateral portals were used and the portal sizes were 5.5 x 5.9 cm .

METASTASIS TO LYMPH NODES IN THE NECK
FROM AN UNKNOWN PRIMARY SITE

Diagnostic workup Not infrequently, patients present with a mass in mid- or upper neck and at initial examination, no primary site is found. These patients are admitted for examination of the mucosal surface of the head and neck region under general anesthesia. Biopsies are taken from suspicious areas and from normal appearing mucosa in the nasopharynx, tonsils, base of tongue and pyriform sinus. In many cases the primary site is found.

However, if the primary site is not found, the neck mass is biopsied. A diagnosis of adenocarcinoma or squamous cell carcinoma involving midjugular or upper neck nodes implies that a small hidden head and neck primary is present. If disease involves lower neck or supraclavicular lymph nodes the primary site may be below the clavicle and the patient should be evaluated for a lung, pancreas, esophagus or gastrointestinal primary. If lymphoma is diagnosed, a staging workup for lymphomas is indicated.

Treatment The choice of treatment for the patient in whom no primary site is found depends upon the histology of the disease in the neck mass, the location

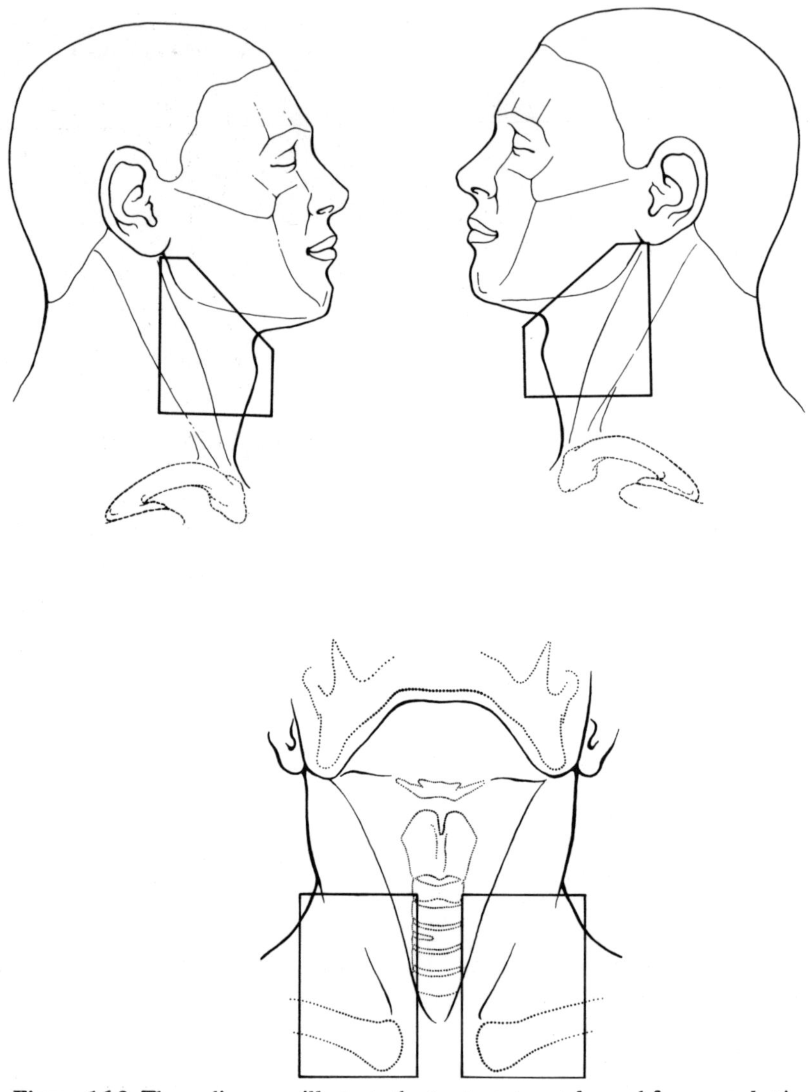

Figure 16.9 These diagrams illustrate the treatment portals used for supraglottic carcinomas.

of the mass and the stage of disease:

1)   Patients presenting with small upper jugular nodes or posterior cervical nodes receive radiotherapy to the nasopharynx, tonsillar fossae, base of tongue and both sides of the neck. The radiation dose for areas irradiated for microscopic disease is 50 to 60 Gy and higher doses are used for neck masses.

2) Surgery is the preferred treatment for patients with a single node in the submaxillary region or in the midjugular region. Postoperative radiation is given to the neck if the disease in the node is extensive.

3) Palliative RT to the neck is indicated for patients presenting with supraclavicular adenopathy.

Fletcher et al, obtained a 3 year survival rate of 50% for 184 patients treated for carcinoma metastatic to lymph nodes in the neck from an unknown primary site.[8]

SALIVARY GLAND TUMORS

Anatomy The salivary glands include the parotid, submaxillary and sublingual glands.

Distribution of cases Only 3% of head and neck tumors originate in the salivary glands. Approximately 80% of all salivary gland tumors occur in the parotid glands, and, of these, 30% are malignant; 15% occur in the submandibular glands and 5% in sublingual or minor salivary glands.

Histopathology Numerous histologic varieties of carcinomas occur in the salivary glands and the 4 most common are mucoepidermoid carcinoma, adenocarcinoma, adenois cystic carcinoma and malignant mixed tumor.

Treatment Surgery is the treatment of choice for most salivary gland tumors. Postoperative radiotherapy is indicated if 1) the tumor is high grade; 2) there is invasion of muscle, bone, skin, nerve or other tissue beyond the gland; 3) regional lymph node metastases are present; 4) there is evidence of residual disease postoperatively.

Radiotherapy techniques and doses The parotid and submaxillary regions can be treated with anterior and posterior portals utilizing wedges. Techniques combining direct electron and photon beams are also used. The lower neck on the side of the primary is usually treated. The dose for the upper portals is 60 Gy and for the lower neck 45 Gy. Sites of residual disease are boosted.

CANCER OF THE THYROID GLAND

Etiology and epidemiology The incidence of thyroid cancer is low; only about 10,000 cases are seen each year in the U.S. The disease is more common in females. A high incidence of thyroid cancer in endemic areas for nodular goiter, such as the Great Lakes region of the U.S. has been noted. This suggests that long-standing stimulation of the thyroid gland by thyrotrophic hormone, due to inadequate iodine intake, can lead to thyroid cancer. Other studies dispute this view. Radiation to the thyroid region is associated with an increased risk since children and adolescents exposed to radiotherapy for benign conditions and persons exposed to radioactive fallout have a high incidence of thyroid cancer. Genetic factors are involved in the etiology of medullary carcinoma.

Pathology There are four histologic types of thyroid carcinoma: papillary, 60% of cases, follicular, 20%, anaplastic, 15% and medullary, 5%. Primary lymphomas of the thyroid are also seen.

Treatment Surgery is the treatment of choice for thyroid carcinoma. Radioactive iodine-131 is often effective treatment for patients with papillary or follicular carcinomas having lymph node metastasis and/or distant metastasis when tumor cells concentrate iodine. Endocrine therapy, with thyroid hormone to suppress functioning tumor cells, is also effective for patients with papillary or follicular tumors.

External beam is rarely used in thyroid carcinoma. However, it is occasionally indicated in patients with residual or recurrent disease in the neck following surgery when the tumor does not concentrate radioactive iodine, i.e., medullary or anaplastic carcinomas. In general, however, thyroid carcinomas are not known to be radiosensitive. Ten year survival rates according to histology are shown in Table 16.10.

Table 16.10 Results of treatment of thyroid carcinoma according to histology (Mayo Clinic)[9]

Histology	Prognostic factor	No. Patients	10 year survival
Papillary	Age < 40	175	95%
	Age > 40	240	73%
Follicular	No vascular invasion	100	85%
	Vascular invasion	98	34%
Medullary	No node metastasis	36	83%
	Node metastasis	41	40%
Anaplastic		160	0%

ESTHESIONEUROBLASTOMA

Esthesioneuroblastomas are rare malignant tumors thought to originate from the olfactory nerve in the olfactory region of the nasal cavity. They are usually slow growing and locally invasive. They are moderately radionsensitive and radiotherapy usually plays a role in treatment. Large tumors are treated with radiotherapy alone (60 Gy); when surgery is the initial treatment, postoperative radiotherapy (50-60 Gy) is indicated. Reported 5 year survival rates range from 20% to 45%.

BENIGN HEAD AND NECK TUMORS
OCCASIONALLY TREATED WITH RADIATION

Juvenile nasopharyngeal angiofibroma These are rare benign vascular tumors which occur primarily in adolescent males. Nasal obstruction and hemorrhage are the usual presenting symptoms. Surgical excision is the preferred treatment but occasionally the tumor is too large or inaccessible. Radiotherapy is often effective in inducing tumor regression in these patients. Thirty Gy in three weeks is the recommended dose.[10]

Chemodectoma of the temporal bone Chemodectomas are rare benign tumors that originate from chemoreceptor tissue in the head and neck. They can arise in the neck from the carotid body (carotid body tumor), from chemoreceptors along the course of the jugular bulb in the temporal bone (glomus jugular tumor), or along the course of the tympanic nerve in the middle ear. They are usually treated surgically but, occasionally, those originating in the temporal bone are so large that surgical excision is impossible. Radiotherapy is often effective in preventing further growth and reducing symptoms. Anterior and posterior or superior and inferior angled wedged portals are used and tumor doses of 45-50 Gy are administered. Local control rates in the range of 65%-85% have been reported following RT for chemodectomas.

DENTAL CARE IN THE IRRADIATED PATIENT

Radiotherapy to the salivary glands causes dryness of the mouth, due to reduced production of saliva, which leads to increased susceptibility to dental caries. Therefore, dentulous patients are evaluated by a dentist prior to initiation of radiotherapy. Those whose teeth are in poor condition and beyond repair have their remaining teeth extracted. Radiotherapy is not initiated for 2 weeks following extraction to allow healing of the sockets. Patients whose teeth are in fair or good condition have their teeth cleaned and repaired. They begin a program of daily fluoride applications to prevent radiation-induced caries. The fluoride applications are continued indefinitely because the decay process will begin if the fluoride is discontinued. Therefore, close follow-up by the dentist is essential to ensure proper oral hygiene and correct dental problems early.

SUPPORTIVE CARE DURING RADIOTHERAPY

Smoking and alcohol These habits should be discontinued to improve tolerance to treatment, prevent complication and reduce the risk of a second primary carcinoma in the head and neck region or lung.

Mucositis Radiation-induced inflammation of the mucous membranes often cause pain on swallowing and reduced nutrient intake. Salt and soda irrigations (1 teaspoon table salt and 1 teaspoon of baking soda and 1 quart water) help to reduce pain and provide cleansing and lubrication of the oral cavity. Pain medication (codeine) and local anesthetics (viscous xylocaine) are helpful in relieving discomfort. Dentures should not be worn to prevent injury to underlying soft tissue.

Xerostomia Dry mouth is a troublesome side effect and if 50 Gy or more are given to the salivary glands, loss of function is likely to be permanent. Sugar-free chewing gum and oral irrigations with water and/or artificial saliva preparations are helpful in improving lubrication.

Nutrition Weight loss is a common side effect. Nutritional evaluation and treatment should be a routine part of the management of every patient. Foods can be blended to assist chewing; commercially available food supplements and home-made preparations such as eggnogs, milk shakes and custard provide extra calories and proteins. Nasogastric tube feedings and intravenous hyperalimentation will occasionally be required. Professional dieticians can provide valuable assistance with nutritional problems developing during radiotherapy.

SALIVARY GLAND TUMORS

Anatomy The salivary glands include the parotid, submaxillary and sublingual glands.

Distribution of cases Only 3% of head and neck tumors originate in the salivary glands. Approximately 80% of all salivary gland tumors occur in the parotid glands, and, of these, 30% are malignant; 15% occur in the submandibular glands and 5% in sublingual or minor salivary glands.

Histopathology Numerous histologic varieties of carcinomas occur in the salivary glands and the 4 most common are mucoepidermoid carcinoma, adenocarcinoma, adenois cystic carcinoma and malignant mixed tumor.

Treatment Surgery is the treatment of choice for most salivary gland tumors. Postoperative radiotherapy is indicated if 1) the tumor is high grade; 2) there is invasion of muscle, bone, skin, nerve or other tissue beyond the gland; 3) regional lymph node metastases are present; 4) there is evidence of residual disease postoperatively.

Radiotherapy techniques and doses The parotid and submaxillary regions can be treated with anterior and posterior portals utilizing wedges. Techniques combining direct electron and photon beams are also used. The lower neck on the side of the primary is usually treated. The dose for the upper portals is 60 Gy and for the lower neck 45 Gy. Sites of residual disease are boosted.

REFERENCES

1. Strong EW, Spiro RH. Chapter 14, Cancer of the oral cavity, In Cancer of the Head and Neck, Eds. Suen JY, Myers EN, Churchill Livingstone, Edinburgh, Scotland 1981, pp 301-304.

2. Shah JP, Endon RA, Farr HW, Strong EW. Carcinoma of the oral cavity, Am J Surg 132:504-507, 1976.

3. Lindberg RD, Fletcher. The role of irradiation in the management of head and neck cancer: Analysis of results and causes of failure, Tumori 64:313-325, 1978.

4. Fletcher GH, Jesse RH, Healey JE, Thoma GW. Chapter 6, Oropharynx, In Cancer of the Head and Neck, Eds. MacComb WS, Fletcher GH, Williams & Wilkins, Baltimore, 1967, pp 179-212.

5. C. C. Wang. Chapter 13, Carcinoma of the nasopharynx, In Radiation Therapy for Head and Neck Neoplasms, Second edition, Yearbook Medical Publishers, Inc, 1990, pp 261-283.

6. Mesic JB, et al. Megavoltage irradiation of epithelial tumors of the nasopharynx, In J Radiation Oncology Biol Phys 6:1735-1738, 1980.

7. Petrovich Z, et al. Advanced carcinoma of the nasopharynx, Radiology 144:905-908, 1982.

8. Jesse RH, Perez CA. Chapter 3, Head and neck cervical lymph node metastasis: Unknown primary cancer, In Textbook of Radiotherapy, Ed. Fletcher GH, Lea & Febiger, 1980, pp 400-407.

9. Beahrs OH, Kiernan PD, Hubert JP. Chapter 23, Cancer of the thyroid gland, In Cancer of the Head and Neck, Eds. Suen JY, Myers EN, Churchill Livingstone, Edinburgh, Scotland ,1981, pp 599-632.

10. Fields JN, Halverson KJ, Devineni VR, et al. Juvenile nasopharyngeal angiofibroma: Efficacy of radiation therapy, Radiology 176: 263-265, 1990.

Chapter 17

EYE AND ORBIT

LIDS AND CONJUNCTIVA

Basal and squamous carcinoma of eyelids See Chapter 15.

Pterygium This is not a true neoplasm, but a wing-shaped fibrovascular proliferation of the bulbar conjunctiva occurring at the limbus (see glossary at end of chapter) on the nasal side. Pterygia are thought to be caused by excessive exposure to ultraviolet light since they are common in the southern U.S. and in individuals who spend a great deal of time outdoors. If untreated, they can grow slowly over the cornea to cause visual and cosmetic impairment.

Surgical excision is the mainstay of treatment but recurrence following surgery alone is common. Post-operative radiotherapy is often used after re-excision of recurrent lesions to prevent further recurrence.[1] Radiotherapy is administered with beta rays from a strontium-90 applicator (Figure 17.1). The beta rays of 0.9 MeV energy have a short range of only 3.9 mm in tissue. Therefore, the conjunctiva is irradiated without significantly irradiating the underlying lens.

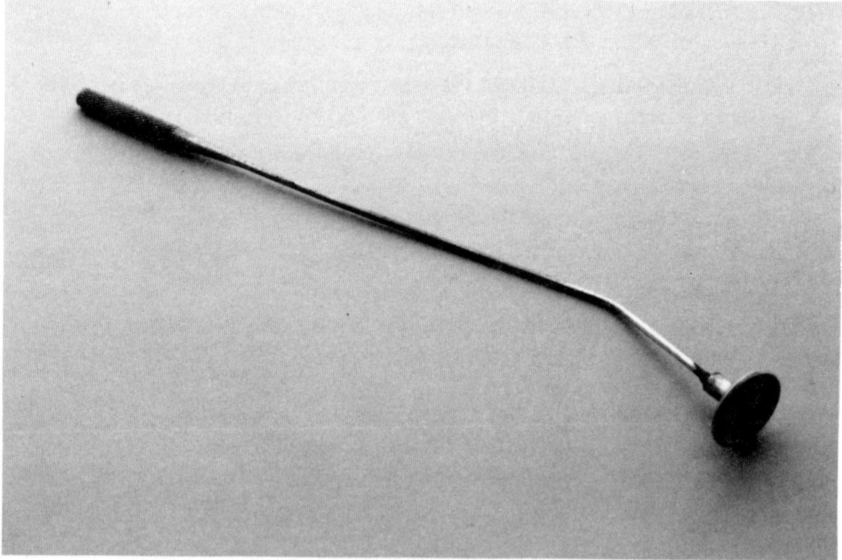

Figure 17.1 This is a strontium-90 applicator used to treat pterygium postoperatively. The eye is anesthetized with drops prior to use.

The initial treatment is delivered the same day that the pterygium is excised. Eight Gy is given to the surface of the eye and this is repeated on days 7 and 14 to bring the total dose to 24 Gy. The recurrence rate is less than 2% following surgery and strontium-90 therapy.[2].

THE EYE

Primary tumors of the eye are uncommon. It is estimated that there were only 1800 new cases diagnosed in the U.S. in 1980.

Malignant melanoma of the choroid This is the most common primary malignant tumor of the eye. Nearly all cases occur after age 30 and the peak incidence is the sixth decade. The choroid is the most common intra-ocular site but melanomas can originate from the ciliary body and the iris.

Enucleation is the treatment of choice for large tumors causing visual impairment. Small melanomas need not be treated, unless there is evidence of growth, because they may not grow significantly for many years. If there is definite evidence of growth, small melanomas can be treated by photocoagulation or cryotherapy.

Radiotherapy is being used with increasing frequency for melanomas of the choroid. They are not very radiosensitive and conventional external beam techniques are not effective. Narrow beams of cyclotron produced protons are being used in some centers to treat melanomas of the choroid.[3] However, the most commonly used approach is to suture a radiation source, usually a cobalt-60 or iodine-125 plaque, to the sclera at the base of the tumor. With this technique high doses in the range of 100 Gy to the apex of the tumor can be given.4

Retinoblastoma This malignant congenital tumor occurs predominantly in children and most are diagnosed prior to age 2. The disease occurs once in every 34,000 births and is often hereditary. Retinoblastomas originate from the photoreceptive cells of the retina and may arise multicentrically in one or both eyes.

These tumors should be treated in specialized treatment centers having a large experience in treating them. The aims of treatment are to eradicate the tumor and to maintain vision. Small tumors can be treated by cryotherapy or photocoagulation. Patients having multiple tumors in one eye or a single tumor located near the macula or optic disc receive external radiotherapy. The eye is enucleated only when there is massive disease with infiltration of the optic nerve and no chance to preserve useful vision.

Retinoblastomas are relatively radiosensitive and can be eradicated with doses in the range of 35 to 50 Gy delivered in 17 to 25 fractions over 4 to 5 weeks.[5] The children are usually treated under anesthesia since complete immobilization is essential to avoid irradiation of the lens. A high-energy x-ray beam with little side scatter is required and a single 3 x 4 cm lateral temporal portal is used to cover the entire retina.

The results of treatment are excellent with an overall cure rate of nearly 90%.[6] However, the presence of extensive local disease or distant metastasis carries a poor prognosis.

Metastasis to the choroid of the eye Metastatic cancer to the eye is the most common intra-ocular malignant process and the choroid is the most commonly involved site in the eye. Breast and lung are the most common primary tumors that metastasize to the eye. Radiotherapy is the treatment of choice for most choroidal metastasis. A single lateral portal posterior to the lens is the most commonly used technique (Figure 17.2).

Doses in the range of 30 Gy in 15 fractions are usually sufficient to induce tumor regression. Seventy to 90% of patients experience improvement in vision following irradiation.

THE ORBIT

Lacrimal gland carcinoma These are rare tumors of adulthood. The histologic types are similar to those occurring in the salivary glands. Surgery is the usual treatment but post-operative radiotherapy may be indicated if the resection is incomplete. The outlook for the patient is poor.

Embryonal rhabodomyosarcoma These are uncommon, rapidly growing tumors of childhood. The majority occur in the head and neck region and the orbit is the most common head and neck site. Modern therapy requires a multidisciplinary approach and patients should be treated in an institution having a pediatric oncology unit.

Radiotherapy is used to treat the orbital tumor and most can be controlled with 50-60 Gy. Chemotherapy is usually started prior to radiotherapy and continued for 2 years. The most popular chemotherapy regimen consists of dactinomycin, vincristine and cyclophosphamide (VAC). The addition of chemotherapy has markedly improved prognosis for children with this disease and the 2 year survival rate now exceeds 80%.

Optic nerve glioma These are rare tumors of childhood The patients experience slowly progressive deterioration of vision with proptosis. Because of their slow growth rate, some require no treatment. However, if there is evidence of tumor growth, surgical resection may be required. Radiotherapy is occasionally used for inoperable or incompletely excised tumors, particularly if vision is threatened.

Lymphoma Malignant lymphomas can originate in the orbit or become involved in the late stages of the disease. In any case, radiotherapy is nearly always used and 30 Gy in 3 weeks is effective in controlling the orbital tumor.

Metastasis to the orbit The orbit can occasionally be the site of metastasis from tumors originating elsewhere in the body. In adults, breast and lung tumors can metastasize to the orbit, whereas in children, neuroblastoma is the most

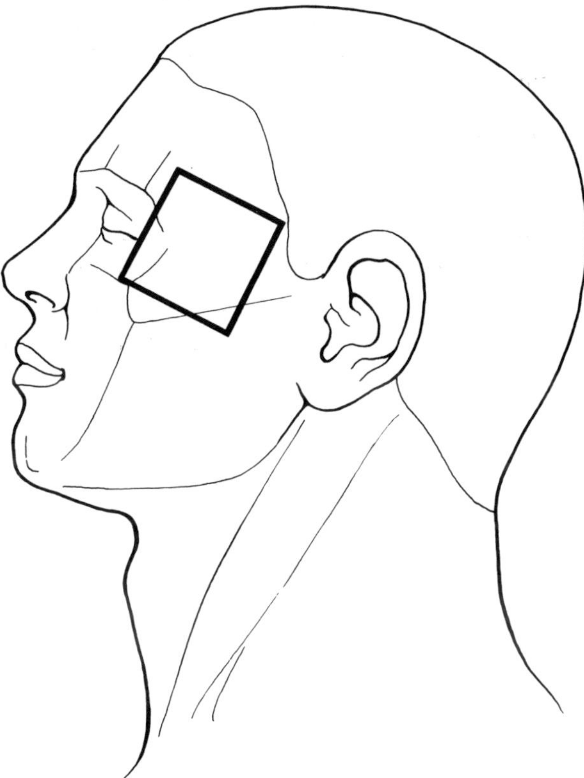

Figure 17.2 Metastases to the choroid are treated with a single lateral 5 X 5 cm portal, angled 3 degrees posteriorly to protect the opposite lens. The anterior margin of the portal is the lateral margin of the orbit.

common histology. Radiotherapy is usually used and 30 to 40 Gy is effective in controlling the orbital mass.

Exophthalmus of hyperthyroidism Exophthalmus can occur as a complication of hyperthyroidism, thyroiditis, nodular goiter and carcinoma of the thyroid gland. It is thought to be an autoimmune reaction because there is massive accumulation of lymphocytes, plasma cells and interstitial fluid in the orbital tissue. Corticosteroids are usually effective in treatment, but radiotherapy is considered in cases having marked proptosis with interference with mobility of the extra-ocular muscles, corneal ulceration and/or optic nerve involvement and failure of corticosteroids to control the disease.[7]

Treatment of the orbits is given with opposing 5 X 5 cm lateral portals, angled 5 degrees posteriorly to protect the lenses. Twenty Gy in 10 treatments is usually effective. A radiation beam having minimal penumbra and side scatter is used. The rapid response in most patients results from destruction of radiosensitive collections of lymphocytes and plasma cells with reduction in orbital tissue volume and edema.

EFFECTS OF RADIATION ON THE EYE

The effects of radiation on the anatomical structures of the eye and the dose thresholds are shown in Table 17.1.

Table 17.1 Effects of radiation on the eye[8]

Tissue	Effect	Threshold Dose (2 Gy/fraction)
Lid skin	Erythema	12
	Moist desquamation	50
Lid margin	Epilation	10
Conjunctiva	Hyperemia	12
	Conjunctivitis	30
Cornea	Keratitis	30
	Ulceration	40
Iris	Edema	60
Retina	Edema	60
Late effects		
Lid skin	Telangiectasis	40
Lid tarsus	Ectropion	60
	Entropion	
Lacrimal gland	Atrophy	50
Lacrimal duct	Stenosis of puncta	50
Cornea	Thinning	30
	Scarring	60
Ciliary body	Glaucoma	60
Lens	Cataract	2
Retina	Hemorrhages	30
	Degeneration	60
	Vascular occlusion	60
Optic nerve	Atrophy	60

GLOSSARY OF TERMS

Canthus --Angle formed by the junction of the upper and lower eyelids

Choroid--A thin, highly vascular membrane which invests the posterior five-sixths of the eyeball. It is loosely connected to the sclera and internally is intimately attached to the retina.

Ciliary body--The wedge-shaped ring structure located between the outer edge of the iris and the choroid. It consists primarily of the ciliary muscle.

Conjunctiva--The thin, transparent membrane that lines the inner surface of the eyelids (palpebral conjunctiva) and the exposed surface of the eye (bulbar conjunctiva)

Ectropion--Eversion or outward displacement of the margin of an eyelid

Entropion--Inversion or inward displacement of the margin of an eyelid

Enucleation--Removal of the eye

Exopthalmus--Abnormal protrusion of the eye

Extraocular--Extending outside the globe of the eye

Hyperemia--Vascular congestion

Intraocular--Within the globe of the eye

Iritis--Inflammation of the cornea

Lacrimal puncta--Opening of the lacrimal duct on the margin of each lower lid at the inner canthus

Limbus--The junction of the cornea and sclera

Macula--A yellowish area on the posterior pole of the eye in the center of which is a depression called the fovea centralis. The fovea centralis is the portion of the retina which provides the greatest visual acuity. It is the part of the retina on which light rays are focused.

Optic disc--The area at the posterior pole of the eye which is the site of emergence of the optic nerve and the blood vessels of the eye

Orbit--The bony cavities in the skull which contain the eyes

Proptosis--Protrusion of the eye

REFERENCES

1. Cooper JS. Postoperative irradiation of pterygia: Ten more years of experience. Radiology 128:753-756, 1978.

2. Van den Brenk HAS. Results of prophylactic postoperative irradiation in 1300 cases of pterygium. Am J Roentgenol 103:723-733, 1968.

3. Gradoudas ES, Seddon JM, Egan K, et al. Long-term results of proton beam irradiated uveal melanomas. Opthalmology 94:4:349-353, 1987.

4. Beitler JJ, McCormick B, Ellsworth RM, et al. Ocular melanoma: Total dose and dose rate effects with Co-60 plaque therapy, Radiology 176:275-278, 1990.

5. Pizzo PA, Horowitz ME, Poplack DG, Hays DM, Kun LE. Chapter 47, Solid tumors of childhood, In Cancer: Principles and Practice of Oncology, 34rd Edition, Eds. DeVita VT, Hellman S, Rosenberg SA. J.B. Lippincott Co., Philadelphia, 1989, pp 1612-1670.

6. Cassady JR, et al. Radiation therapy in retinoblastoma, Radiology 93:405-509, 1969.

7. Covington EE, Lobes L. Sudarsanam A. Radiation therapy for exophthalmus: Report of seven cases. Radiology 122:797-799, 1977.

8. Merriam GR, Szechter A, Focht, EF. The effects of ionizing radiations on the eye. In Frontiers of Radiation Therapy and Oncology, Volume 6. Ed. Vaeth JM, University Park Press, Baltimore, 1972 pp.346-385.

Chapter 18

CENTRAL NERVOUS SYSTEM

EPIDEMIOLOGY

Primary brain tumors constitute less than 2% of all cancer in the U.S. There are two age peaks in incidence The first, between ages 5 and 9, is accounted for by cerebellar astrocytomas, medulloblastomas and ependymomas, the second, between stages 65 and 69, is accounted for primarily by malignant gliomas, meningiomas and pituitary adenomas.[1] It is estimated that 15,600 new central nervous system (CNS) tumors were diagnosed in 1990.[2]

PATHOLOGIC CLASSIFICATION

A pathologic classification for neoplasms of the CNS is shown in Table 18.1. Intracranial tumors in children are medulloblastoma 25%, astrocytoma 20%, glioblastoma 20%, ependymoma 7% and craniopharyngioma 5%. In adults, the five most common primary intracranial tumors are glioblastoma 50%, meningioma 20%, astrocytoma 10%, chromophobe adenoma 5% and hemangioma 2%.

DIAGNOSIS

Brain tumors *History* Headache, usually worse in the morning on awakening, is the most common complaint. Seizures, visual symptoms, untidiness, poor memory, personality changes and weakness or numbness of the extremities are also common symptoms.

Neurologic examination A decreased level of alertness and poor memory are common findings. Hyperactive reflexes, muscle weakness in extremities, visual field defects and cranial nerve abnormalities are also common signs. Frequently there is no objective neurologic deficit.

Radiographic studies Computerized tomography (CT) and magnetic resonance imaging (MRI) have revolutionized the diagnosis of brain tumors. Tumors of 2 cm or more in size can be localized with CT scanning. Arteriograms are needed to determine the vascular supply of tumors prior to surgery.

Spinal cord tumors The neurologic examination is important in the diagnosis of spinal cord tumors; tests of sensory function such as touch, temperature, pain and proprioception are often abnormal. MRI scans are rapidly replacing contrast myelography in the diagnosis and localization of spinal cord tumors.

Table 18.1 Classification of central nervous system neoplasms[3]	
Tissue of origin	**Tumor type**
Neuroglia (supporting cells)	Astrocytoma, grades 1 and 2
	Glioblastoma, grades 3 and 4
	Oligodendroglioma
	Ependymoma
Neurons and primitive bipontential precursors	Medulloblastoma
	Neuroblastoma
Mesoderm (covering cells)	Meningioma
	Sarcoma
Nerve roots	Neurofibroma, schwannoma
Pituitary gland	Adenoma (chromophobe, acidophilic,basophilic)
Pineal gland	Germ cell origin (Germinoma)
	Pinocytoma
Choroid plexus	Papilloma
Remnant cells (developmental)	Chordoma
	Craniopharyngioma
	Teratoma
Blood vessels	Hemangioblastoma
Lymphoreticular	Lymphoma

TREATMENT

Surgery Surgical removal is the treatment of choice for brain and spinal cord tumors. Benign brain tumors such as meningiomas, pituitary adenomas cystic astrocytomas, schwannomas of the eighth cranial nerve, optic nerve gliomas, pinealomas and craniopharyngiomas can often be totally excised. Recently developed neurosurgical techniques employ a low-power microscope to aid the neurosurgeon in visualizing the tumor and normal structures in the operatave fields have yielded improved results for many tumors.

Malignant tumors such as glioblastomas and medulloblastomas cannot be completed excised because they invade brain tissue extensively. Nevertheless, surgical removal of as much tumor as can safely be removed is beneficial because intracranial pressure is reduced resulting in rapid neurological improvement. Occasionally, however, astrocytomas originating deep in the brain (brain stem) cannot be safely removed or biopsied and are treated without tissue diagnosis. Metastatic brain tumors are removed if there is only a single metastasis near the brain surface without other known sites of metastasis.

Spinal cord tumors are difficult to remove completely, but surgery is required to obtain tissue for diagnosis and to relieve pressure on the entrapped spinal cord.

Radiotherapy Our modality has a major role in the treatment of brain and spinal cord tumors. Radiation can be curative for a small number of patients, i.e., medulloblastomas and pineal area tumors. It is used palliatively following surgery for most malignant gliomas and for benign tumors that cannot be totally excised, i.e., pituitary adenomas, craniopharyngiomas and meningiomas. In addition, radiation is the mainstay of palliative treatment for most metastatic tumors to the brain and spinal cord.

Chemotherapy Improved chemotherapy for brain tumors is greatly needed. Currently, the most active drug is carmustine (BCNU). However, survival time for patients with glioblastoma multiforma given BCNU, following completion of RT, is only a few months longer than with RT alone. The combination of procarbazene, lomustine (CCNU) and vincristine yields short-term responses in most patients treated for recurrent medulloblastoma.

Corticosteriods Systemic corticosteroid administration is an accepted method of symptom palliation in patients with brain tumors. The mechanism of action of steroids is thought to be the reduction of edema surrounding the tumor. Reduction in intracranial pressure and improved regional blood flow have been documented following corticosteroid administration. Steroids are administered orally every 6 hours and dexamethasone (methylprednisolone) is most frequently prescribed.

The daily dexamethasone dose is usually 16 mg/24 hours. Side effects of long-term steroid administration include abnormal glucose metabolism, gastric ulceration, muscle weakness and atrophy, osteoporosis and reduced immune function. Therefore, whenever possible, steroid use is curtailed as symptoms improve with RT.

RADIOTHERAPY TECHNIQUES, DOSES AND

RESULTS FOR SPECIFIC TUMORS

Astrocytoma (Grades I and II) of the brain Radiotherapy is indicated following subtotal removal. Techniques are used which irradiate the original tumor volume with an adequate margin. The dose is 50-60 Gy in 5 to 6 weeks. In one series, survival for patients treated with radiation following incomplete removal was 46% at 5 years, 35% at 10 years and 23% at 20 years.[4]

Malignant gliomas of the brain Patients having grade III and IVastrocytomas are treated postoperatively utilizing parallel opposing lateral portals which cover the whole brain (Figure 18.1). The whole brain must be irradiated because malignant gliomas can infiltrate the brain extensively, often beyond the volume seen on CT or MRI scans. The whole brain dose is 40-50 Gy/ 2.0 Gy per fraction followed by a boost to the tumor volume of 15-20 Gy. Five year survival rates for grade III gliomas range from 15% to 25% ; in most series there are no 5 year survivors for grade IV gliomas.

Interstitial brachytherapy In an attempt to improve treatment results for

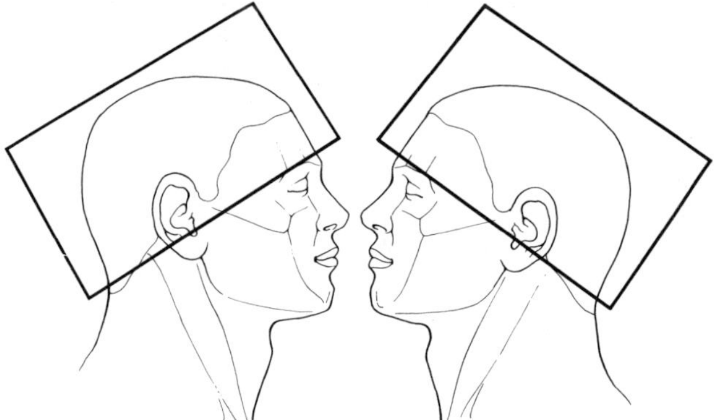

Figure 18.1 These are the treatment portals used for whole brain irradiation for malignant brain tumors.

malignant gliomas, interstitial brachytherapy is combined with external beam therapy in a number of centers. Stereotaxic neurosurgical techniques are used to guide the surgeon during source placement. Iridium-192 is the source material most commonly employed for removable implants and iodine-125 for permanent implants.[5]

Medulloblastoma These are radiosensitive tumors of the cerebellum, accounting for 20-25% of brain tumors in children. They tend to invade the subarachnoid space to metastasize in the cerebrospinal fluid (CSF). For this reason the entire cerebrospinal axis must be treated .The brain and upper cervical spine is treated with parallel opposing lateral portals (Figure 18.2); the spinal canal is treated down to the level of the third sacral vertebra.

The entire brain and upper cord receive 35 to 45 Gy/1.7-2.0 Gy per fraction and the posterior fossa is boosted to bring the tumor dose to the cerebellum to 50-

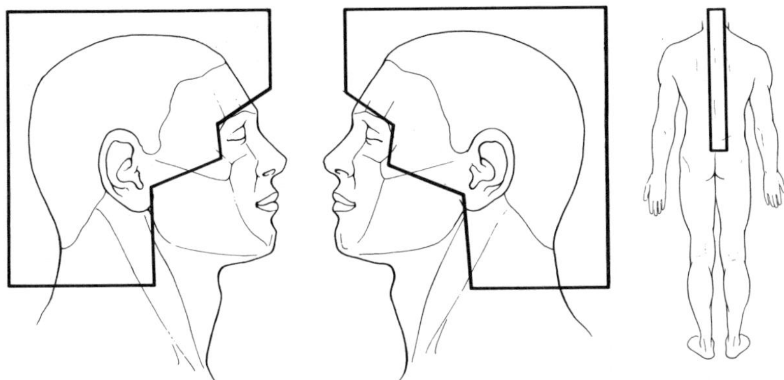

Figure 18.2 These are the treatment portals used for patients with medulloblastoma.

55 Gy. The spinal cord receives 35-40 Gy/1.5-1.8 Gy per fraction. "Hot spots" at the junction between the cranial and spinal portals are prevented with gap calculations and/or moving the junction line half-way through the treatment course. Five year survival rates reported in the literature range from 20% to 70%.[6] Children treated for medulloblastoma may suffer mental impairment as a complication of the tumor and its therapy.[7] The most severely affected children are those irradiated at less than 8 years of age.

Ependymoma These are uncommon tumors. They can arise supratentorially, infratentorially, in the spinal cord or in the cauda equina. Infratentorial ependymomas are seen most commonly in children. Ependymomas are classified as high-grade or low-grade and the grade has an important influence on prognosis and treatment.

The usual treatment for ependymomas is surgical removal and postoperative radiotherapy. High-grade ependymomas metastasize via the CSF and require RT to the entire cerebrospinal axis for medulloblastoma. Low-grade tumors receive RT to the tumor site only (45-50 Gy). Treatment results for spinal cord and cauda equina tumors are superior to the treatment results for supratentorial and infratentorial tumors because spinal cord lesions are, as a group, lower in grade than intracranial tumors.

Pinealoma Tumors of the pineal area are rare. Sixty percent of pineal tumors are germinomas, a tumor similar in histologic appearance to seminoma of the testis. Benign and malignant teratomas and pineal parenchymal tumors occur less commonly in the pineal gland. Germinomas are highly radiosensitive tumors and cure rates in the range of 60% to 85% are reported following RT.[8]

Germinomas occasionally metastasize via the CSF and some authorities recommend RT to the entire cerebrospinal axis, particularly if the CSF cytology is positive. All authorities agree, however, that the entire ventricular system of the brain should be treated and the dose recommended is 45-50 Gy in 5-6 weeks.

Brain stem tumors The brain stem consists of the thalamus, midbrain, pons and medulla oblongata. Most brain stem tumors are gliomas and occur in children. Tumors of the brain stem are occasionally treated by RT alone without a tissue diagnosis. The primary site with a few centimeters margin is treated to 40 to 50 Gy/4-6 weeks. Most authors report 5 year survival rates in the range of 30%.[9]

Oligodendroglioma These tumors grow slowly and have a long natural history. Postoperative radiotherapy to the tumor site improves 5 and 10 year survival rates. Survival rates ranging from 30% to 55% at 10 years have been reported following surgery and postoperative RT.[4]

Chordoma These rare malignant tumors are derived from the primitive notochord. The notochord is a supporting column of cells in the embryo which is eventually replaced by the skull and vertebral column. Chordomas can arise anywhere along the spinal column but are most common in the sacrum and base of skull. They are slow growing and have a long clinical course. Surgical excision and postoperative RT (60-65 Gy) offer the best chance of long-term disease control. In unresectable cases, RT alone (70-75 Gy) is used.

Meningioma These benign tumors are usually treated by surgery alone. However, clinical studies suggest that incompletely excised meningiomas should be given postoperative RT (50 Gy).[10]

Craniopharyngioma These rare benign cystic tumors arise from residual embryonic gut tissue, called Rathke's pouch, in the pituitary region. They are usually diagnosed in childhood. The preferred treatment, whenever possible is total excision under magnified vision. This will lead to long-term control in 75% of cases.[11] However, for large tumors, the risk of surgical complication is great and in these, partial excision followed by RT is used.

Intracavitary brachytherapy A technique for intracavitary therapy for cystic craniopharyngiomas has been developed.[12] Yttrium-90, a beta emitting isotope is instilled into the cyst under stereotaxic control to deliver 200 Gy to the cyst wall.

Brain metastasis The most frequent neoplasm involving the brain is metastasis. Lung carcinoma is the most common primary site followed by breast carcinoma. Brain metastases are treated with whole brain irradiation. The standard regimen is 30 Gy in 10 fractions over 2 weeks. The patients are given oral steriods during treatment to prevent brain edema and increase the rapidity of neurologic improvement. Fifty to 80% of patients experience neurologic improvement following RT.[13] However, the median survival following RT is only 15 weeks.

Patients with a single metastasis to the brain may be candidates for surgical excision of the metastasis. Surgery reduces tumor bulk, decreases edema and

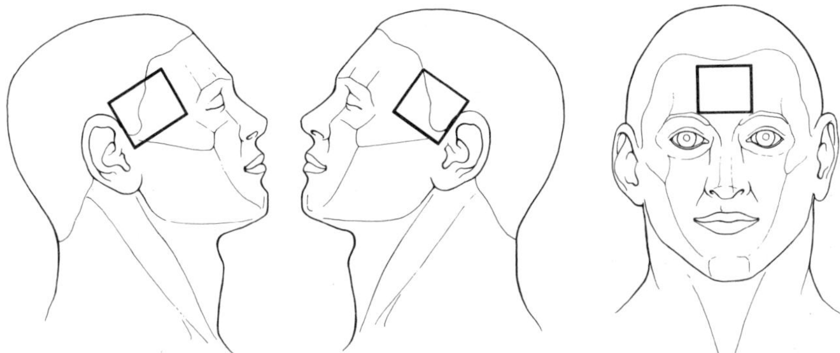

Figure 18.3 These are the treatment portals used to treat pituitary adenomas. sually the tumor is easily encompassed by 5 x 5 cm portals.

relieves obstruction to flow of CSF resulting in improved neurologic function. Whole brain irradiation is given following surgery for the purpose of eradicating microsocpic foci of metastasis.

Pituitary adenoma *Non-hormone secreting tumors* Adenomas which do not secrete hormones may be large when discovered and the patients often present with visual impairment due to encroachment of the tumor on the optic chiasm. Most are treated initially with surgery via a trans-sphenoidal approach to the tumor through the nasal cavity. Postoperative radiotherapy is recommended and most tumors can be treated with three small 5 X 5 cm portals (Figure 18.3, 18.4, and 18.5). The standard regimen is 45 Gy/25 fractions/5 weeks. Brain necrosis and blindness due to injury to the optic nerves have been observed following RT, but these complications are uncommon with doses below 50 Gy.[14]

Hormone secreting tumors Small hormone-producing adenomas, called microadenomas are usually removed by trans-sphenoidal microsurgery which allows normal pituitary tissues to be preserved. The patients are followed with hormone studies and RT is not given unless there is evidence of persistence or recurrence. If radiation is required conventional RT is usually given. However, cyclotron-produced high energy proton beams are used in some centers because a higher radiation dose can be given to the tumor without significant risk of brain or optic nerve injury while preserving normal pituitary function.[15]

Spinal cord *Primary intramedullary tumors* Spinal cord tumors (usually astrocytomas or ependymomas) are treated by laminectomy (removal of the posterior arch of the vertebra) to provide decompression and tumor removal. Postoperative RT (45-50 Gy/5-6 weeks) is usually indicated.

Metastatic extradural tumors Metastasis to the epidural space with compression of the spinal cord is a common clinical problem. The epidural metastasis usually develops by direct extension from adjacent vertebral bodies. This is the usual mode of the spinal cord invovlement from lung, breast and prostate primaries. However, the epidural metastasis can develop by direct tumor growth through intervetrebral foramina from abdominal or mediastinal lymph nodes. This type of spread can be seen with lymphoma in adults and neuroblastoma in children.

Most patients with cord compression have severe back pain and sensory deficit is often detectable. Motor deficit can proceed rapidly to total paralysis and may be associated with loss of bowel and bladder control. Early diagnosis is essential and MRI or lumbar myelography should be obtained if cord compression is suspected, because if total loss of motor function develops, return of function is unlikely.[16]

Current standard therapy for malignant spinal cord compression is oral

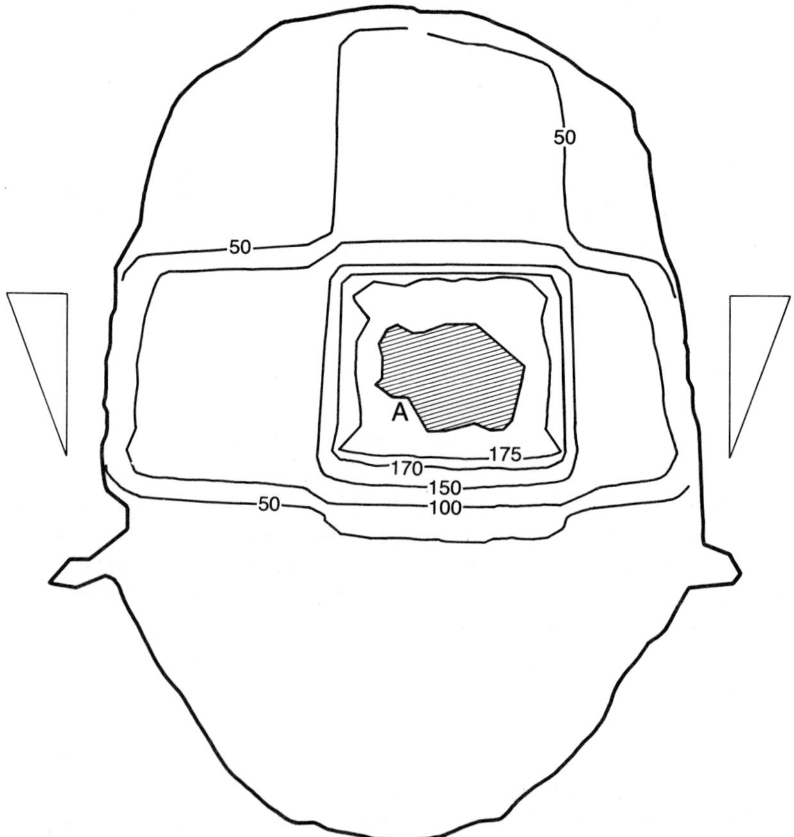

Figure 18.4 This is the computer plan for a patient treated for a large pituitary adenoma. A single anterior and right and left lateral wedged (15 degree) portals were used.

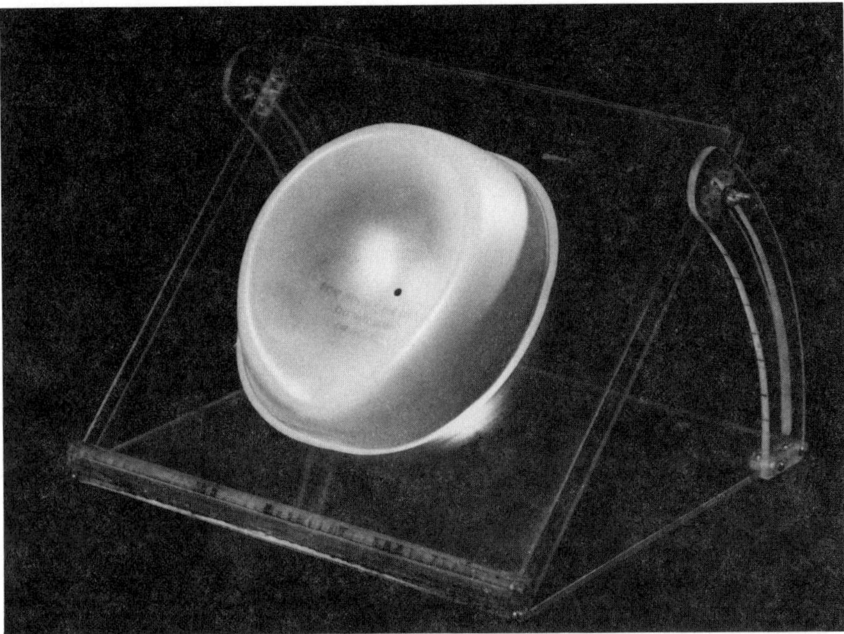

Figure 18.5 This is the head holder that we use for patients treated for pituitary adenoma. It flexes the neck and elevates the head to ensure that the anterior beam passes superior to the eyes.

steroids (dexamethasone 16-64 mg/day), radiotherapy (25 to 45 Gy) and chemotherapy. Surgery is reserved for those whose disease fails to respond to nonsurgical therapy.

STEREOTAXIC RADIOSURGERY

Arteriovenous malformations of the brain (AVM) are clusters of abnormal arteries and veins that shunt blood from the arterial to the venous system. The abnormal vessels are prone to spontaneous bleeding. Surgery is the treatment of choice for small lesions, but some AVMs cannot safely be approached surgically. It is for these that special techniques for stereotaxic radiosurgery have been developed to treat small (<1 cm) lesions in the brain with one large radiation dose (15-25 Gy).

The first unit, known as the Gamma Unit, was built by Leksell in Sweden.[17] This unit employs narrow beams of gamma rays from multiple cobalt-60 sources fixed in a helmet-like collimating device. The gamma ray beams cross-fire the AVM which is localized with stereotaxic techniques. High single doses in the range of 15 to 25 Gy produce sclerosing lesions in the AVM thus preventing future hemorrhage.

Gamma Units are expensive and are not very practical since they are not adaptable for other uses. In the U.S., therefore, radiosurgery is performed with narrow x-ray beams from linear accelerators or cyclotron-produced proton beams.[18, 19]

COMPLICATIONS OF RADIOTHERAPY

Delayed radiation necrosis of the brain Necrosis is the most important complication of brain irradiation. The onset of brain necrosis may be several months to years after treatment and the lesion is usually irreversible, progressive and often fatal. The histologic characteristic of brain necrosis is damage to white matter. The signs and symptoms of brain necrosis depend on the site and volume irradiated but often are consistent with an intracranial mass. For this reason, the lesion is often mistaken for recurrent tumor.

Radiation myelopathy This is the most feared complication of radiotherapy. In affected patients the onset of spinal cord dysfunction is usually delayed for months to years post-treatment. The lesion is progressive and there is no known treatment. The incidence of myelopathy depends upon the dose-time-fractionation schedule used and the length of cord irradiated. When the length of the cord irradiated extends over 3 to 5 vertebral segments the tolerance to conventional treamtent is 50 Gy/25 fractions/35 days.[20] However, when a longer segment is irradiated, i.e., 6-7 vertebrae, the tolerance is only 45 Gy.

The pathogenesis for radiation myelopathy is unknown, but probably results from white matter or vascular injury since white matter necrosis and vascular damage are the predominate patholgoic alteration seen.

Soft tissue injury Patients irradiated for a primary brain or pituitary tumor often experience radiation-induced soft tissue injuries invovling the scalp and ears.[21] Forty percent experience complete and permanent epilation, 6% have scalp swelling, 6% external otitis, 5% otitis media and 4% ear swelling. The frequency of soft tissue injury is greatest among patients receiving whole brain irradiation, whereas patients treated with small portals have few soft tissue injuries.

REFERENCES

1. Schoenberg BS. Chapter,1, The epidemiology of central nervous system tumors, In Oncolgoy of the Nervous System, Ed. Walk MD. Martinus Nijhoff Publishers, Boston, 1983, pp 1-29.

2. Silverberg BS, Boring CC, Squires TS. Cancer statistics, 1990, CA-A Cancer Journal for Clinicians 40:9-26. 1990.

3. Rubinstein LJ. Tumors of the Central Nervous System, Fascicle 6 of Atlas of Tumor Pathology, Armed Forces Institute of Pathology, Washington, 1972.

5. Wu A, Chun M, Kasdon D, et al. Interstitial iridium-192 implantation for malignant brain tumors, Brit J. Radiol 623:154-157, 1989.

6. Bloom HJG. Intracranial tumors: Response and resistance to therapeutic endeavors, 1970-1980, Int J Radiat Oncol Biol Physi 8:1082-1113, 1982.

7. Silverman CL et al. Late effects of radiotherapy of patients with cerebellar medulloblastoma, Cancer 54:825-829, 1984.

8. Amendola BE, et al. Pineal region tumors: Analysis of treatment results, Int J Radiat Oncol Biol Phys 10:991-997, 1984.

9. Ryoo MC, et al. Irradiation of primary brain stem tumors, Radiology 131:503-5076, 1979.

10. Wara WM, Sheline GE, Newman H, et al. Radiaiton therapy of meningiomas, Am J Roentengol 123:453-458, 1975.

11. Danoff BF, et al. Childhood craniopharyngioma survival, local control, endocrine and neuorologic function following radiotherapy, Int J Radiat Oncol Biol Phys 9:171-175, 1983.

12. Strauss L, et al. Radioisotope therapy of cystic craniopharyngiomas, Int J Radiat Oncol Biol Phys 8:1581-1585, 1982.

13. Borgelt B, et al. The palliation of brain metastases: Final results of the first two studies by the Radiation Therapy Oncology Group, Int J Radiat Oncol Biol Phys 6:1-9,. 1980.

14. Aristizabal S, Caldwell WL, Avila JH. The relationship of time-dose-fractionation factors to complications in the treatment of pituitary tumors by irradiation, Int J Radiat Oncol Biol Phys 2:667-673, 1977.

15. Kjellberg RN, Shintani A, Frantz AG, Kliman B. Proton-beam therapy in acromegaly, N. Engl J Med 278:689-695, 1968.

16. Kim RY, Spencer SA, Meredith RF, et al Extradural spinal cord compression: Analysis of factors determining functional prognosis-prospective study, Radiology 176:279-282, 1990.

17. Leksell L. Stereotactic radiosurgery, J Neurol Neurosurg, and Psychiat 46:797-803, 1983.

18. Kejllberg RN, Hanamura T, Davis KR, et al. Bragg-peak proton beam therapy for arteriovenous malformations of the brain, N.Engl J Med 309:269-274, 1983.

19. Saunders WM, Winston KR, Siddon RL, et al Radiosurgery for arteriovenous malformations of the brain using a standard linear accelerator: Rationale and technique, Int J Radiat Oncol Biol Phys 15:441-447. 1988.

20. Lambert PM. Radiation myelopathy of the thoracic spinal cord in long-term survivors treated with radical radiotherapy using conventional fractionation, Cancer 41:1751-

1760, 1978.

21. Baglan RJ, Marks JE. Soft-tissue reactions following irradiation of primary brain and pituitary tumors, Int J Radiat Oncol Biol Phys 7:455-459, 1981.

Chapter 19

BREAST CANCER

ETIOLOGY AND EPIDEMIOLOGY

Breast cancer is the second most common cause of death from cancer among women in the U.S. [1] It is estimated that in 1990, 150,000 new cases were diagnosed and 44,000 women died of breast cancer. As shown in Table 19.1, ovarian function seems to have a role in the development of breast cancer suggesting a role for estrogen hormones in etiology. It has been suggested that the western diet, which is high in fat, is important in the etiology of breast cancer but the data are inconclusive. Viruses are known to cause breast cancer in animals, but there is not conclusive evidence that viruses cause breast cancer in humans.

Table 19.1 Risk Factors associated with breast cancer

Increased risk of breast cancer

Early menarche and late menopause

Late or no childbearing

Long-term estrogen administration

Family history of breast cancer

History of benign breast disease

Exposure of breast to radiation

Decreased risk

Castration

Early childbearing

PATHOLOGY

Histologic types Breast cancers arise from the epithelium of large, medium or small-sized ducts. If tumor growth is confined entirely to the duct lumena, the process is termed intraductal carcinoma. However, if there is penetration of the basement membrane of the ducts, the tumor is an invasive or infiltrating carcinoma. Breast cancers are classified according to their microscopic pattern of growth. The classification scheme and the incidence of each type is shown in Table 19.2. The prognosis for patients having papillary, medullary, tubular or mucinous carcinoma is better than for those having infiltrating duct carcinoma. A variety of nonepithelial tumors occur rarely in the breast including sarcomas and lymphomas. Cystosarcoma phyllodes is an uncommon breast tumor which is partially epithelial and partially nonepithelial.

Table 19.2 Pathologic classification of breast cancer and relative
incidence of each type

Type	Incidence
Infiltrating duct	53.0%
Medullary	6.0%
Lobular invasive	5.0%
Mucinous (colloid)	2.0%
Tubular	1.0%
Adenocystic	.4%
Papillary	.3%
Carcinosarcoma	.1%
Paget's disease	2.0%
With intraductal	.2%
With infiltrating	1.1%
With other types	.3%
Combinations with infiltrating duct	28.0%
Combinations with other types	2.0%

Paget's disease This clinical entity occurs in 2% of patients with breast cancer. Patients with Paget's disease present with eczema-like skin changes involving the nipple of one breast associated with itching, oozing and bleeding of the nipple. The nipple changes are associated with an underlying intraductal or invasive carcinoma. Microscopically, the nipple epithelium contains nests of tumor cells. The prognosis is that of the histologic type of the underlying carcinoma.

Inflammatory carcinoma This clinical syndrome is characterized by redness, edema and increased heat of the skin of one breast. These changes are associated with an underlying rapidly growing carcinoma and the skin changes result from the presence in the skin of undifferentiated cancer cells which cause obstruction of the lymphatics of the skin. The prognosis for patients with this clinical type is poor.

The primary Forty-eight percent of breast cancers arise in the upper outer quadrant of the breast, 15% in the upper inner quadrant, 11% in the lower quadrant, 6 % in the lower inner quadrant, 17% in the central regions, and 3% arisein multiple sites in the breast

Breast cancers spread locally by direct infiltration into breast parenchyma, grow along ducts and through breast lymphatics. If untreated, direct spread to the overlying skin and/or deep to the pectoral fascia occurs. Tumor size is important in prognosis because large tumors are frequently associated with axillary nodal metastasis. Minimal breast cancer is cancer that is discovered at an early stage of 5 mm or less in size. The prognosis for minimal breast cancer is good.

Microscopic tumor characteristics which are of prognostic importance include: 1) histologic grade (degree of tubule formation, size of cells and nuclei, degree of hyperchromatism, number of mitoses); 2) nuclear grade (degree of anaplasia of nuclei); 3) the presence of an infiltrate of lymphocytes in the tumor improves prognosis; 4) invasion of lymphatic and blood vessels has a negative effect; 5) multiple sites of breast cancer in one breast, which is seen in 13% of cases, may adversely affect prognosis.

Estrogen receptors Hormone receptors are proteins, present in the cytoplasm of cells, which bind and transfer specific hormones to the nuclei where the hormone functions. These receptors can be measured in normal tissue and some tumors. The most frequently measured receptor is the estrogen receptor protein (ER). The ER levels in the primary tumor are measured in the tumor following removal. About 50% of breast cancers are ER+. ER (+) tumors have a better overall prognosis than ER (-) tumors. Response to endocrine therapy usually occurs only in tumors containing estrogen receptors.

Lymph nodes The routes of regional spread of breast cancer are to the axillary, internal mammary and supraclavicular lymph nodes. Axillary lymph nodes metastasis are present in 40-50% of patients at the time of diagnosis. The incidence of (+) nodes increases as the size of the primary increases. The prognosis correlates with the number of (+) axillary nodes at the time of surgery (Table 19.3).

Internal mammary lymph node metastasis occurs less commonly than axillary lymph node metastasis. The incidence of internal mammary spread is

Table 19.3 Survival according to the number of positive axillary nodes[3]	
No. nodes (+)	**5 year survival**
0	83%
1-3	73%
4-6	54%
7-12	50%
13	28%

related to the location of the primary; with central and inner quadrant primaries the incidence is 30% versus 15% for outer quadrant primaries. Also, when the axillary nodes are involved, the incidence of internal mammary spread is 45%

compared to only 15% when the axillary nodes are negative.

Supraclavicular lymph nodes are usually involved only if the axillary or internal mammary nodes are involved. Supraclavicular lymph node metastasis carries a grave prognosis.

Distant metastasis Current information suggests that most patients with breast cancer have disseminated disease by the time the diagnosis is established. A tumor 1 cm in size is already "advanced"because it has progressed through 30 cell doublings. Forty cell doublings would theoretically be lethal. Even though some patients are apparently cured, it is probable that local treatment does not eradicate every cancer cell and host factors undoubtedly play a role in killing residual cancer cells.

DIAGNOSIS OF BREAST CANCER

History Many breast cancers are found by the patient. The most common presenting symptom is that the patient has discovered a painless "lump" in her breast. Less frequent presenting symptoms include pain in the breast, nipple discharge and skin changes. Symptoms of advanced cancer include changes in breast size, inflammatory changes in the breast and bone pain.

Physical examination A complete physical examination is carried out. The examination includes inspection and palpation of both breasts, axillae and both supraclavicular fossae. The breast is inspected for nipple discharge or skin crusting or ulceration. The breasts are palpated in search of masses; masses 1 cm in size or larger can usually be detected by palpation.

Mammography This test is used in screening for detection of minimal breast cancer. Mammography is also used to assist the surgeon and radiologist in performing needle directed biopsy of suspicious lesions.

Biopsy The true nature of all breast masses must be established. This is usually accomplished by excisional biopsy, but needle and aspiration biopsies are also frequently used. In addition to breast cancer, a number of benign conditions can present as a breast mass i.e., cystic disease of the breast and fibroadenoma.

STAGING

The staging classification used for breast cancer is shown in abbreviated form in Table 19.4. Clinical data from physical examination and radiographic studies, i.e., bone and liver scans, and pathologic findings in removed tissues are used in staging.

SURGICAL TREATMENT

Criteria of operability In Table 19.5 are listed criteria of operability used

Table 19.4 Staging of breast cancer-abbreviated version

T1	Tumor 2 cm or less in greatest dimension
T2	Tumor more than 2 cm but not more than 5 cm
T3	Tumor more than 5 cm in greatest dimension
T4	Tumor of any size with extension to chest wall or skin
N0	No palpable axillary nodes
N1	Palpable enlarged but not fixed nodes
N2	Palpable nodes fixed to one another or to other structures
N3	Metastasis to internal mammary lymph nodes
M0	No evidence of distant metastasis
M1	Distant metastasis present (includes supraclavicular lymph node metastasis)

Stage grouping

I	T1N0M0
IIA	T1N1M0 or T2N0M0
IIB	T2N1M0 or T3N0M0
IIIA	T1N2M0, T2N2M0 or T3N0, N1 or N2
IIIB	T4 + any N and M0 or any T + N3M0
IV	any T + any N + M1

by surgeons as a guide to determine the suitability of patients for surgical therapy.

Radical mastectomy This operation was used in the past for stage I and II tumors. In it the entire breast, the skin overlying the tumor, the pectoralis major and minor, and the contents of the axilla are removed. Morbidity associated with the procedure includes deformity of the chest, arm edema and loss of normal arm function. This operation has been replaced by modified radical mastectomy in the surgical armamentarium.

Modified radical mastectomy The pectoralis major and minor muscles are preserved resulting in less morbidity and a superior cosmetic result compared to radical mastectomy.

Extended radical mastectomy This operation was used in some centers to treat central and inner quadrant tumors. In it, the internal mammary lymph nodes and, in some cases, even the supraclavicular and mediastinal nodes were removed. Since cure rates are not significantly better with this operation than

Table 19..5 Criteria of operability [5]

Surgery not indicated if any of the following are present

Extensive edema of skin over breast

Satellite tumor nodules in skin over breast

Inflammatory carcinoma

Parasternal mass (internal mammary node metastasis)

Supraclavicular lymph node metastases

Edema of arm

Distant metastasis

Two or more of the following grave signs:

    Ulceration of skin

    Edema of skin of limited extent

    Fixation of tumor to chest wall

    Axillary lymph nodes 2.5 cm in size or greater

    Fixation of axillary lymph nodes to skin or deep tissue

with lesser procedures, it is rarely performed today.

Total or simple mastectomy The entire breast is removed but the pectoral muscles and axillary lymph nodes are not dissected. In one large ongoing study by the National Surgical Adjuvant Project (NSABP), comparing total mastectomy to modified radical mastectomy in treatment of early breast cancer, no difference in survival rates between the two procedures was found.

Segmental mastectomy (lumpectomy) The primary tumor and a generous portion of surrounding breast tissue are removed. It should be combined with an axillary dissection to determine histologic status of lymph nodes.

RADIATION THERAPY IN OPERABLE BREAST CANCER

Radiation combined with lumpectomy The idea of combining a conservative surgical procedure with radiotherapy is not new.[6] However, the method only recently gained acceptance in the U.S. as an alternative therapy for women who do not want the cosmetic deformity associated with a modified radical mastectomy. Patients choosing this treatment usually have stage T1N0 or T2N0 disease. They will have undergone a local excision of the primary and many will have had an axillary lymph node dissection. Results from numerous institutions around the world suggest that cure rates following this treatment are equivalent to those seen with a more radical surgical procedure.[7]

Technique To ensure a reproducible treatment position a mold is made for each patient prior to simulation (Figures 19.1 and 19.2). The breast is treated with tangential fields (Figure 19.3). Wedge filters are used to provide a homogeneous dose in the breast. Bolus is not used. The axillary lymph nodes are not treated if the axillary dissection fails to reveal nodal metastasis. The dose is 45 Gy/25 fractions/5 weeks. If the surgical margins are close to the tumor, the primary site is boosted with an electron beam (10-15 Gy) or an interstitial iridium-192 implant.

If an axillary dissection has not been carried out, the axilla is irradiated with an anterior portal which covers the axilla and the supraclavicular region (Figure 19.4). The portal is angled 15 degrees to reduce exposure to the esophagus and

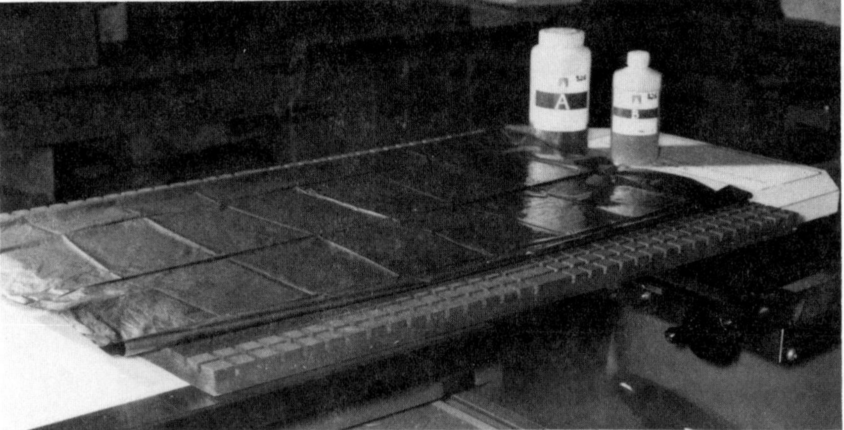

Figure 19.1 To immobilize the patient and ensure reproducibility of setups, a body mold (Alpha Cradle) is made. The chemicals are mixed and placed in the plastic bag. The chemicals and materials can be obtained from Smithers Medical Products.

spinal cord. A cerrobend beam splitting lung shield is constructed to ensure that the supraclavicular area is irradiated only by the upper half of the portal. This reduces the amount of underlying lung irradiated. The dose to the axilla is 45 Gy at 5 cm depth/25 fractions.

Furthermore, cerrobend shields are used at the junction line between the tangential portals and the supraclavicular portal for the purpose of reducing beam divergence at the junction line (Figure 19.5). This prevents the occurrence of subcutaneous fibrosis along the junction line.

Modified radical mastectomy + Postoperative radiotherapy

The role of postoperative radiotherapy is controversial. Radiotherapy can eliminate residual foci of cancer cells on the chest wall and in regional lymphatics but it has not been shown convincingly that such treatment improves survival. The traditional indications for postoperative radiotherapy are shown in Table 19.6.

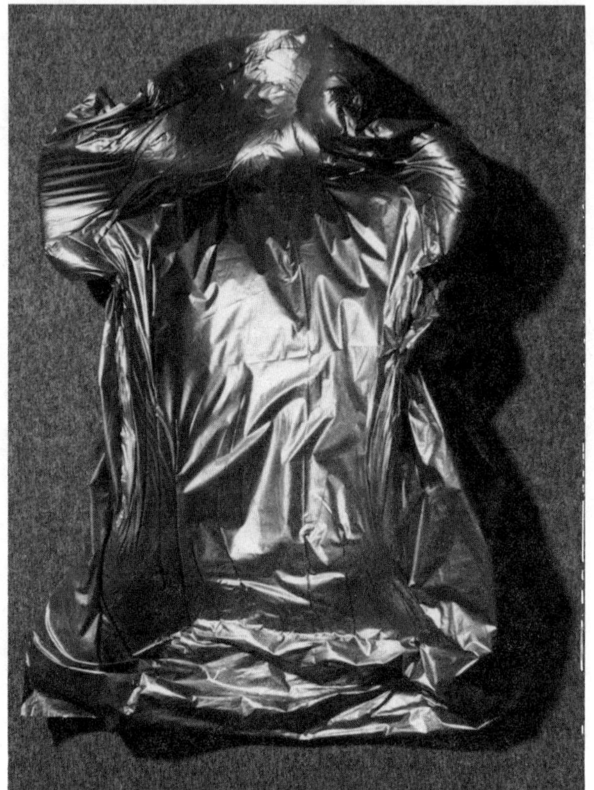

Figure 19.2 This is the appearance of a completed Alpha Cradle.

Technique If the chest wall is covered by a thick layer of soft tissue it is treated with parallel opposing tangential portals. The tumor dose is 45-50 Gy/25 fractions/5 weeks. Tissue equivalent bolus material is used to increase the skin dose on the chest wall. The axilla and supraclavicular regions are irradiated with a separate anterior portal as described above.

If the chest wall is thin with little subcutaneous tissue overlying the ribs a single large 6 MeV electron beam portal can be used to irradiate the chest wall.

Table 19.6 Indications for postoperative radiotherapy following modified radical mastectomy [8]

Indications	Treatment volume
Large primary (>5 cm in size)	Chest wall and lymphatics
>20% axillary nodes (+)	Chest wall and lymphatics
Close surgical margin	Chest wall and lymphatics

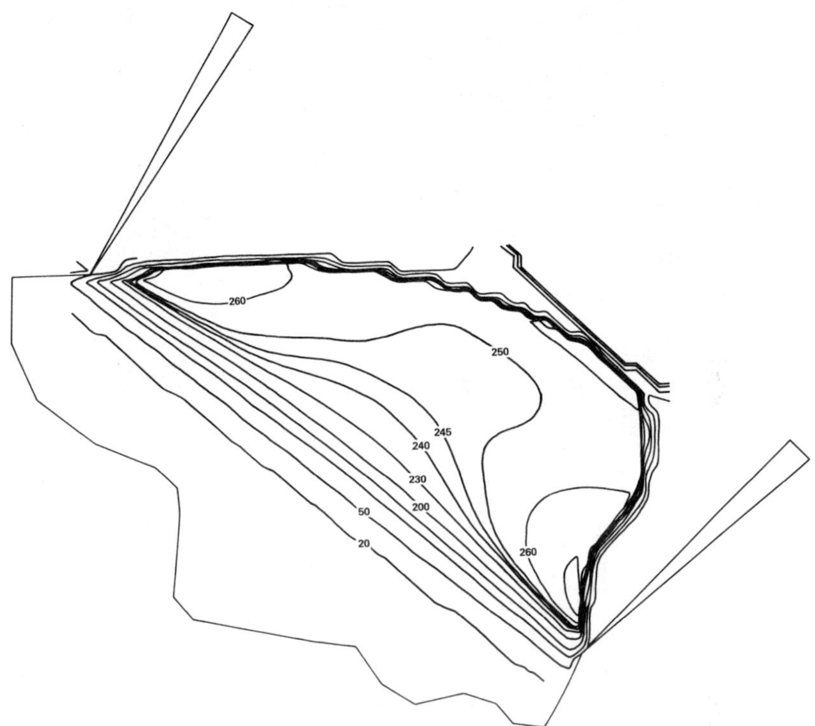

Figure 19.3 A computer plan for a patient treated following lumpectomy.

RADIOTHERAPY FOR INOPERABLE BREAST CANCER

Current treatment for locally advanced breast cancer employs surgery, radiotherapy and chemotherapy in planned combination. Treatment is usually initiated with chemotherapy to reduce tumor size and treat subclinical micrometastasis. If feasible, a mastectomy is then carried out to eradicate bulky local disease and radiotherapy to the chest wall and nodes is given. However, if a simple mastectomy is not possible, RT alone is given to the breast and nodes. Local control rates as high as 75% can be achieved with radiation combined with surgery and chemotherapy, with 5 and 10 year survival rates in the range of 40% and 20% respectively.[9]

RADIOTHERAPY FOR LOCALLY RECURRENT DISEASE

Patients who develop local chest wall recurrence following modified radical mastectomy usually receive electron beam treatment to the chest wall in combination with systemic therapy. The radiation portals and doses are similar

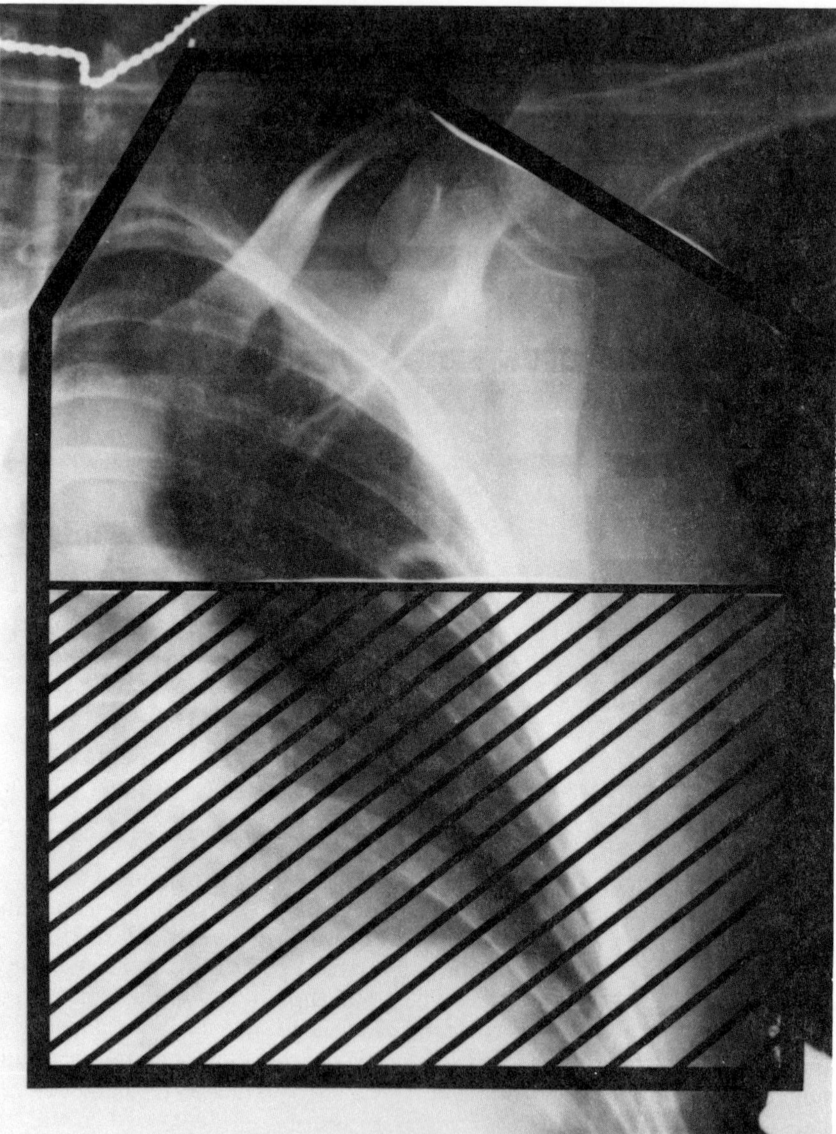

Figure 19.4 If the axilla and supraclavicular region are treated, steps must be taken to ensure a homogenous dose along the match line between the supraclavicular portal and the tangential portals. This is particularly important if a linear accelerator is used. This special attention to match-line is necessary to prevent radiation fibrosis along the line. A cerrobend shield is used to block the lower half of the beam. This prevents divergent radiation from reaching the tangentially treated area.

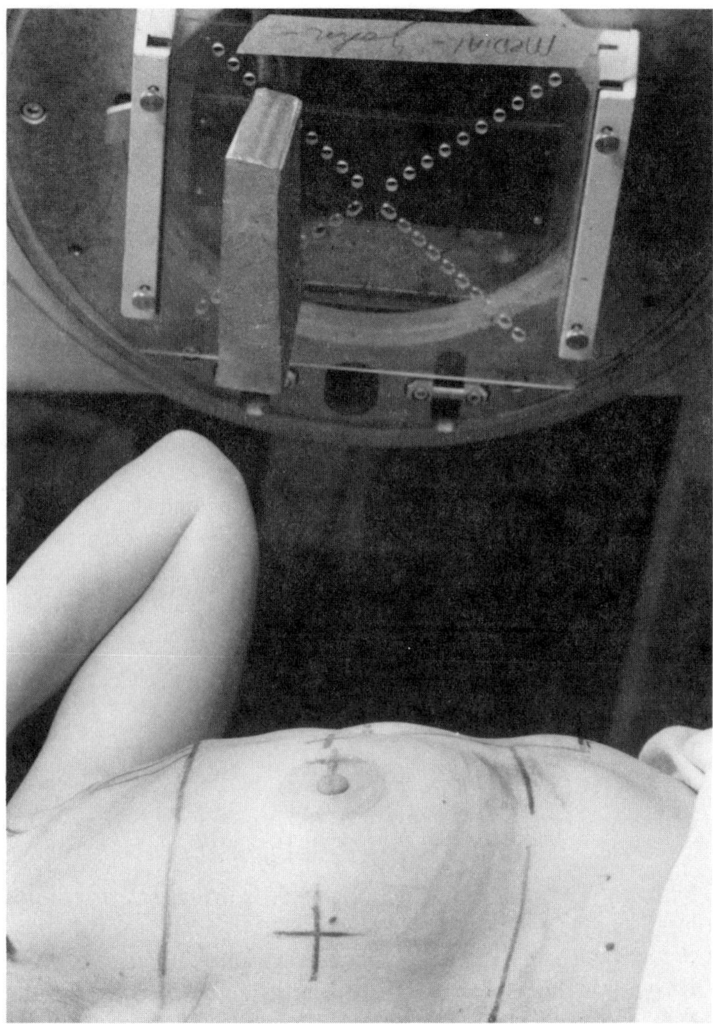

Figure 19.5 This is the treatment setup for the medial tangential portal. Note the cerrobend shield for the match-line, which prevents divergent radiation from reaching the supraclavicular area.

to those used for postoperative treatment. The site of recurrence is usually boosted with electrons. Unfortunately, the treatment for locally recurrent breast cancer is not very satisfactory.[10] The patients frequently develop re-recurrence and subsequent distant metastasis occurs in the majority of patients.

RADIOTHERAPY FOR DISTANT METASTASIS

Radiotherapy is effective in the palliative treatment of distant metastasis. Bone metastasis is the most common indication for RT and doses of 20 Gy/5 fractions or 30 Gy/10 fractions are effective in pain relief in 80% of cases. Brain metastasis is also common and usually responds to 30 Gy/10 fractions to the whole brain.

CHEMOTHERAPY FOR BREAST CANCER

Metastastic disease A number of drugs have activity against breast cancer. Most regimes employ combinations of agents. The most popular regimens are the Cooper regimen (cyclophosphamide, 5-fluorouracil, methotrexate, vincristine and prednisone), CMF (cyclophosphamide, methotrexate and 5-FU) and FAC (5-FU, cyclophosphamide and oxorubicin or adriamycin). These regimens are capable of producing tumor responses in 50-80% of patients for mediandurations ranging from 8 to 15 months.

Adjuvant chemotherapy A number of large clinical trials are underway evaluating elective chemotherapy following surgery for patients with positive axillary nodes. Early results from these trials suggest that disease-free survival time is improved for premenopausal patients but not for postmenopausal patients. In premenopausal patients the improvement is greatest in those with only 1 to 3 positive nodes and not as great in those with more than 4 positive nodes. Currently, the most widely used regimen is CMF. In the Milan trial, 66% of premenopausal patients with Stage II breast cancer were surviving free of disease 5 years after receiving surgery + CMF versus only 43% for controls receiving surgery alone.[11]

ENDOCRINE THERAPY

This method was traditionally used primarily in Stage IV disease but its role in earlier disease is under investigation.

Castration Bilateral oophorectomy is the usual method but ovarian irradiation (20 Gy/10 fractions) is also effective in reducing estrogen production.

Medical adrenalectomy Aminoglutethamide is a drug which suppresses steroid synthesis by the adrenal glands resulting in reduced estrogen production.

Antiestrogens These are drugs which block uptake of estrogen in target tissues by binding to estrogen receptors. Tamoxifen, nafoxidine and clomiphene are antiestrogens which have significant antitumor activity.

Adjuvant endocrine therapy Data from large clinical trials suggest that adjuvant tamoxifen therapy following surgery fo rStage I and II breast cancer increases disease free survival for premenopausal and postmenopausal patients.[12]

BREAST CANCER IN PREGNANCY

Breast cancer occasionally develops in pregnant patients. The prognosis depends on the stage of disease at the time of diagnosis. Unfortunately, there is often a delay in diagnosis and many patients already have advanced local disease when finally diagnosed. Surgery can be accomplished during pregnancy, but radiotherapy and chemotherapy are usually withheld until the postpartum period.

BREAST CANCER IN MALES

Breast cancer in males accounts for only 1% of cases of breast cancer. The common presenting symptoms include the presence of a breast mass, bloody nipple discharge, nipple retraction, axillary mass and bone pain. The histologic characteristics of breast cancer in males are similar to that seen in females. The treatment of the primary and the prognosis are also similar. Ten year, disease free survival rates for patients without axillary metastasis is 70% versus only 35% for those with positive nodes.[13]

REFERENCES

1. Silverberg E, Boring CC, Squires TS. Cancer statistics, 1990, CA-A Cancer Journal for Clinicians 40:9-26, 1990.

2. Henderson IC, Harris JR, Kinne DW, Hellman S. Chapter 38, Cancer of the breast, In Cancer: Principles and Practice of Oncology, 3rd Edition, Eds. DeVita VT, Hellman S, Rosenberg SA, J. B. Lippincott Company, Philadelphia, 1989, pp 1197-1268.

3. Fisher B, et al. Relationship of number of positive axillary nodes to the prognosis of patients with primary breast cancer: An NSA P update, Cancer 52:1551-1557, 1983.

4. Chapter 23, Breast, In Manual for Staging of Cancer, Third edition, Eds. Beahrs OH, Henson DE, Hutter RVP, Myers MN, J.B. Lippincott Company, Philadelphia, 1988, pp 145-150.

5. Haagensen CD, Stout AP. Carcinoma of the breast: Criteria of operability, Ann Surg 118:1032, 1943.

6. Keynes G. Conservative treatment of breast carcinoma, Brit Med J., 2:6543-647, 1937.

7. Harris JR, Hellman S. Chapter 6, The results of primary radiation therapy for early breast cancer at the Joint Center for Radiation Therapy, In Conservative Management of Breast Cancer, Ed., Harris JR, Hellman S, Silan W, J. B. Lippincott Company, Philadelphia, 1983, pp 47-52.

8. Fletcher GH, Montague ED, Tapley N, Barker JL. Chapter 6, Breast, In Textbook of Radiotherapy, 3rd Edition, Ed. Fletcher GH, Lea & Febriger, 1980, pp 527-583.

9. Lopirinzi CL, et al. Aggressive combined modality therapy for advanced local-regional breast cancer, J Clin Oncol 2:157-163, 1984.

10. Toonkel LM, et al. The significance of local recurrence of carcinoma of the breast, Int J Radiat Oncol Biol Phys 9:33-39, 1983.

11. Bonnadonna G, Valagussa P. Chemotherapy of breast cancer: Current views and results, Int J Radiat Oncol Biol Phys 9:279-297, 1983.

12. Ribeiro G, Palmer MK. Adjuvant tamoxifen for operable carcinoma of the breast: Report of clinical trial by the Christie Hospital and Holt Radium Institute, Brit Med J 286:827-830, 1983.

13. Robison R, Montague ED. Treatment results in males with breast cancer, Cancer 49:403-406, 1982.

Chapter 20

THE THORAX

LUNG CANCER

ETIOLOGY AND EPIDEMIOLOGY

Lung cancer is a major health problem. In the U.S. it is the leading cause of death from cancer in men and women.[1] The sex ratio in incidence is about 3:1 for males:females. The highest incidence rates are along the east coast from metropolitan New York to Florida. Florida has the highest rate in the nation. Among nations, Scotland, England and Wales have the highest rates and Japan and Mexico have the lowest.

At least 80% of lung cancer is believed to be caused by exposure to carcinogens. The major factor in etiology is cigarette smoking, but there are carcinogens in polluted air such as 3,4 benzpyrene, copper, lead, nickel, zinc, coal and tar. Also, there are occupational carcinogens such as radioactivity, asbestos, arsenic, nickel, iron oxides, chromium, chloromethyl methyl ether and vinyl chloride.

PATHOLOGY

Histologic types Most lung cancers originate in the epithelium of the bronchial tree. The incidence of the four major histologic types is shown in Table 20.1. The disease arises in response to repeated injury and chronic inflammation and the process may take 10-20 years.

Table 20.1 Incidence and prognosis of the histologic types of lung carcinoma[2]		
Histologic type	**Incidence**	**5 year survival**
Squamous cell	45%	25%
Adenocarcinoma	22%	12%
Small cell	19%	1%
Large cell	11%	13%
Other	3%	

Pathogenesis Initially, exposure to carcinogens causes non-specific inflammation followed by proliferation of the basal cells in the bronchial mucosa. With further injury, the normal columnar epithelium undergoes metaplasia and is replaced by stratified squamous epithelium. Eventually, the epithelium becomes disorganized with nuclear atypia and mitosis in the basal layer. With further injury the process extends through the full thickness of the mucosa and is called carcinoma in situ. Finally, the basement membrane is penetrated by the neoplastic cells becoming an invasive carcinoma.

Lymph node metastasis Regional lymph node metastasis is found in nearly 50% of patients at the time of surgery. The incidence is highest in small cell carcinoma (70%). Periobronchial, hilar and mediastinal lymph nodes on the same side as the primary are involved most frequently.

Distant metastasis Distant metastasis is common in patients with lung cancer. The liver, bones and brain are the most common sites and the highest incidence is seen with small cell carcinoma.

SYMPTOMS

Ninety-five percent of patients with lung cancer have symptoms at the time of diagnosis and there is a wide spectrum of possible symptoms. The symptoms may be caused by the primary tumor, regional or distant metastasis or there may be only systemic symptoms such as anorexia, weight loss and fatigue. Cough is the most common symptom related to the primary but hemoptysis, dyspnea, pneumonitis, chest pain and hoarseness of the voice are frequent symptoms. Swelling of the face, neck and arms due to obstruction of the superior vena cava by mediastinal lymph node metastasis, called superior vena cava syndrome, is the presenting symptom in about 5% of cases.

Thirty percent of patients present with symptoms of distant metastasis. Brain metastasis can present as convulsions, headaches, nausea, personality changes and hemiplegia. Liver metastasis can cause abdominal pain and bone metastasis also causes pain. Occasionally, spinal cord compression due to vertebral metastasis is the presenting symptom.

DIAGNOSIS AND STAGING

The initial step is a complete history and physical examination. Enlarged supraclavicular lymph nodes or other peripheral masses can be biopsied. Chest x-rays are obtained on all patients. Lesions as small as 1 cm in size can be seen on a chest x-ray. Pleural effusions seen on the chest x-ray are removed for cytologic examination.

Cytologic examination of sputum is a sensitive method for detecting lung cancer and the sputum is positive in 85% of patients with lung cancer. Fiber-optic bronchoscopy is the best method of identifying the exact location of cancers in the tracheobronchial tree. Visible lesions are biopsied through bronchoscope and washings and brushings are taken for cytologic examination. Lesions located in the periphery of the lung can often be diagnosed by transthoracic fine needle aspiration biopsy.

Patients with lung cancer require an assessment of the extent of disease prior to attempt at surgical excision. Mediastinoscopy, performed through a small suprasternal incision is an important technique used to assess the status of the mediastinal lymph nodes. Patients having a positive mediastinal lymph node biopsy are usually not candidates for surgery. Scans of the chest are useful preoperative assessments of the mediastinum.

Patients having symptoms of distant metastasis require appropriate scans. Bone, brain and liver scans are often obtained prior to surgery as part of the base line staging evaluation. The staging classification is presented in abbreviated form in Table 20.2.

Table 20.2 TNM Classification for lung cancer[2]	
T1	A tumor 3.0 cm or less in greatest dimension surrounded by lung without invasison more proximal than the lobar bronchus (not in the main bronchus)
T2	A tumor more than 3.0 cm in greatest dimension or a tumor of any size that invades the main bronchus or the pleura or is associated with atelectasis or obstructive pneumonitis
T3	Tumor of any size that invades chest wall, diaphragm, mediastinal pleura, pericardium or tumor of main bronchus less than 2 cm from carina or atelectasis or obstructive pneumonitis of entire lung
T4	Tumor that invades mediastinum, heart, great vessels, trachea, esophagus, vertebral body, carina, or tumor with malignant pleural effusion
N0	No regional lymph node metastasis
N1	Metastasis in ipsilateral periobronchial and/or hilar lymph nodes
N2	Metastasis in ipsilateral mediastinal nodes
N3	Metastasis in contralateral mediastinal nodes or supraclavicular nodes
M0	No distant metastasis; M1 Distant metastasis

Stage grouping

Stage I T1N0M0 or T2N0M0; Stage II T1N1M0 or T2N1M0

Stage IIIA T1N2M0 or T2N2M0 or T3N0, N1, N2M0

Stage IIIB any T+N3M0 or T4+ any NM0; Stage IV any T+any N+M1

TREATMENT OF NON-SMALL CELL LUNG CANCER

Surgery Surgical excision offers patients with non-small cell lung cancer the best chance for cure. Therefore, all patients with non-small cell lung cancer undergo thoracotomy except those with the contraindications shown in Table 20.3. Surgical resection will not be successful in patients with these findings. The assessment of pulmonary function is important to determine the extent of lung resection that will be tolerated.

About 45% of patients with lung cancer undergo thoracotomy and 35%

have a resection for cure. Thirty percent of patients undergoing resection survive for 5 years, 15% for 10 years. However, in the small group of patients who have a resection for pathologic Stage I disease, long-term survival rates in the range of 80% to 90% are seen.[3]

Table 20.3 Contraindications to surgery for lung cancer[3]

Small cell carcinoma

Distant metastasis

Superior vena cava syndrome

Pleural effusion containing malignant cells

Involvement of the heart

Vocal cord paralysis

Tumor located less than 2 cm from carina

Meatastasis to opposite lung

Bilateral lung primaries

Involvement of main pulmonary artery

Metastasis to mediastinal lymph nodes on side opposite primary

Metastasis to supraclavicualr lymph nodes

Severe pulmonary or cardiac disease

Radiotherapy for non-small cell lung cancer *Stages I and II*

RT alone A small number of patients with early lung cancer are candidates for an attempt at cure with radiotherapy alone. Patients who are inoperable because of lung or heart disease fall into this group. Small portals are used and tumor doses in the range of 55-65 Gy are given (Figure 20.1). Five year cure rates as high as 20% have been reported following RT.

Postoperative RT Patients who undergo surgical resection and who have positive lymph nodes in the specimen are given postoperative RT to the mediastinum (45 Gy/23-25 fractions/4.5-5 weeks) for the purpose of preventing mediastinal recurrence. Postoperative RT is of no value in patients who do not have lymph node metastasis.

Stage III Most patients referred for radiotherapy have inoperable or unresectable disease. In these the primary and mediastinum are irradiated with parallel opposing portals (60-65 Gy/30-35 fractions/6-7 weeks). The mediastinum is shielded at 40-45 Gy to protect the spinal cord. The supraclavicular region is treated if there is palpable supraclavicular adenopathy. Five year survival rates of 5-10% are seen for such patients.

Interstitial brachytherapy Several centers use interstitial brachytherapy in patients who undergo thoracotomy and are found to have unresectable disease. Iodine-125 is the radioactive source most frequently used. The implant is usually

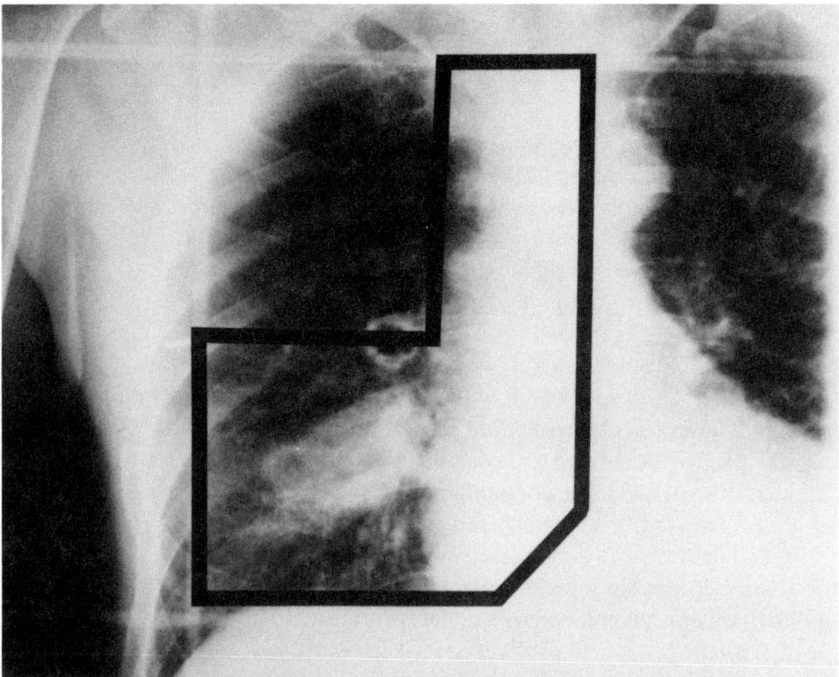

Figure 20.1 Simulator film on patient with lung carcinoma. The mediastinum and spinal cord are shielded at 40 Gy.

combined with external beam therapy to the mediastinum. Improved local control rates are reported for implanted patients compared to those treated with external beam alone.

Transbronchial brachytherapy One of the newer techniques used to palliate patients with locally recurrent disease following external therapy is transbronchial brachytherapy. The radioactive source is placed through a large-channel flexible fiberoptic bronchoscope.[5] Low or high intensity sources can be used. This method is of greatest use when the disease is predominately intrabronchial. Recurrent intrabronchial tumors can also be treated with transbronchial laser beam surgery.

Superior sulcus (Pancoast) tumors Patients with locally advanced tumors originating in the upper lobe of the lung often present with severe pain in the shoulder or back due to tumor invasion of the chest wall. External beam therapy (60 Gy/6 weeks) is effective in giving symptomatic relief in a high percentage of patients, with a 5 year survival rate in the range of 20%.[6] Small superior sulcus tumors can be treated with surgical excision combined with pre-operative RT (50 Gy/5 weeks) yielding similar long-term results.

Palliative RT for metastatic disease Radiotherapy is a valuable method of palliation for patients having metastatic lung cancer. Painful bone metastasis usually responds to 20 Gy/1 week or 30 Gy/2 weeks; brain metastasis responds to 30 Gy/2 weeks.

Side effects and complications Radiation esophagitis develops in all patients receiving radiotherapy to the mediastinum. The discomfort on swallowing begins after 2 weeks of treatment, is usually not severe and resolves within 1-2 weeks following completion of mediastinal irradiation. In a few patients, stricture of the esophagus develops as a late effect of treatment.

Radiation pneumonitis develops in the irradiated lung in some patients beginning 6-22 weeks following completion of treatment. Usually the symptoms are not severe and consist mainly of cough. If a large volume of lung was treated there may also be dyspnea and, in these, corticosteroid administration may be beneficial. These acute symptoms resolve after a few months and the only residual is fibrosis confined to the irradiated lung volume as seen on chest x-ray. The severity of radiation pneumonitis can be minimized by restricting the radiation to the tumor volume as much as possible.

Chemotherapy *Preoperative chemotherapy and radiation* In an attempt to improve cure rates for patients with Stage III lung cancer several groups have used chemotherapy combined with radiation in an attempt to improve resectability rates.[7] Cisplatin and 5-FU infusions and concurrently administered thoracic radiation (30 Gy/15 fractions) is the combination frequently used. One group has reported an improvement in survival time with preoperative chemoradiotherapy.[8]

Advanced disease A number of agents have activity against non-small cell lung cancer including cisplatin, ifosfamide, mitomycin-c, vinblastine, vindestine and etoposide (VP-16). Drugs with less activity include cyclophosphamide, doxorubicin, lomustine (CCNU), 5-FU and methotrexate. These drugs have been used as single agents or in combination in trials and clinical benefits such as symptomatic improvement for many patients have been demonstrated. However, few studies have shown increased survival for treated patients.

TREATMENT OF SMALL CELL LUNG CANCER

Significant improvements in survival rates have been demonstrated with chemotherapy for patients with small cell lung cancer. The most active drugs include cyclophosphamide, nitrogen mustard, doxorubicin, methotrexate, hexamethylmelamine, carboplatin, VP-16 and vincristine. Most patients are treated with 3 or 4 drug combinations.

Current treatment protocols for small cell lung cancer limited to the thorax, employ both chemotherapy and radiotherapy in planned combination. Chemotherapy is given initially for 6-8 weeks followed by radiotherapy to the primary and mediastinum (30-50 Gy in a continuous or split course). Chemotherapy is continued following RT for 12 months to 2 years.

Small cell lung cancer frequently metastasizes to the brain and studies have shown that prophylatic brain irradiation (24-30 Gy/8-10 fractions) can reduce the incidence of relapse in the brain. Therefore, prophylactic cranial irradiation is usually given during the time that the chest is being irradiated.

Data from clinical trials, involving patients with disease limited to the chest indicate that aggressive combination of therapy yields overall response rates of 85-95%, complete response rates of 50-60%, median survival times of 12-16 months and 2 year disease-free survival rates of 15-20%.

CANCER OF THE ESOPHAGUS: ETIOLOGY AND EPIDEMIOLOGY

In the U.S. esophageal cancer accounts for only 1.5% of all cancers. The disease is more common in men with reported sex ratios ranging from 2:1 to 6:1. The incidence rates among blacks is significantly higher than among whites.

There are wide variations in incidence rates among countries and geographic regions. The highest incidence is in Iran and the USSR around the Caspian sea. High incidence rates are found in some northern provinces of China. The disease is common in France, Chile, Switzerland and Japan.

In western countries tobacco and alcohol abuse are etiologic factors but other nutritional factors have been implicated. For example, nitrosamines have been in high concentrations in the food in northern China. The disease is common in women with long-standing iron deficiency anemia, glossitis and esophagitis, a clinical entity called Plummer-Vinson syndrome. Heavy seasoning of foods, hot foods and liquids, the use of betel nut, tannin-rich foods, contamination of foods with silica particles and deficiencies of trace metals and vitamins in foods have all been implicated as possible nutritional factors.

Several benign disorders of the esophagus are associated with a high incidence. The disease is more common among patients with achalasia, lye stricture, diaphragmatic hernia, previous gastric surgery and esophageal webs. Each of these conditions is often associated with chronic inflammation due to repeated regurgitation or obstruction, suggesting that chronic irritation is an etiologic factor.

PATHOLOGY

The esophagus is arbitrarily sub-divided into three anatomic areas: 1) the cervical esophagus extends from the phayrngoesophageal junction to the thoracic inlet; 2) the upper and midthoracic esophagus extends from the thoracic inlet to a point 10 cm above the gastroesophageal junction and; 3) the lower esophagus consists of the distal 10 cm of the esophagus. Cancers of the esophagus develop least commonly in the cervical esophagus (10% of cases); 40% originate in the upper half of the thoracic esophagus and 50% in the lower half.

Most esophageal malignancies arise from the epithelial lining of the esophagus. Squamous cell carcinoma is the most common histologic type accounting for 98% of cases; adenocarcinomas account for 2% of cases. In the past, many series of patients with esophageal cancer included patients with adenocarcinoma of the stomach extending upward to the esophagus. Most authorities now agree that adenocarcinomas which involve the lower esophagus are stomach primaries and should be classified as such.

Esophageal carcinomas often metastasize to regional lymph nodes. Tumors of the upper esophagus spread primarily to cervical and supraclavicular lymph nodes, whereas tumors of the lower esophagus spread primarily to gastric, celiac and para-aortic nodes. Distant metastasis to the liver and lungs is common.

TREATMENT OF CARCINOMA OF THE ESOPHAGUS

Surgery Fifty percent of patients with esophageal cancer are candidates for surgery. Many patients are rejected because of poor cardiac and/or lung function because of advanced disease. Of those that actually have a radical excision, the 5 year survival rate is only 10% with an operative mortality rate of 20%.

Total or subtotal esophagectomy is the recommended surgical procedures and several methods of reconstruction are used to restore the continuity of the gastrointestinal tract. The most commonly used reconstruction is to place the stomach into the thorax (esophagogastrostomy), but a portion of the colon (colon interposition) can also be used. For tumors of the cervical esophagus, skin tubes and grafts are constructed to restore continuity.

Surgical techniques are frequently required to maintain patency of the esophagus in palliative treatment. Various types of intraluminal tubes can be inserted through the tumor and endoscopic laser beam therapy can provide an opening to allow passage of nutrients.

Radiotherapy RT is frequently used for palliative and curative treatment. For curative treatment RT can be used alone or in combination with surgery. The only contraindication to RT is the presence of a tracheoesophageal fistula due to extensive local tumor.

Tumors of the thoracic esophagus are usually treated with three portals (Figure 20.2). Tumor doses in the range of 50 Gy/20 fractions/4 weeks to 65 Gy/33 fractions/6.5 weeks are well-tolerated. The dose to the spinal cord should not exceed 45 Gy.

Tumors of the cervical esophagus are technically difficult to irradiate because of the close proximity of the spinal cord, but 2 anterior oblique wedged

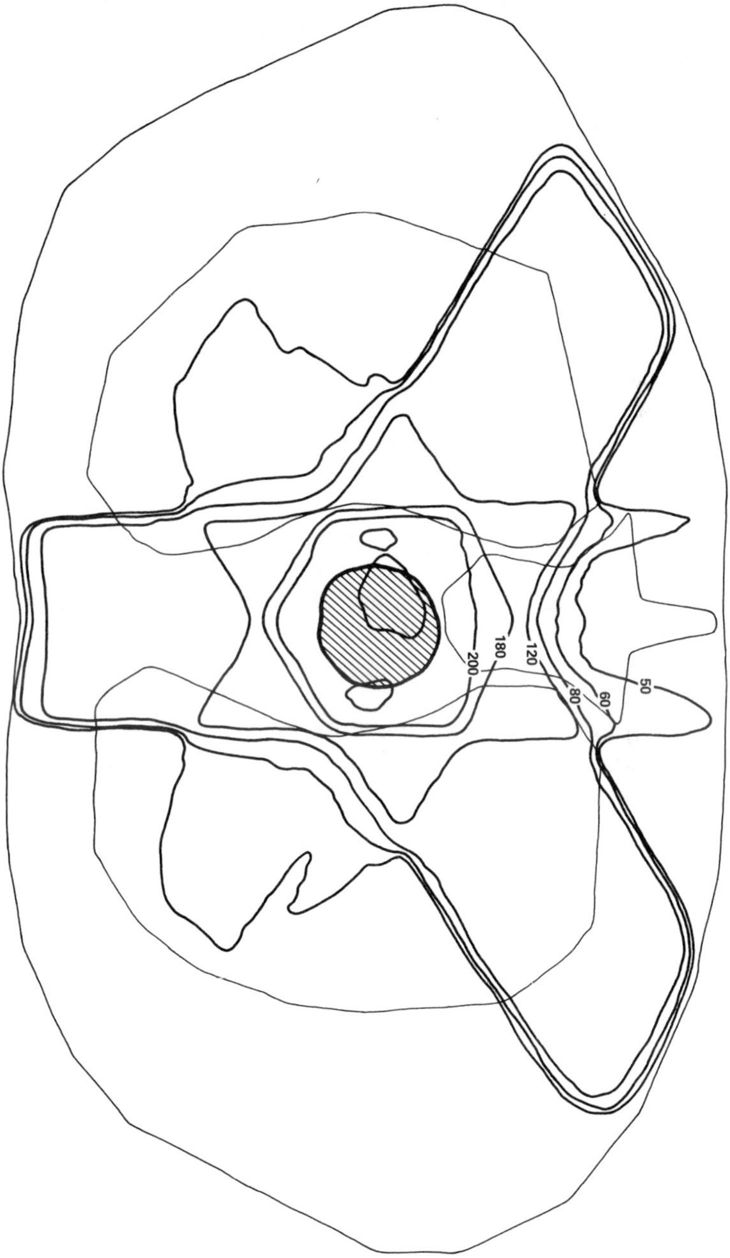

Figure 20.2 This is the computer plan for a patient with squamous cell carcinoma of the middle 1/3 of the esophagus who was treated with 3 portals.

portals usually yield an adequate dose distribution. Mendenhall, et al, described an innovative 4 portal box technique which employs beeswax to compensate for the difference in tissue thickness between the shoulders and neck.[9]

Results of RT for cancer of the esophagus are discouraging. The survival experience reported from 49 publications over a 25 year period (1954-1979) in which RT alone was used for squamous carcinoma of the esophagus, was recently reviewed.[10] The total number of patients treated was 8499 and the overall 5 year survival rate was 6%.

Patients treated by RT alone often develop esophageal stricture as a late effect and dilation may be required to maintain patency. Other complications such as radiation pneumonitis, carditis and spinal cord injury are uncommon with modern techniques.

Brachytherapy Inability to control local disease is the main reason for the ineffectiveness of external RT. For many years, therefore, intracavitary brachytherapy has been used in an attempt to administer a higher local dose. Radium tubes were used in earlier attempts, but afterloading techniques, utilizing low-intensity or high-intensity sources, have been employed more recently.[11,12]

Preoperative RT Surgical resection combined with preoperative RT (20-60 Gy/2-6 weeks) has been used in a number of centers. However, results from studies combining radiation and surgery fail to show consistent improvement in cure rates compared to RT alone.

Postoperative RT The mediastinum is irradiated (40-50 Gy/4-5 weeks) when: 1) the resection margins are histologically positive; 2) there is known tumor remaining in the mediastinum or; 3) the lymph nodes are positive. Few reports of the results of postop RT in esophageal cancer have appeared.

Preop chemotherapy+radiation Research protocols evaluating the combination of drugs such as cisplatin+5FU administered concurrently with RT prior to surgery have appeared.[13] At this time no significant benefit from adjuvant chemotherapy+radiotherapy has been established.

MEDIASTINAL TUMORS

ANATOMY

The anatomic boundaries of the mediastinum are: the diaphragm inferiorly; the thoracic inlet superiorly (the first thoracic vertebra and first ribs); the sternum anteriorly; the vertebral column and adjacent ribs posteriorly; the pleura laterally.

The mediastinum has four compartments: the superior mediastinum contains the aortic arch and the thymus gland; the anterior mediastinum contains the ascending aorta, vena cava, thymus, lymph nodes, fat and connective tissue; the posterior mediastinum contains the sympathetic nerves, esophagus, thoracic duct, lymph nodes and descending aorta; the middle mediastinum contains the heart, trachea and major bronchi, pulmonary vessels, lymph nodes, fat and connective tissue.

PATHOLOGY

A large number of benign and malignant neoplasms originate in the mediastinum but they are uncommon and only 50% are malignant. The relative incidence of mediastinal tumors and cysts is shown in Table 20.4. Ninety percent of thyomas are located in the anterior or superior compartments; 80% of neurogenic tumors arise in the posterior mediastinum; 50% of lymphomas are in the middle compartment.

Thymoma The thymus gland is classified as a lymphoid organ but it originated embryologically from the epithelium of the third pharyngeal pouches.

Table 20.4 Relative incidence of mediastianal tumors and cysts		
	All patients	**Children**
Thymomas	21%	--
Neurogenic tumors	20%	38%
Lymphoma	12%	19%
Germ cell neoplams	11%	12%
Cysts	19%	17%
Other	17%	14%

It is from the epithelial components that most thymomas arise. Thymomas are classified histologically as lymphocytic, epithelial or mixed depending upon the predominate cell type. Most thymomas are benign, but about 35% are invasive and infiltrate into adjacent structures in the thorax. Metastasis to regional lymph nodes or distant sites are uncommon.

Seventy percent of thymomas are associated with systemic syndromes such as autoimmune phenomena, endocrine disorders, cancer and severe infections. The most common syndrome associated with thymoma is an autoimmune neuromuscular disorder called myasthenia gravis.

Thymectomy is curative for benign thymomas but invasive thymomas often recur locally after surgery alone. Therefore, postoperative RT to the mediastinum and supraclavicular region is indicated in all invasive thymomas. Following complete removal, 45 Gy/5 weeks is given, but incompletely excised or inoperable tumors require 55-60 Gy. Reported overall 5 year survival rates range from 25-60%.

Germ cell tumors All types of germ cell tumors found in the testis have been found in the mediastinum. Germ cell tumors arise in the thymus gland and are classified as pure seminoma (germinoma) or non-seminomas. Seminomas have a better prognosis and are most responsive to treatment than non-seminomas. Seminomas of the mediastinum usually occur in men age 20-40 but 5% occur in women. Surgical excision is carried out initially and postoperative mediastinal irradiation (35-40 Gy) is given. Chemotherapy is reserved for patients with metastasis. Cure rates in the range of 50-75% have been reported.

Neurogenic tumors These tumors usually arise from intercoastal nerves of sympathetic ganglia in the posterior mediastinum. In children they are the most common mediastinal neoplasms. Most are benign and can be removed. However, malignant neurogenic tumors are often not completely removed and postoperative RT may be required. The treatment of malignant neurogenic tumors will be considered again in Chapter 26.

MALIGNANT MESOTHELIOMA

ETIOLOGY AND EPIDEMIOLOGY

Malignant mesothelioma is a primary tumor of the pleura or peritoneum. It is a rare disease accounting for only 1000 new cases in the U.S. annually. The male:female ratio is 2:1 to 4:1. In 80% of cases there is a history of asbestos exposure and the exposure to asbestos fibers is often occupational. The delay between first exposure to asbestos and onset of mesothelioma is 15-40 years.

PATHOLOGY

The pleura is the primary site more frequently than the peritoneum. The tumor spreads over serosal surfaces and may involve the entire pleura, diaphragm, mediastinum and pericardium. Peritoneal cases involve the omentum, mesentery, serosal surface of the large and small intestine, liver and spleen. Regional lymph nodes are frequently involved and distant metastasis is common.

DIAGNOSIS

Chest pain, dyspnea, weight loss, cough and fever are common in pleural cases. Abdominal pain and distention due to ascites are common symptoms in peritoneal cases. Pleural effusion is present in 80% of pleural cases and chest x-rays show fluid and pleural thickening or nodules. Thoracotomy with pleural biopsy is the best diagnostic procedure. Laparotomy with biopsy is the usual method of diagnosis for peritoneal cases.

TREATMENT

Current therapies for pleural mesothelioma are ineffective and new methods of treatment are needed. Removal of the pleura (total pleurectomy), in cases in which the disease appears to be localized to the pleura, is possible. However, most cases are not amenable to surgery because the tumor is invading the mediastinum, chest wall or other adjacent structures. In these cases radiotherapy is often tried. Techniques have been developed to irradiate the entire pleural space with a combination of electrons and photons (40/60 Gy) while shielding underlying normal lung. Palliation of pain following RT is seen in most cases. Few reports evaluating RT for peritoneal cases have appeared.

Because surgery and radiotherapy alone have produced few long-term survivors combined modality approaches are needed. Response rates of 30-40% for doxorubicin or cisplatin containing drug regimenshave been reported. Protocols combining chemotherapy with surgery and/or RT are under study. The prognosis for patients with malignant pleural mesothelioma is only 12 months and for peritoneal cases, 10 months.

REFERENCES

1. Silverberg E, Boring CC, Squires RS. Cancer statistics, 1990, CA-A Cancer Journal from Clinicians 40:9-226, 1990.

2. Chapter 18, Lung, In Manual for Staging of Cancer, Third Edition, Eds. Beahrs OH, Henson DE, Hutter, RV, Myers MH, J.B. Lippincott Company, Philadelphia, 1988, pp 115-121.

3. Minna JD, Pass H, Glastein E, Ihde DC, Chapter 22, Cancer of the lung, In Cancer-Principles and Practice of Oncology, 3rd Edition, Eds. DeVita VT, Hellman S, Rosenberg SA, J.B. Lippincott Company, Philadelphia, 1989, pp 591-705.

4. Hilaris BS, et al. Value of perioperative brachytherapy in the management of non-oat cell carcinoma of the lung, Int J Radiat Oncol Biol Phy 89:1161-1166, 1983.

5. Moylan D, et al. Transbrochnial brachytherapy of recurret bronchogenic carcinoma: A new approach using the flexible fiberoptic bronchoscope, Radiology 147:253-354. 1983.

6. Komaki R, et al. Superior sulcus tumors, Cancer 48:1563-1568, 1981.

7. Weiden PL, Piantoadosi S. Preoperative chemotherapy (cisplatin and fluorouracil) and radiation therapy in stage III non-small-cell lung Cancer: A phase II study of the Lung Cancer Study Group, J Nat Cancer Inst 83:266-272, 1991.

8. Dillman RO, et al. A randomized trial of induction chemotherapy plus high dose radiation versus radiation alone in stage III non-small-cell lung cancer, N Engl J Med 323:940-945, 1990.

9. Mendenhall WM, et al. Carcinoma of the cervical esophagus treated with radiation therapy using a four-field box technique, Int J Radiat Oncol Biol Phys 8:14535-1439, 1982.

10. Earlam R., Cunha-Melo JR. Oesophageal squamous cell carcinoma: A critical review of radiotherpy, Brit J Surg 67:457-461, 1980.

11. Rider WD, Mendozza R. Some opinions on the treatment of cancer of the esophagus, Am J Roentgenol 105:514-, 1969.

12.George FW. Radiation managemnt in esophageal cancer, Am J Surg 139:795-804, 1980./

13. Leichman L, et al. Preoperative chemotherapy and radiation therapy for patients with cancer of the esophagus: A potentially curative approach , J Clin Oncol 2:"75-79, 1984.

Chapter 21

GASTROINTESTINAL TRACT

STOMACH CANCER

ETIOLOGY AND EPIDEMIOLOGY

It is estimated that 13,700 people died of stomach carcinoma in the U.S. in 1990.[1] The disease is more common in men by a ratio of 3:2 and it is more common among low socioeconomic groups. There has been a progressive reduction in incidence and mortality from stomach cancer in the U.S. since 1930. No cause for this reduction has been found.

The incidence of stomach cancer is very high in Japan and Chile. The etiology of stomach cancer is unknown but it is likely that dietary carcinogens are involved. Dietary factors that have been implicated include smoked foods, heavily salted foods and foods contaminated with aflatoxin.

PATHOLOGY

Approximately 95% of gastric cancers are adenocarcinomas but lymphomas and sarcomas also occur. Fifty percent of adenocarcinomas develop in the pylorus and antrum, 20% in the body, 15% on the lesser curvature, 10% in the cardia and 5% on the greater curvature. The spread of gastric cancer is by direct extension to neighboring structure, lymphatic, vascular and trans-peritoneal metastasis.

DIAGNOSIS

Abdominal discomfort is the earliest and most common symptom. This is usually a vague epigastric discomfort that the patient attempts to relieve with antacids and dietary alteration. Loss of appetite, easy filling and weight loss are also common symptoms.

STAGING

The TNM classification for gastric cancer is shown in Table 21.1

TREATMENT

Surgery This is the only known curative treatment of gastric cancer, but only 50% of patients are candidates for attempt at curative surgery. Radical subtotal gastrectomy is the preferred operation. The overall 5 year survival rate following surgery is only 10%. Survival rates are better (30%) for patients who have no lymph node metastasis.

Table 21.1. The staging of gastric cancer[2]

T1	Tumor invades lamina propria or submucosa
T2	Tumor invades the muscularis propria or subserosa
T3	Tumor penetrates the serosa without invasion of adjacent structures
T4	Tumor invades adjacent structures
N0	No lymph node metastasis
N1	Metastasis in perigastric lymph node(s) within 3 cm of the edge of the primary tumor
N2	Metastasis in perigastric lymph node(s) more than 3 cm from edge of the primary tumor
M0	No distant metastasis
M1	Distant metastasis

Stage grouping

IA	T1N0M0
IB	T1N1M0 or T2N0M0
II	T1N2M0 or T2N1M0 or T3N0M0
IIIA	T2N2M0 or T3N1M0 or T4N0M0
IIIB	TN2M0 or T4N1M0
IV	T4N2M0 or any T+ any NM1

RT+chemotherapy RT alone is ineffective for gastric cancer. However, there is evidence that radiation combined with chemotherapy improves survival for patients with locally advanced and inoperable disease. For example, a clinical trial at the Mayo Clinic evaluated RT (37.5 Gy/4 weeks) plus placebo, versus RT plus intravenous 5-FU for patients with unresectable disease and found that the mean survival time for the placebo patients was 6 months versus 14 months for the 5-FU patients.[5] There are also data from other clinical trials that support the use of radiation+chemotherapy in gastric cancer. Therefore, patients with inoperable or incompletely resected disease are treated with RT to the stomach and regional lymphatics in combination with concurrently administered 5-FU.

Postoperative RT Local recurrence is a significant problem for patients treated with surgery alone.[4] Therefore, postop RT (40-45 Gy/4-5 weeks) combined with chemotherapy is under investigation for patients with gastric cancer at high risk for local recurrence (extensive local tumor and/or nodes positive).

Chemotherapy Drugs which have shown activity against gastric cancer include 5-FU, doxorubicin, BCNU, methotrexate, mitomycin C and methyl - CCNU. Responses occur in 20-25% of patients with advanced disease but the responses are of short duration. The most active current regimen is known as FAM (5-FU, doxorubicin, mitomycin C) with more than 40% of patients responding.

CANCER OF THE PANCREAS

ETIOLOGY AND EPIDEMIOLOGY.

Cancer of the pancreas ranks fourth as a cause of death from cancer in the U.S. In 1990, 28,100 new cases were diagnosed and 25,000 deaths occurred from cancer of the pancreas. The incidence of the disease has been increasing since 1930, but a portion of the apparent increase is due to improved methods of detection rather than a real increase in incidence. The disease is more common in males (2:1) and blacks. The median age at onset is 69. High rates of pancreatic cancer are seen in Canada, South Africa, Sweden, Denmark, Finland and Scotland. The disease is uncommon in Japan.

The etiology of pancreatic cancer is unknown, but factors which appear to be associated with an increased risk are diabetes, smoking and dietary factors. In one study the risk was six times greater in diabetic women than non-diabetic women but was not increased in diabetic men. Smokers have twice the risk of non-smokers and the disease is more common in affluent countries where diets high in meat and fat are consumed, suggesting that high fat diets may be etiologic. Other factors which have been implicated are alcohol abuse and excessive coffee drinking.

PATHOLOGY

Ninety-five percent of pancreatic cancers are adenocarcinomas which arise from the pancreatic ducts or acinar cells. Tumors of the islet cells are rare. Seventy percent arise in the head of the pancreas, 20% in the body and 10% in the tail.

Pancreatic cancers grow by direct extension to involve neighboring structures such as the common bile duct, duodenum and stomach. Metastasis to regional lymph nodes and distant sites occurs early in the course of the disease. The liver is the distant site most commonly involved.

DIAGNOSIS

Pain is the presenting symptom in the majority of cases. The pain may be confined to the upper abdomen or radiate to the back. Weight loss occurs in most patients and change in bowel habit or jaundice are common symptoms.

CT scanning is the preferred method of evaluating the pancreas in symptomatic patients. Ultrasound scanning is a useful screening technique and arteriography is of value in selected patients to localize the lesion. Each of these imaging techniques can be used as a guide for fine needle aspiration biopsy. Endoscopic retrograde cholangiopancreatography (ERCP) is often used to evaluate the patency of the biliary ducts and collect pancreatic fluid for cytology. Tumor markers such as carcinoembryonic antigen (CEA) and alpha-fetoprotein are frequently elevated in the serum and can be used to follow therapeutic response.

STAGING

The TNM staging classification is shown in Table 21.2.

Table 21.2 The staging of pancreatic cancer[2]

T1 Tumor limited to the pancreas

  T1a Tumor 2 cm or less in diameter

  T1b Tumor more than 2 cm in diameter

T2 Tumor extends to the duodenum, bile duct or peripancreatic tissue

T3 Tumor extends to the stomach, spleen, colon or adjacent large vessels

N0 No regional lymph node metastasis

N1 Regional lymph node metastasis

M0 No distant metastasis

M1 Distant metastasis

Stage grouping

I T1N0M0 or T2N0M0

II T3N0M0

III any TN1M0

IV any T any NM1

TREATMENT

Surgery Curative surgery is possible for only 10-25% of patients who are explored. The two surgical procedures used for cancer of the pancreas are the Whipple operation, and total pancreatectomy. The Whipple operation is an extensive procedure which involves resection of the head of the pancreas, the duodenum and antrum of the stomach, end-to-end pancreaticojejunostomy, end-to-end choledochojejunostomy and gastrojejunostomy. The operative mortality rate is 15-20% and the 5 year survival rate is only 8%.

There is less experience with total pancreatectomy and the major disadvantage is the management of the problems resulting from total removal of the pancreas. Surgery is also of value in palliation in patients with biliary and/or duodenal obstruction.

Radiotherapy *RT+chemotherapy* RT alone does not improve quality of life or survival time for patients with advanced pancreatic carcinoma. Therefore, clinical trials are evaluating the role of combined modality therapy. For example, the Gastrointestinal Tumor Study Group completed a clinical trial in which patients with localized unresectable disease received either high-dose RT alone (60 Gy in 3 courses of 20 Gy/2 weeks with each course separated by a week's rest), moderate dose radiation (40 Gy in 2 courses) + 5-FU (500mg/m^2/day IV on the first 3 days of each course) or high dose RT + 5-FU.[6]

The median survival time was significantly better for the combined modality patients compared to the RT alone patients; at 1 year 40% of the combined treatment patients were surviving versus only 10% for the RT alone patients. However, at 2 years, the survival rate for all patients was nearly 0%. There was not a significant difference in survival between the 40 Gy+5-FU and 60 Gy+5-FU groups.

A three field technique is used for unresectable pancreas tumor is with an anterior open portal and right and left lateral wedged portals. Forty to 60 Gy can be given with this technique but care must be taken to avoid excessive radiation to radiosensitive organs including small bowel, stomach, liver, kidneys and spinal cord.

Intraoperative irradiation Conventional external beam therapy yields a very high local failure rate. A technique which has recently been adopted for the treatment of unresectable pancreatic carcinoma in an attempt to administer a higher local radiation dose is intraoperative radiotherapy (IORT).[7] In this technique, an exploratory laparotomy is carried out in the radiotherapy department in a specially constructed OR suite/treatment room.

The tumor is located and isolated from the surrounding bowel, an electron beam applicator is applied to the tumor under sterile conditions and a single large electron beam treatment (15-20 Gy) is given with 15-30 MeV electrons. In most institutions, the IORT is combined with conventional RT alone or with chemotherapy. Early results suggest that local control is improved with IORT but overall survival rates are not improved.

Brachytherapy Permanent interstitial iodine-125 seed implants, performed at the time of exploratory surgery, are another means of administering a higher local tumor dose.[8] As with IORT, brachytherapy is usually combined with external beam therapy and chemotherapy. Also, as with IORT, early results suggest that local tumor control rates, but not survival rates, are improved with brachytherapy. High-LET particle therapy with neutron, pi-meson or proton beams is also under investigation for pancreatic carcinoma.

Chemotherapy The results of chemotherapy for metastatic pancreatic cancer are poor. 5-FU is the most active drug but only 15% of patients respond and the duration of responses is short (2.5 months). Current studies are evaluating 5-FU, semustine (methyl-CCNU), carmustine (BCNU), mitomycin C, doxorubicin and streptozotocin in 2-4 drug combinations.

THE LIVER

In the U.S. primary cancers of the liver are rare. The most common type is hepatoma (hepatocellular carcinoma) which accounts for 90% of cases; 5-10% are cholangiocarcinomas and 2-5% are mixed liver cell and ductal carcinomas.

ETIOLOGY AND EPIDEMIOLOGY

Approximately 2500 deaths occur annually in the U.S. from hepatoma. The disease is more common in males by a ratio of 3:2. In some African and Oriental countries hepatoma is the most common internal cancer in men.

The etiology of hepatoma is unknown, but 50% of cases occur in patients with cirrhosis of the liver and about 5% of patients with cirrhosis eventually develop hepatoma. Hepatitis-B virus may also be an etiologic factor in hepatoma.

A number of carcinogens have been implicated; in Africa aflatoxin present in common plants has been implicated; in China and Thailand parasitic infections may be etiologic. Nutritional diseases such as kwashiorkor may predispose to hepatoma and in the U.S. oral contraceptive use has been implicated because of reports of hepatoma in young women taking oral contraceptives.

PATHOLOGY

Hepatomas usually do not invade neighboring structures and death results from liver failure due to massive tumor growth. However, metastasis to regional lymph nodes and distant sites can occur and the lungs are the most commonly involved distant site.

Cholangiocarcinomas can originate from intrahepatic bile ducts or bile ductules. Cirrhosis of the liver is present in 20% of cases. They tend to metastasize more frequently to regional lymph nodes than hepatomas.

TREATMENT

The 5 year survival rates for patients with hepatomas is nearly 0%, but a small number of cures have been reported following surgical resection for small tumors confined to a single lobe. Radiotherapy has not found a role in the treatment of hepatomas but systemic chemotherapy has produced short-term responses and the most active agents are 5-FU and doxorubicin. Infusion of chemotherapeutic agents directly into the liver via the hepatic artery has been of value in palliation for some patients.

GALLBLADDER CARCINOMA

ETIOLOGY AND EPIDEMIOLOGY

It is estimated that approximately 6000 cases of primary gallbladder carcinoma occur annually in the U.S. Women are affected more commonly than men by a ratio of 4:1 . The average age of onset is 60. The etiology is unknown but gallstones are present in the gallbladder in 90% of cases, suggesting that chronic irritation from gallstones causes cancer.

PATHOLOGY

Ninety-five percent of gallbladder carcinomas are adenocarcinomas but squamous carcinomas can occur. Direct extension to the liver is common and regional lymph node metastases are present in 50% of cases. Distant metastasis is common and transperitoneal spread can occur.

DIAGNOSIS

Right upper quadrant pain, jaundice and a palpable mass are present in the majority of cases. The serum alkaline phosphatase level is nearly always elevated, the oral cholecystogram may show a non-functioning gallbladder and the intravenous cholangiogram may reveal an obstructed cystic duct. In most cases, however, the diagnosis is not made until the time of abdominal exploration.

TREATMENT

Surgery is the only hope for cure but nearly 90% of cases are unresectable. Even in resected cases the outlook is grim and 5 year survival is seen in only 5% of cases. However, surgery has definite palliative value in providing diversion of bile in jaundiced patients. Radiotherapy is occasionally used in palliation but successes following RT are few. There are few reports of responses to chemotherapy.

CARCINOMA OF THE EXTRAHEPATIC BILE DUCTS

ETIOLOGY AND EPIDEMIOLOGY

Carcinomas of the extrahepatic bile ducts are uncommon. The disease is slightly more common in males and the average age is 65. The etiology is unknown but gallstones are present in 20-30% of cases. Normal hepatic metabolites such as bile acids may be etiologic in patients who have delayed biliary drainage due to benign cysts of the bile ducts. In Asian countries, bile duct carcinoma occurs in association with infestation of the biliary system by parasites.

PATHOLOGY

Nearly all bile duct carcinomas are adenocarcinomas. Fifty percent originate in the distal common bile duct, 30% in the proximal common bile duct and hepatic ducts and 20% in the porta hepatis. Local infiltration with biliary obstruction occurs in all cases and regional lymph node and distant metastasis are common.

DIAGNOSIS

Jaundice occurs in all patients and many experience epigastric or right upper quadrant pain. The serum bilirubin and alkaline phosphatase levels are elevated. Ultrasonography demonstrates dilated bile ducts and thin needle transhepatic cholangiography demonstrates the site of obstruction. However, the true nature of the obstruction is usually not established until the time of surgery.

TREATMENT

Surgical removal is the only hope for cure, but only 10% of patients have resectable disease and less than 5% of patients survive 5 years after surgery. Nevertheless, even in incurable disease, surgery has an important palliative role in relieving biliary obstruction.

Radiotherapy is of little proven value in bile duct carcinoma but there is enthusiasm among some radiotherapists for brachytherapy via iridium-192 ribbons inserted through a biliary drainage catheter.[9] The brachytherapy is combined with external beam therapy.

CANCER OF THE SMALL INTESTINE

ETIOLOGY AND EPIDEMIOLOGY

Malignant tumors of the small intestine are uncommon, accounting for only 1% of gastrointestinal tract malignancies. They are more common among males and the average age is 57. They occur with increased frequency in persons with inherited diseases of the small intestine such as familial polyposis, Gardner's syndrome, Peutz-Jegher's syndrome, Crohn's disease, celiac disease and neurofibromatosis.

PATHOLOGY

Fifty percent of neoplasms developing in the small intestine are benign. Leiomyomas, adenomatous polyps, lipomas, and hemangiomas are the most common benign tumors. Fifty percent of small bowel malignancies are adenocarcinomas, 30% are carcinoid tumors, 18% leiomyosarcomas, 1% non-Hodgkin's lymphomas and 1% miscellaneous. Adenocarcinomas arise most commonly in the duodenum or jejunum, whereas carcinoids are most commonly in the ileum.

DIAGNOSIS

Abdominal pain and weight loss are the most common symptoms and intestinal obstruction occurs in 35% of cases. Radiographic studies are useful in diagnosis and endoscopy can be used in duodenal tumors. In most patients, however, the diagnosis is established at the time of surgery.

TREATMENT

Surgery is indicated for all patients. When the tumor has been completely resected radiotherapy and chemotherapy have no established role if the histology is adenocarcinoma, carcinoid or leiomyosarcoma. For patients with malignant lymphoma, however, most authorities recommend postoperative RT to the abdomen and/or chemotherapy.

RT and chemotherapy are indicated in unresectable or recurrent disease but the results are discouraging, except in malignant lymphoma where long-term survival following palliative treatment is occasionally seen.

The 5 year survival rate following surgical resection for adenocarcinoma and carcinoid is 20%, for leiomyosarcoma 50% and for lymphoma 40%. For unresectable lymphoma the 5 year survival rate is 25%.

CARCINOMAS OF THE COLON AND RECTUM

ETIOLOGY AND EPIDEMIOLOGY

Cancer of the large bowel is the second most commonly occurring internal malignancy in the U.S. In 1990, 155,000 new cases were diagnosed and 61,000 persons died of carcinoma of the colon and rectum. The risk of developing colorectal cancer is the same for males and females. The incidence begins to rise between ages 40-45 and increases during each decade reaching a peak at age 75.

Among countries, high incidence rates are seen in North America, northwest Europe and other anglo-saxon countries. Low incidence rates are seen in Africa, Asia, Mexico and Central and South America. In the U.S., low incidence rates are seen among Seventh-Day Adventists, Mormons and vegetarians.

The cause of colorectal cancer is unknown, but diets high in fat and low in fiber are associated with a high incidence of the disease. A number of risk factors have been identified and these are listed in Table 21.3. The genetic diseases associated with a high-risk of colorectal cancer are listed in the Table. However,

---

Table 21.3. Risk factors for colorectal cancer[10]

Genetic

    Familial adenomatous polyposis syndrome

    Gardner, Oldfield, or Turcot syndrome

    Peutz-Jegher syndrome

Familial

    Familial colorectal cancer syndrome

    Hereditary adenocarcinomatosis syndrome

    Family history of colorectal cancer

Preexisting disease

    Inflammatory bowel disease

    Colorectal cancer

    Pelvic cancer post irradiation

    Neoplastic colorectal polyps

General

    All men and women over age of 40

---

for the majority of colorectal cancer patients, even those without genetic or familial disease, there is an increased incidence among family members.

DIAGNOSIS

Symptoms The most common presenting symptom of colorectal cancer is rectal bleeding; change in bowel habits, narrowing of stool caliber, abdominal pain and unexplained anemia are also common presenting complaints.

Physical examination Rectal examination is important in rectal cancer because 75% of rectal cancers are within reach of the examining finger. Tumors of the right or left colon can often be palpated as an abdominal mass.

Endoscopy Flexible fiberoptic endoscopy is rapidly replacing barium enemas for the evaluation of suspected lesions of the colon. Colonoscopy and proctosigmoidoscopy are the procedures most commonly used and if a lesion is seen it can be biopsied endoscopically.

Roentgenologic examination Contrast studies are still widely used in the evaluation of colon lesions. CT scanning is also useful in evaluating local disease extent and looking for liver metastasis.

Carcinoembryonic antigen (CEA) This is a circulating tumor-associated antigen that is frequently found in the serum of patients with colorectal cancer.

The test is not specific for colorectal cancer and occasionally patients with lung, breast, prostate, stomach and bladder cancer have elevated CEA levels. The test is not of value in detecting early bowel tumors but is useful in following patients post-treatment.

Screening The early detection of colorectal carcinoma may result in a reduction in mortality rates from the disease. Most authorities recommend that screening for the disease begin at age 40. Fecal testing for occult blood should be performed each year and sigmoidoscopy every 3 to 5 years. Individuals with positive stool tests for occult blood require additional diagnostic study.

PATHOLOGY

Ninety five percent of large bowel cancers are adenocarcinomas. Carcinoid tumors, other types of epithelial tumors, lymphomas, and nonepithelial tumors occur rarely. Adenocarcinomas can arise de novo or from pre-existing benign villous adenomas or adenomatous polyps.

Adenocarcinomas spread by local extension, lymphatic and hematogenous metastasis and trans-peritoneal implantation. They spread within the bowel wall causing constriction and narrowing of the lumen. There is also progressive invasion through the muscular layer with eventual penetration of the serosa and involvement of neighboring structures. Regional lymph node metastases is found in more than 50% of cases and the most common distant site is the liver.

STAGING

The staging of colorectal carcinoma is based on the pathologic findings at the time of surgery. The original staging system was introduced by Dukes at St. Mark's Hospital, London, England in 1928. In the Dukes classification, a Dukes A tumor is limited to the bowel wall and the 5 year survival rate is 60-80%; a Dukes B tumor extends deeply through the bowel to involve serosal fat and the 5 year survival rate is 40-60%; a Dukes C tumor has metastasized to regional lymph nodes with a 5 year survival rate of 5-30%.

Most modern systems are variations of the Dukes system and the TMN classification of the American Joint Committee is shown with the corresponding Dukes stages in Table 21.4.

TREATMENT

Surgery Surgical resection is the standard treatment for colorectal carcinoma. The primary and regional lymph nodes and anastomosis of the cut ends of the bowel. Rectal tumors located within 5 cm of the anus must be treated by abdominoperineal (AP) resection and permanent colostomy.

Radiotherapy Local recurrence following surgery for colorectal cancer is

Table 21.4 Staging of colorectal cancer[11]		
T1	Carcinoma invades submucosa	
T2	Tumor invades muscularis propria	
T3	Tumor invades through the muscularis propria into the subserosa, or into pericolic or perirectal tissue	
T4	Tumor perforates the visceral peritoneum or invades other organs or structures	
N0	No regional lymph node metastasis	
N1	Metasitasis in 1 to 3 periocolic or perirectal nodes	
N2	Metastasis in 4 or more pericolic or perirectal nodes	
N3	Metastasis in any lymph node along the course of a named vascular trunk	
M0	No distant metastasis	
M1	Distant metastasis	
Stage grouping		
I	T1N0M0 or T2N0M0	Dukes A
II	T3N0M0 or T4N0M0	Dukes B
III	Any TN1M0 or any TN2, N3M0	Dukes C
IV	Any T any NM1	

common. The incidence of local recurrence is higher for rectal tumors than for those arising elsewhere in the colon and the recurrence rate increases with increasing stage. In one series the local recurrence rate for Dukes C rectal cancer was 68%.[12]

It is for this reason that adjuvant RT +/- chemotherapy has become widely accepted, especially for rectal carcinoma. Radiation has been used preoperatively, postoperatively and both pre- and post operatively (sandwich technique) for patients with Dukes B and C rectal carcinoma. In addition, some authorities recommend postoperative RT for selected high-risk cases of colon carcinoma, but few reports of treatment results for adjuvant RT for colon carcinoma have appeared.

Preoperative RT for rectal carcinoma Various doses and techniques have been studied . Although the results of pre-op RT were promising the method did not gain wide acceptance because it is not possible to accurately assess the stage of disease preoperatively, especially the status of the lymph nodes. However, for selected patients with locally advanced, inoperable rectal cancer, it is possible to convert the tumor to an operable condition with pre-op RT.[13]

Postoperative RT This method has gained wider acceptance among surgeons because it allows selection of patients at high risk for recurrence on the basis of operative and pathologic findings. The major indication for postop RT is Dukes C disease, but patients with extensive B lesions and those in whom surgical margins are inadequate are also candidates.

The dose usually recommended is 45 Gy/5 weeks utilizing APPA portals or a three field technique (posterior and right and left lateral). The major risk of postop RT is injury to the small bowel portions of which may become fixed in the pelvis postoperatively. The risk of small bowel injury can be minimized with small bowel shielding (Figure 21.1). Other techniques to minimize small bowel toxicity have been described.[14] These include surgical procedures such as pelvic reconstruction to exclude small bowel loops from the pelvis, and radiation techniques such as treating the patient in the prone position on a special treatment board (Figure 21.2).

Results from non-randomized and randomized studies suggest that local failure rates are reduced with postop RT in stage B and C disease particularly for tumors located within 6 cm of the anus. However, no significant improvements in 5 year survival have been seen with adjuvant postop RT alone.

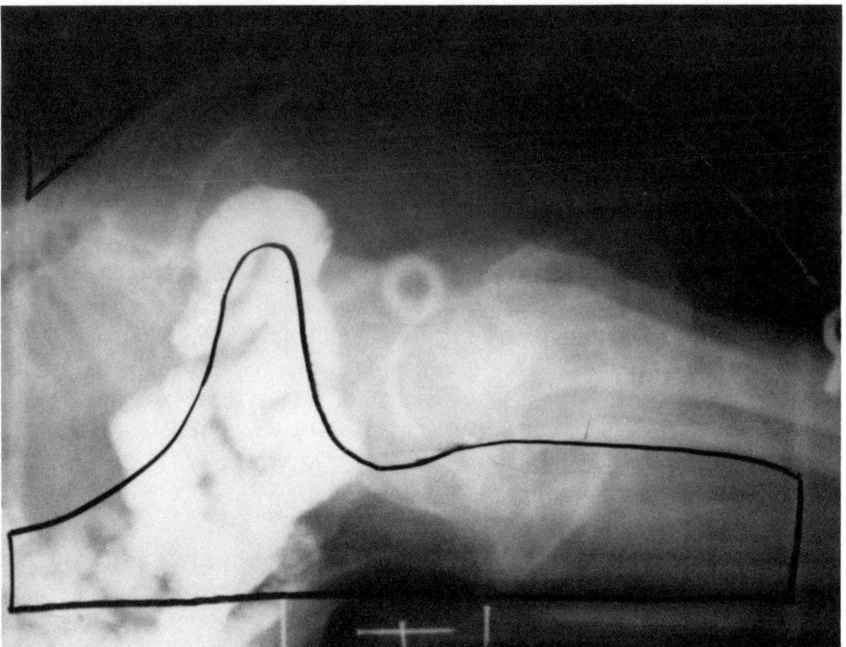

Figure 21.1 This is the lateral simulator film on a patient with rectal carcinoma who had an abdomino-perineal resection. She was given barium orally one hour previously which opacified the loops of small bowel in the pelvis. The black lines on the film were used to make cerrobend small bowel shields. She was treated in the prone position via a portal technqiue with a posterior and right and left lateral portals.

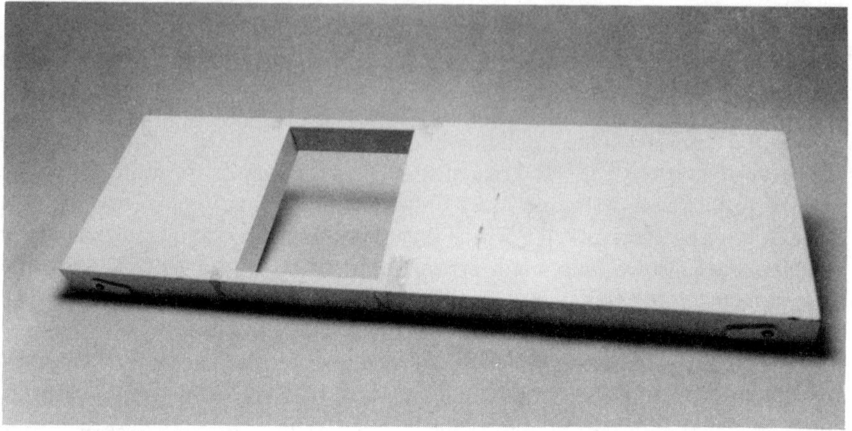

Figure 21.2 This is the rectal board, measuring 5 feet in length, on which the patient is positioned during RT. It has an opening for the abdomen which allows the bowel to fall out of the pelvis thus providing additional protection for the small bowel.

Adjuvant RT+chemotherapy Several clinical trials have been completed which demonstrate that local control and survival rates are improved for patients with TNM Stage II and III rectal cancer following postop radiation and chemotherapy. [15,16] All of the protocols employ radiation doses of at least 45 Gy and 5-FU plus the investigational drug methyl-CCNU (semustine).

Long-term administration of semustine can cause significant toxicity such as leukemia and kidney damage and there is controversy whether the drug really improves results compared to RT+5-FU alone. Therefore, the National Cancer Institute published a clinical announcement indicating that appropriate current treatment for Stage II and III rectal cancer should include both RT and 5-FU. [17] Treatment should be initiated one to two months after surgery. In weeks one and five 5-FU (500Mg/M^2/day) is administered for 5 days. In week nine RT to the tumor area and regional nodes is started (45 Gy/4-6 weeks) followed by a boost to the tumor bed (5.4 Gy/3 fractions). 5-FU (500 Mg/M^2/day) X 3 days is given during the first and last weeks of RT. 5-FU (450 mg/M^2/day) X 5 days is again given in weeks 4 and 8 following completion of RT.

Endocavitary radiotherapy RT alone has never found a role in the U.S. for operable rectal cancer. However, in France, a technique known as endocavitary radiotherapy has been used by Papillon for selected patients with rectal cancer. [18] In this technique a Philips superficial x-ray machine is used to deliver 50 KV x-rays through a proctoscope. Treatment is given every 2-3 weeks and the total dose is 90-125 Gy over 7-8 weeks. The treatment is indicated for Dukes A rectal carcinomas which are no larger than 5 cm in diameter and located within 10 cm of the anus.

The advantages of endocavitary radiotherapy are that hospitalization is not required, colostomy is not needed, patients who are surgical risks can be treated, there is little morbidity or mortality associated with the procedure and surgery can be used for failures. The authors achieved a local control rate of 95% among 37 patients treated.

Intraoperative RT In a number of centers IORT is being used in combination with conventional external beam therapy for selected patients with unresectable or recurrent colorectal carcinoma. [19] Treatment is initiated with external beam (45-50 Gy/5-6 weeks). Three to 6 weeks following completion of external beam therapy a laparotomy is carried out and the tumor site is exposed. The patient is transported to the irradiation area where an electron beam cone is inserted into the wound and a single 10-15 Gy fraction is given. At this time it is too early to determine whether IORT will be a significant advance in the treatment of colorectal cancer.

Palliative RT Pelvic RT is of value in palliation of painful local recurrence following surgery for rectal cancer.[20] Fifty-five percent of patients experience symptomatic benefit following doses of 35-50 Gy, but only 5% of patients survive 3 years.

Low-dose RT (15-30 Gy) to the liver has been used in several institutions as palliative treatment for liver metastasis from colorectal cancer.[21] Improvement in symptoms such as abdominal pain, nausea, fever and night sweats, weakness, jaundice, abdominal distention, anorexia and ascites has been seen following hepatic RT. Infusion of chemotherapeutic agents into the hepatic artery in combination with low-dose hepatic irradiation is under investigation.[22]

Chemotherapy Systemic therapy has not yielded improved survival rates for patients with metastatic colorectal cancer. Nevertheless, objective responses can produce an advanced disease and 5-FU is the most active drug. Objective responses are seen in 17% of patients treated with 5-FU and a larger number report symptomatic benefit without objective tumor responses.[23] Current protocols are investigating 5-FU combined with drugs such as semustine or biologic response modifiers such as levamisole, interferons, interleukins or monoclonal antibodies.

CANCER OF THE ANUS

ETIOLOGY AND EPIDEMIOLOGY

Malignant neoplasms of the anus are uncommon, occurring only 1/30th as frequently as rectal carcinoma. Carcinomas of the anus occur more frequently in females by a 3:2 ratio and the mean age at diagnosis is 65. Any condition that causes chronic irritation in the anal region can be associated with anal carcinoma. Among these are hemorrhoids, fissures, fistulae, scars, abscesses and previous irradiation.

PATHOLOGY

Ninety percent of cancers of the anal canal and perianal skin are squamous cell carcinomas or variants of squamous carcinoma. Local spread occurs by infiltration of perianal tissues and regional lymph node metastasis is common. Tumors of the proximal anal canal tend to metastasize upward to pelvic lymph nodes, whereas tumors of the distal canal and perianal region metastasize to inguinal lymph nodes. Blood-borne metastasis to liver, lungs and bone is common in locally advanced disease.

TREATMENT

Surgery Small tumors can be excised locally but large tumors require an AP resection. Five year survival rates following local excision range from 70-90% and following AP resection, 45-65%.

Radiotherapy Squamous cell carcinomas of the anal region are moderately radiosensitive and potentially radiocurable. Small tumors can be treated with RT alone using external beam techniques, interstitial brachytherapy, or external beam combined with interstitial brachytherapy.[24]

Locally advanced tumors, which in the past, would have required AP resection, are treated by preoperative RT and concurrent chemotherapy. 5-FU +mitomycin C combined with 30 Gy/3 weeks is the combination most commonly used.[25] Surgical resection is carried out 4-6 weeks later. The data indicate that in many cases the chemotherapy +RT are effective in reducing the size of the primary to an extent that a sphincter-saving operation can be performed.

REFERENCES

1.Silverberg E, Boring CC, Squires TS, Cancer Statistics 1990, CA-A Cancer J for clin 450:9-26, 1990.

2. Chapter 10, Stomach, In Manual for Staging of Cancer, Third Edition, Eds. Beahrs OH, Henson DE, Hutter RVP, Myers MH, J.B. Lippincott Company, Philadelphia, 1988, pp 69-73.

3. Moertel CG, Childs DS, Reitemeier RJ, et al. Combined 5-fluorouracil and supervoltage radiation therapy of locally unresectable gastrointestinal cancer, Lancet 2:865-867, 1969.

4. Gunderson LL, Sosin H. Adenocarcinoma of the stomach: Areas of failure in a re-operation series (second or symptomatic look) clinicopathologic correlations and implications for adjuvant therapy, Int J Radiat Oncol Biol Phy 8:1-11, 1982.

5. Chapter 17, Endocrine pancreas, In Manual for Staging of Cancer, Third Edition, Eds. Beahrs OH, Henson DE, Hutter RVP, Myers MH J. B. Lippincott Company, Philadelphia, 1988, pp 109-113.

6. Moertel CG, Fytak S, Hahn RG, et al. Therapy of locally unresectable pancreatic carcinoma: A random comparison of High dose (6000 rads) radiation alone, moderate dose radiation (4000 rads + 5-fluorouracil), and high dose radiation +5 fluorouracil, Cancer 48:1705-1710, 1981.

7. Wood WC, Shipley WU, Gunderson LL, et al. Intraoperative irradiation for unresectable pancreatic carcinoma, Cancer 49:1272-1275, 1982.

8. Syed AM, Puthawala AA, Neblett DL, et al. Interstitial iodine-125 implant in the management of unresectable pancreatic carcinoma, Cancer 52:808--813, 1983.

9. Herskovic A, Heaston D, Engler MJ, et al, Irradiation of biliary carcinoma, Radiology 139:219-222, 1981.

10. Cohen AM, Shank B, Friedman MA. Chapter 29, Colorectal cancer, In Cancer-Principles & Practice of Oncology, 3rd Edition, Eds. DeVita VT, Hellman S, Rosenberg SA, J.B. Lippincott Company, Philadelphia, 1989, pp 895-964.

11. Chapter 11, Colon and rectum, In Manual for Staging of Cancer, Third Edition, Eds. Beahrs OH, Henson DE, Hutter RVP, Myers MH, J. B. Lippincott Company, Philadelphia, 1988, pp 75-80.

12. Mendenhall WM, Million RR, Pfaff WW. Patterns of recurrence in adenocarcinoma of the rectum and rectosigmoid treated with surgery alone: Implications in treatment planning with adjuvant radiation therapy, In J Radiat Oncol Biol Phys 9:977-985, 1983.

13. Dosoretz DE, Gunderson LL, Hedberg S, et al. Preoperative irradiation for unresectable rectal and rectosigmoid carcinomas, Cancer 52:814-818, 1983.

14. Gunderson LL, Russell AH, Llewellyn HJ , et al. Treatment planning for colorectal cancer: Radiation and surgical techniques and value of small-bowel films, Int J Radiat Oncol Biol Phys 11:1379-1393 1985.

15. NIH Consensus Conference of adjuvant therapy for patients with colon and rectal cancer. JAMA 2264:1444-1450, 1990.

16. Krook JE, Moertel CG, Gunderson LL, et al. Effective surgical adjuvant therapy for high risk rectal carcinoma, N Engl J Med 324:709-715, 1991.

17. Clinical Announcement: Adjuvant therapy of rectal cancer March 14, 1991, National Cancer Institute, U.S. Department of Health and Human Services, Public Health Service, National Institutes of Heatlh, Bethesda, Maryland.

18. Papillon J. Endocavitary irradiation in the curative treatment of early rectal cancer, Dis Colon & Rectum 17:172-180, 1974.

19. Gunderson LL, Cohen AC, Dosoretz DD, et al. Residual, unrsectable or recurrent colorectal cancer: External beam irradiation and intraoperative electron beam boost +/- resection, Int J Rdiat Oncol Biol Phys 9:1597-1606, 1983.

20. Ciatto S, Pacini P. Radiation therapy of recurrences of carcinoma of the rectum and sigmoid after surgery, Acta Radiol Oncol 21:105-109, (Fasc 2), 1982.

21. Borgelt BB, Gelber R, Brady LW, et al. The palliation of hepatic metastasis: Results of the Radiation Therapy Oncology Group pilot study, Int J Radiat Oncol Biol Phys 7:587-591, 1981.

22. Barone RM, Byfield JE, Goldfarb PB, et al. Intra-arterial chemotherapy using an implantable infusion pump and liver irradiation for the treatment of hepatic metastasis, Cancer 50:850-862, 1982.

23. Moertel CG, Thynne GS. Chapter 25, Large bowel, In Cancer Medicine, 2nd Edition, Eds. Holland JF, Frei E, Lea & Febiger, Philadelphia, 1982, pp 1830-1859.

24. Papillon J, Mayer M, Montonbon JE, et al. A new approach to the management of epidermoid carcinoma of the anal canal, Cancer 51:1830-1837, 1983.

25. Nigro ND, Seydel HG, Considine B, et al. Combined preoperative radiation and chemotherapy in squamous cell carcinoma of the anal canal, Cancer 51:1826--1829, 1983.

Chapter 22

GENITOURINARY TRACT

KIDNEY

ETIOLOGY AND EPIDEMIOLOGY

Eighty percent of renal tumors are renal cell carcinomas and 5% are carcinomas of the renal pelvis. There are about 18,000 renal cell carcinomas diagnosed in adults each year and about 9,000 persons die of the disease.[1] Renal cell carcinomas occur more commonly in men (2:1) as do carcinomas of the renal pelvis (4:1). Most renal cell carcinomas occur in persons aged 50 to 70.

The etiology of cancer of the kidney is unknown, but renal cell carcinoma and carcinoma of the renal pelvis are more common in smokers than in nonsmokers. Chemical carcinogens seem to play a role in some patients since there is a high incidence of the disease in persons with a long history of abuse of the analgesic phenacetin. In women, obesity is associated with an increased risk.

A number of occupational factors has been identified. The incidence of the disease is increased in leather tanners, shoe workers and asbestos workers. Exposure to cadmium is associated with increased risk as is exposure to petroleum, tar and pitch products. Chronic exposure to thorotrast, a radioactive material that was used as a contrast agent in radiology, is associated with an increased risk. Finally, there are genetic factors in renal cell carcinoma since there are pedigrees with familial renal cell carcinoma.

PATHOLOGY

Renal cell carcinomas, also known as hypernephromas, are adenocarcinomas. Spread of renal cell carcinoma occurs by direct extension to the renal capsule and the renal vein. Regional lymph node and distant metastasis are common. The lungs, bones, and liver are the most frequent sites of metastasis. Ninety percent of carcinomas of the renal pelvis are transitional cell carcinomas and 7% are squamous cell carcinomas. Carcinomas of the renal pelvis spread locally, metastasize to regional lymph nodes and disseminate via the blood stream. Transitional cell carcinomas of the renal pelvis tend to be associated with other carcinomas of the urinary tract.

DIAGNOSIS AND STAGING

Symptoms The most common presenting symptom in patients with cancer of the kidney is hematuria. Pain in the flank is also a common symptom. Thirty percent of patients present with symptoms caused by tumor metastasis. Fever, fatigue, and weight loss may be presenting symptoms.

Radiographic studies Intravenous pyelography, ultrasound, abdominal CT scans, renal arteriography and magnetic resonance imaging (MRI) are useful tests in evaluating and staging patients suspected of having renal cell carcinoma. These studies suggest the correct diagnosis in over 90% of cases.

Carcinomas of the renal pelvis are more difficult to diagnose. Intravenous pyelography, CT scanning and arteriography are usually successful in delineating the lesion.

Staging The TNM staging classification for renal cell carcinoma is shown in Table 22.1.

Table 22.1 Staging of kidney cancer[2]

T1 Tumor 2.5 cm or less in diameter and limited to kidney

T2 Tumor more than 2.5 cm in diameter and limited to kidney

T3 Tumor extends to major veins or invades adrenal gland or perinephric tissues but not beyond Gerota's fascia

T4 Tumor invades beyond Gerota's fascia

N0 No regional lymph node metastasis

N1 Metastasis in a single node 2 cm or less in diameter

N2 Metastasis in a single node more than 2 cm in diameter but none more than 5 cm, or multiple nodes none more than 5 cm

N3 Nodes more than 5 cm in diameter

M0 No distant metastasis

M1 Distant metastasis

Stage grouping

I	T1N0M0	III T1N1M0, T2N1M0, T3N0, N1M0
II	T2N0M0	IV T4, any NM0, any TN2, N3M0, any T any NM1

TREATMENT

Surgery Radical nephrectomy with or without regional lymph node dissection is the standard treatment for renal cell carcinoma. The operation involves removal of the kidney, the adrenal gland, the perinephric fat, Gerota's fascia and the regional lymph nodes.

The standard treatment for carcinoma of the renal pelvis is radical nephroureterectomy with excision of a cuff of bladder.

Radiotherapy RT alone has not found a role in renal cell carcinoma or carcinoma of the renal pelvis. Preoperative and postoperative RT has been studied in clinical trials for renal cell carcinoma and the results are inconclusive. Therefore, adjuvant RT is not routinely used.

On the other hand, RT has role in the palliation of metastasis. Metastases to bone and brain often respond to RT. A single brain metastasis can occasionally be removed surgically if there are no other sites of active disease. In these cases, postop RT is given to the brain.

Chemotherapy No effective chemotherapy regimens are available for renal cell carcinoma. The disease is occasionally responsive to hormones such as progestin, testosterone or an antiestrogen. Current clinical research studies are evaluating the role of biologic response modifier therapy in renal cell carcinoma. For example, adoptive cellular therapy with lymphokine-activated (LAK) cells plus interleukin-2 (IL-2) has produced objective responses in 30% of patients with metastatic renal cell carcinoma.[3] Interferon used alone or in a combination with IL-2 produces responses in 20% of patients.

Prognosis Reported 5 year survival rates for patients with Stage I renal cell carcinoma range from 65-95%; for Stage II disease, 45-65%, for Stage III, 35-50%, and for Stage IV, 0-18%.

Overall 5 year survival rates for renal pelvis carcinomas range from 30-40%.

CARCINOMA OF THE URETER

Cancer of the ureter is an uncommon disease accounting for only 1% of neoplasms of the upper urinary tract. It occurs in older age groups and is more common in men (2:1). Ninety percent are transitional cell carcinomas. Nephroureterectomy is the standard treatment for cancer of the ureter and RT has traditionally had little role in management. However, one report described encouraging results with postop RT (40-50 Gy) for patients with locally advanced carcinoma of the ureter.[4] The overall 5 year survival rate is about 40%.

CARCINOMA OF THE BLADDER

ETIOLOGY AND EPIDEMIOLOGY

Bladder cancer is the most common malignant tumor of the urinary tract. About 49,000 new cases were diagnosed in the U.S. in 1990 and 9,700 persons died of the disease. Bladder cancer occurs most commonly in the 50-60 year age group and is more common in men (3:1). The etiology of bladder cancer is unknown but the disease occurs more commonly in smokers. Also, some industrial dyes are known to be etiologic factors. Aniline dye used in the dye, rubber and paint industries, napthylamine and benzidine are examples of known industrial carcinogens. In Egypt and North Africa bladder cancer is associated with chronic infestation of the bladder with Schistosoma hematobium.

PATHOLOGY

Bladder tumors may occur at single or multiple sites in the bladder and grow as papillary, sessile, nodular or ulcerated masses. In the case of in-situ carcinoma, the bladder mucosa has a granular or reddened appearance. Tumors arise most commonly in the trigone area of the bladder or near the ureteral orifices.

To fully assess a bladder tumor microscopically, the pathologist must evaluate the growth pattern, cell type, degree of differentiation and depth of penetration into the bladder wall. The pattern of growth is determined by examination under low microscopic power. The pattern may be papillary, solid or infiltrating, papillary and solid or non-invasive (in-situ). Papillary tumors grow into the lumen of the bladder whereas solid tumors grow into the bladder wall. In papillary and solid tumors both growth patterns are seen. In-situ carcinomas may be multifocal or diffuse. A significant number of in-situ carcinomas eventually become invasive.

The cell type may be transitional, squamous or glandular, but 90% are transitional cell carcinomas. The grade of the carcinoma and the depth of penetration into the bladder wall are important in predicting prognosis; high-grade tumors tend to penetrate the bladder wall more deeply than low-grade tumors and they metastasize more frequently to lymph nodes and distant sites. The lungs, bones and liver are common sites of metastasis.

DIAGNOSIS AND STAGING

Symptoms Hematuria is the presenting symptom in 75% of cases. Dysuria and frequent urination are also common presenting symptoms.

Cystoscopy The diagnosis is established at the time of cystoscopy. The tumor can be visualized directly and biopsied through the cystoscope.

Radiographic studies Intravenous pyelography is used to evaluate the upper urinary tract and CT scanning of the pelvis is of value in determining disease extent.

Staging The Jewett-Marshall staging classification is widely used in the U.S. (Table 22.2)

TREATMENT

Surgery *Stages O and A* Papillary and low-grade superficial tumors can be controlled by transurethral resection or fulgeration. The 5 year survival rate is about 80%.

Stages B_1, B_2 and C Most patients whose tumor invades muscle require radical cystectomy. In males, this operation involves removal of the bladder, prostate, seminal vesicles and the immediately adjacent perivesical tissue. In females, the bladder, uterus, tubes, ovaries, anterior vagina and urethra are

---

Table 22.2 The Jewett-Marshall staging classification for bladder cancer

O   Superficial tumor confined to mucosa (carcinoma in-situ)

A   Superficial infiltration into submucosa

B   Muscle invasion

      B1 Superficial

      B2 Deep

C   Extension through bladder wall to perivesical tissues

D   Metastatic

      D1 Adjacent organs involvved

      D2 Metastasis to regional lymph nodes below aortic bifurcation

      D3 Metastasis to lymph nodes above aortic bifurcation and/or distant metastasis

---

removed. A pelvic lymphadenectomy is often combined with the radical cystectomy.

Radiotherapy *Stages O and A* External RT alone is occasionally recommended for patients with multiple, low-grade tumors. Sixty-five Gy in 6 1/2 to 7 weeks is given to the bladder with small field techniques. Five year survival rates as high as 50% have been reported in this selected group.

Stages B and C External beam RT alone is used for patients who refuse surgery, are elderly or medically unfit for surgery. Sixty-five Gy in 6 1/2 weeks to 70 Gy in 7 to 8 weeks is given with small portals. Treatment results following RT alone in this group are discouraging with 5 year survival rates of <15%.

Results of RT for patients found to have unresectable disease at the time of laparotomy are especially dismal with 2 year survival rates of <10%. Nevertheless, RT can have a palliative benefit for patients with hematuria, pain and/or urinary obstructive symptoms.

In spite of this discouraging data, RT offers the patient an opportunity to preserve bladder function. For this reason, some centers use RT for all patients, reserving surgery for those who do not respond. For example, in one report from Canada, all patients with invasive bladder cancer were given RT (50 Gy or more) and cystectomy was carried out only in patients who did not respond or who developed recurrence.[5] Only 16% of 470 patients, required cystectomy and the overall 5 year survival rate was 38%.

Preoperative RT Preop RT combined with radical cystectomy has been evaluated in numerous studies. Low-dose, high-dose and sandwich (preop + postop) regimen has been used, but as yet, there is not a definitive study demonstrating that local control and survival are improved with preop RT. For this reason adjuvant RT is not used in most institutions.

Interstitial brachytherapy This method has not found wide application in the U.S., but Van der Werf-Messing in Rotterdam has reported outstanding results for selected patients, with radium needle implants.[6] The implants are carried out only on tumors less than 5 cm in diameter without lymph node metastasis. The needles are implanted through an opened bladder. The needles remain in place for 168 hours to deliver 65 Gy. Five and 10 year survival of 75% and 70% respectively were obtained with this technique.

Chemotherapy + RT Clinical trials are ongoing in which RT is combined with chemotherapy in an attempt to preserve bladder function and improve survival rates for patients with invasive bladder cancer. For example, one protocol combines RT (40 Gy) with cisplatin.[7] Patients whose tumor has not responded to this combination undergo cystectomy, whereas those whose tumor has responded receive an additional 20-25 Gy and no cystectomy.

Chemotherapy *Systemic chemotherapy* In recent years improved results for patients with advanced bladder cancer have been reported. Combinations of agents are used and one of the most popular regimens is known as M-VAC (methotrexate, vinblastine, doxorubicin, cisplatin).[8] Complete remission rates as high as 35% have been reported with this regimen. Clinical trials are evaluating the efficacy of M-VAC therapy prior to radical cystectomy in patients with invasive disease.

Intravesical chemotherapy Patients with multiple superficial bladder tumors are often treated, following transurethral resection of as many lesions as possible, with chemotherapeutic agents instilled directly into the bladder. Thiotepa, mitomycin C, doxorlubicin and BCG are the agents which have been most extensively used.

CARCINOMA OF THE PROSTATE

ETIOLOGY AND EPIDEMIOLOGY

Prostate cancer is a very common disease in men over age 60. There were approximately 106,000 new cases and 30,000 deaths from prostate cancer in 1990 in the U.S. It is the most common cancer in males and the third most common cause of death from cancer. Black males in the U.S. have the highest incidence in the world, whereas the incidence in Japan is one of the lowest in the world. The incidence in U.S. blacks is 40 times that in Japan.

The etiology of prostate cancer is unknown. However, a number of studies have shown that prostate cancer occurs with greater frequency in men who have had multiple sexual partners and a history of venereal disease, suggesting a possible viral factor in etiology. No viruses have been established to be etiologic, but herpes virus Type II and a strain of cytomegalovirus have been isolated from human prostatic carcinomas.

Another possible etiologic factor is male hormone. Prostate cancer does not occur in castrated men and the disease is uncommon in men with cirrhosis of the liver, a disease associated with elevated levels of estrogen. The disease tends to run in families and mortality from prostate cancer is three times higher in relatives of prostate cancer patients than in controls.

PATHOLOGY

More than 95% of prostate carcinomas are adenocarcinomas. The tumor grade is closely correlated with prognosis. A grading system used in many hospitals, known as the Gleason system, uses the degree of glandular differentiation and the growth pattern of the tumor in relation to the prostatic stroma to determine the grade which may vary from grade 1 (well-differentiated) to grade 5 (undifferentitated).

Prostate cancer spreads by local extension to the seminal vesicles, bladder, urethra and pelvic sidewalls. Metastasis to pelvic lymph nodes and to the bones of the pelvis and vertebral column is common. Bone metastases tend to be osteoblastic.

DIAGNOSIS AND STAGING

Symptoms An increasing number of cases are discovered at an early asymptomatic Stage by digital rectal examination at the time of routine physical examination. Larger tumors may produce urinary obstructive symptoms such as increased frequency of urination, nocturia, hesitancy and narrow stream. Some patients present with acute complete obstruction due to advanced local disease. In a few cases, the diagnosis is made by the pathologist after examining tissue removed at the time of transurethral resection for what was thought to be benign prostatic hypertrophy. Patients often present with bone pain due to metastasis.

Physical examination On digital rectal examination, an area of firmness or nodularity in the prostate can be palpated in early cases, whereas in locally advanced cases a large firm mass is found.

Transrectal ultrasound and needle biopsy. In the evaluation of prostate nodules transrectal ultrasound imaging has found an important role.[9] Hypoechoic areas in the prostate suggest carcinoma and these can be biopsied via transrectal needle biopsy to establish the diagnosis. Transrectal ultrasound is also being evaluated as a possible screening test for early prostate cancer detection.

Prostate-specific antigen (PSA) This antigen is produced exclusively by normal and neoplastic duct epithelium of the prostate and secreted into the gland lumen.[10] The antigen levels are elevated in the serum of patients with benign prostatic hypertrophy and prostate cancer. Serum PSA is a very sensitive test and levels may become elevated very early in the disease. Therefore, studies are underway to evaluate its' role as a screening test for early prostate cancer. Also, the test is extremely useful in following patients post-treatment.

Staging The American Urologic Association staging system is widely used in the U.S. A comparison of the American Urologic Association and TNM systems is shown in Table 22.3.

Table 22.3 Two staging systems for prostate cancer[11]	
TNM	**American Urological**
T1a Three or fewer microscopic foci	A1 Focal
T1b More than 3 microscopic foci	A2 Diffuse
T2a Tumor 1.5 cm or less in diameter	B1 Small discrete nodule
T2b Tumor >1.5 cm in diameter	B2 Large or multiple nodules
T3 Tumor invades prostatic capsule, bladder, seminal vesicles	C1 No involvement of seminal vesicles
T4 Tumor fixed or invades adjacent organs	C2 Involvement of seminal vesicles
N1 Metastasis in single node <2 cm	D1 Pelvic lymph node metastasis
N2 Metastasis in node >2 cm	D2 Distant metastasis
M1 Distant metastasis	

Staging procedures performed on all patients include serum acid phosphatase and PSA determinations and bone scans. Pelvic CT and MRI scans are of value in detecting local disease extensions. Pelvic lymph node exploration and biopsy is recommended, by some authorities, in patients being considered for local RT. The incidence of pelvic lymph node metastasis is 7% in Stage B_1, 43% in Stage B_2 and 60% in Stage C.[12]

TREATMENT

Surgery Radical prostatectomy is the operation used for the small group (5-10%) of patients having disease limited to the prostate gland. In this operation the prostate, seminal vesicles and a cuff of the bladder neck are removed. The operation can be performed through a perineal or suprapubic incision.

In the past, the major disadvantages of the operation were that many patients experienced urinary incontinence following surgery and nearly 100% of the patients were impotent. However, improvements in the surgical technique have reduced the incidence of incontinence and allowed the nerves to the prostate to be spared thus reducing the incidence of impotence.

Radiotherapy *External beam technique* This is the most commonly used method of treatment for patients with localized disease (Stages A, B, and C). Usually small field techniques are used but some authorities recommend treatment of regional lymph nodes in addition to the primary. Sixty-five Gy in 6 1/2 week to 70 Gy in 7-8 weeks is the dose range most commonly used.

The treatment planing protocol for external beam therapy via the "box" technique is as follows:

1.   A Foley catheter is placed in the bladder and 20 cc of renografin is instilled into the bladder.

2.   A rectal tube is inserted and 100 cc of barium is instilled into the rectum.

3.   Anterior and Posterior and right and left lateral simulator films are taken. Portal sizes of 10 X 10 cm to 12 X 12 cm cover the prostate and seminal vesicles. Cerrobend blocks are made for the lateral portals to shield a portion of the bladder and anus.

4.   A CT scan for treatment planning is obtained. The adequacy of coverage by the simulated fields is assessed and changes made if indicated.

5.   A computerized set of isodose curves is prepared.

Acute side effects Acute radiation proctitis manifested by rectal irritation, tenesmus and diarrahea is experienced by nearly all patients. Agents such as lomotil are usually effective in controlling symptoms, but occasional patients will require a 1-2 week rest to allow the symptoms to subside.

Acute radiation cystitis is also experienced by most patients producing symptoms such as dysuria, frequency of urination and bladder spasms. Pyridium 200 mg. t.i.d. is occasionally helpful in controlling symptoms.

Results and complications The results of external beam therapy for localized prostate cancer at Stanford are shown in Table 22.4. The Stanford data are unique because of the long follow-up for a significant number of patients.

Late complications following external beam RT are an important problem. In one larger series, the type and incidence of late complications was urethral stricture, 5%, proctitis, 4.5% and bladder injury, 3.5%.[14] In the Stanford series 60% of the patients maintained erectile potency for 5 years following RT, 45% for 10 years, 33% for 15 years and 33% for 20 years.[13]

Table 22.4 Stanford data: 15 year survival rates after external beam therapy for prostate cancer[13]			
Stage	**No. Patients**	**Overall**	**Disease-Specific**
T0	69	45%	85%
T1	282	35%	64%
T2	183	33%	45%
T3	348	20%	33%
T4	32	10%	15%

Pelvic lymph node irradiation An important issue in external beam therapy is whether or not the pelvic lymph nodes should be irradiated. In an attempt to answer this question, the Radiation Therapy Oncology Group (RTOG) completed a clinical trial in which patients with Stage A_2 and B disease were randomized to receive RT to the prostate only or RT to the prostate + the pelvic lymph nodes.[15] With at least 5 years follow-up there was not a statistically significant difference between the 2 groups in survival or local recurrence.

Insterstitial brachytherapy For many years radiotherapists have been interested in interstitital brachytherapy for prostate cancer. Early attempts involved the use of radon seeds and colloidal gold-198 ,but more recently iodine-125, gold-198 seeds and iridium-192 have been used.

The most popular current method was developed at Memorial Hospital in New York. [16] The surgeon initially performs a pelvic lymphadenectomy and dissects around the prostate gland to provide easy access for the radiotherapists. The radiotherapist then inserts the iodine-125 seeds into the prostate. One hundred and sixty Gy are delivered to the prostate over the course of 1 year.

Complications developing following pelvic lymphadenectomy and iodine-125 implants are related to the lymphadenectomy and the implant. In general, the complication rate resulting from the radiation is quite low and, as expected, few rectal and bladder injuries are seen compared to external beam therapy. However, the tumor control rate is not great as is seen with external beam therapy. In one series, local recurrence occurred in 29% of patients treated with iodine-125 implant versus only 17% in patients treated with external beam.[17]

The reason for the high incidence of local failure following implants appears to be that a homogenous dose to the prostate is not always obtained resulting in "cold spots" which lead to local recurrence. Also, it is possible that the dose rate with iodine-125 is too low allowing tumor cells to proliferate even while being irradiated.

Therefore, it would appear that another radioactive source to replace iodine-125 will be required. An isotope with a higher gamma ray energy and a shorter half life may yield a more homogenous dose with a more biologically effective dose rate. Palladium-103 is currently under investigation as a replacement for iodine-125. The half-life of palladium-103 is 17 days which is an improvement over iodine-125 (70 days). However, the energy of the gamma ray is only 23KV which is lower than that of iodine (28 KV).

Palliative RT Painful bone metastases usually responds to palliative RT (30 Gy/10 fractions).

Breast irradiation to prevent gynecomastia Patients undergoing estrogen therapy for metastatic prostate carcinoma often develop painful breast enlargement called gynecomastia. The symptoms can be prevented with local irradiation to each breast (4 Gy per day for 3 consecutive days).[18] Breast irradiation is given 2 or 3 days prior to the start of estrogen therapy.

Endocrine therapy Locally advanced and/or metastatic prostatic carcinoma is often responsive to endocrine therapy. Bilateral orchiectomy is usually the initial method used. Plasma testosterone levels are reduced by 90% following orchiectomy. Administration of estrogens is also effective in suppressing testosterone production. Diethylstilbestrol (1-5 mg/day) is the estrogen most often used. Estrogens act by preventing release of luteinizing hormone by the pituitary gland which, in turn, reduces testicular testosterone production.

Inhibitors of androgen synthesis, such as aminoglutethamide, and antiandrogens, such as flutamide, which block the action of androgens at the tumor cell binding sites, are newer methods of endocrine therapy.

Chemotherapy This modality has not improved survival time or cure rates in patients with metastatic prostate cancer. Nevertheless, responses are produced by a number of drugs including hydroxyurea, cisplatin, estramustine phosphate, doxorubicin, 5-U, and cyclophosphamide. Current protocols are evaluating the effectiveness of combinations of agents.

CANCER OF THE TESTIS

ETIOLOGY AND EPIDEMIOLOGY

Cancer of the testis accounts for only 1% of cancers in males but is a leading cause of death from cancer in young adults. The average age at onset is 32. The incidence of testis cancer is increased in cryptorchidism (undescended testis) and in atrophy of the testes which can occur following mumps orchitis. The etiology of testis cancer is unknown and no other etiologic factors have been identified.

PATHOLOGY

Most malignant tumors of the testis originate from germ cells. There are four histopathologic types: seminoma, embryonal carcinoma, teratoma and choricocarcinoma. Each cell type can occur alone or in combination with one or more of the others. In mixed tumors, the prognosis is determined by the component with the worst prognosis. There are three forms of seminoma: classic seminomas the most common type, anaplastic and spermatocytic. Some of the clinical features for each of the major types are shown in Table 22.5.

Lymphatic metastasis occurs via the lymph vessels that accompany the testicular vessels along the spermatic cord through the inguinal canal to terminate in the lumbar lymph nodes around the inferior vena cava and aorta inferior to the renal vessels. Spread from the retroperitoneal nodes occurs via the thoracic duct to the left supraclavicular lymph nodes. Hematogenous metastasis is primarily to the lungs.

DIAGNOSIS AND STAGING

Symptoms The most common presenting symptom is that the patient has discovered a painless enlargement of one testis.

Table 22.5   Major features of germ cell tumors of the testis.

Tumor Type	Clinical features
Classical seminoma	70% of testicular tumors Most common in 4th & 5th decades Mestastasizes predominantly via lymphatics Very radiosensitive
Anaplastic seminoma	Prognosis may be slightly worse
Spermatocytic seminoma	10% of seminomas Excellent prognosis
Embryonal carcinoma	20% of testicular tumors Peak incidence in 2nd and 3rd decades Metastasis via lymphatics and blood
Choriocarcinoma	<1% of testicular tumors Most common in 2nd & 3rd decades Metastasis mostly via blood stream

Physical examination Testicular tumors present as a hard, nontender mass involving the testis.

Inguinal orchiectomy The diagnosis is confirmed by removing the testis through an inguinal incision and histologic study of the specimen.

Staging The TNM staging classification is shown in Table 22.6. Studies used in staging include chest x-rays, lymphangiography, and CT scanning of the abdomen. Pathologic staging in non-seminomatous tumors is accomplished by retroperitoneal lymph node dissection.

The Beta subunit of human chorionic gonadotropin (B-HCG) and alpha-fetoprotein are produced by the majority of non-seminomatous tumors. There-

Table 22.6 The staging classification for testicular tumors [19]

Stage I	Tumor limited to testis
Stage II	Clinical or radiographic evidence of spread to lymph nodes below diaphragm
	IIA Moderate sized metastasis
	IIB Massive retroperitoneal metastasis
Stage III	Metastasis above diaphragm
	IIIA Mediastinal or supraclavicular metastasis
	IIIB Metastasis to lung or other distant sites

fore, if B-HCG and alpha-fetoprotein levels are elevated after the primary is removed, residual disease is likely to be present.

TREATMENT

Surgery Radical inguinal orchiectomy is required in all patients to establish the diagnosis and provide treatment for the primary. Patients having clinical Stage I and II non-seminomatous tumors usually undergo retroperitoneal lymph node dissection as a staging procedure and as treatment for possible lymph node metastasis. Patients found to have lymph node metastasis receive adjuvant chemotherapy, but some authorities give chemotherapy to all patients regardless of lymph node status.

Radiotherapy *Seminoma* In Stage I, the retroperitoneal and iliac lymph nodes on the side of the primary are irradiated with opposing anterior and posterior portals (Figure 22.1). Twenty five Gy in 3 weeks to 30 Gy in 4 weeks is sufficient to eradicate microscopic disease. The cure rate in Stage I approaches 95%.[19]

In Stage IIA, the retroperitoneal and iliac doses on the side of the tumor are treated as in Stage I. However, following completion of the basic treatment, the involved lymph nodes are boosted with an additional 5 to 10 Gy. After a 2 week to 1 month rest, the mediastinum and left supraclavicular region is irradiated electively to a dose of 25 Gy in 3 weeks. Reported cure rates in Stage IIA following RT are in the range of 85%.

Extensive Stage IIB cases require whole abdominal RT and /or chemotherapy. Five year survival rates following RT alone in Stage IIB range from 33% to 62%. Most Stage III cases are treated by chemotherapy alone.

Complications following RT for seminoma are uncommon, occurring in less than 2% of patients. Injuries to the small bowel and stomach are the most frequently reported complications and these are usually seen only in patients receiving a dose to the retroperitoneal nodes in excess of 30 Gy.

Non-seminomatous tumors Most centers in the U.S. do not use radiotherapy for Stage I and II non-seminomatous tumors but rely on surgery and chemotherapy. However, there are data from Europe suggesting that retroperitoneal RT (40-50 Gy in 5 to 6 weeks) is an acceptable alternative to retroperitoneal lymph node dissection.[20]

Chemotherapy Major improvements in treatment results for patients with testicular cancer have been seen in recent years due to advances in chemotherapy. The drugs with activity against the disease are actinomycin D, chlorambucil, methotrexate, vinblastine, bleomycin, mithramycin, etoposide (VP-16) and cisplatin. Current protocols utilize a number of the agents in combination. Two of the most popular regimens are VAB-VI (cyclophospha-

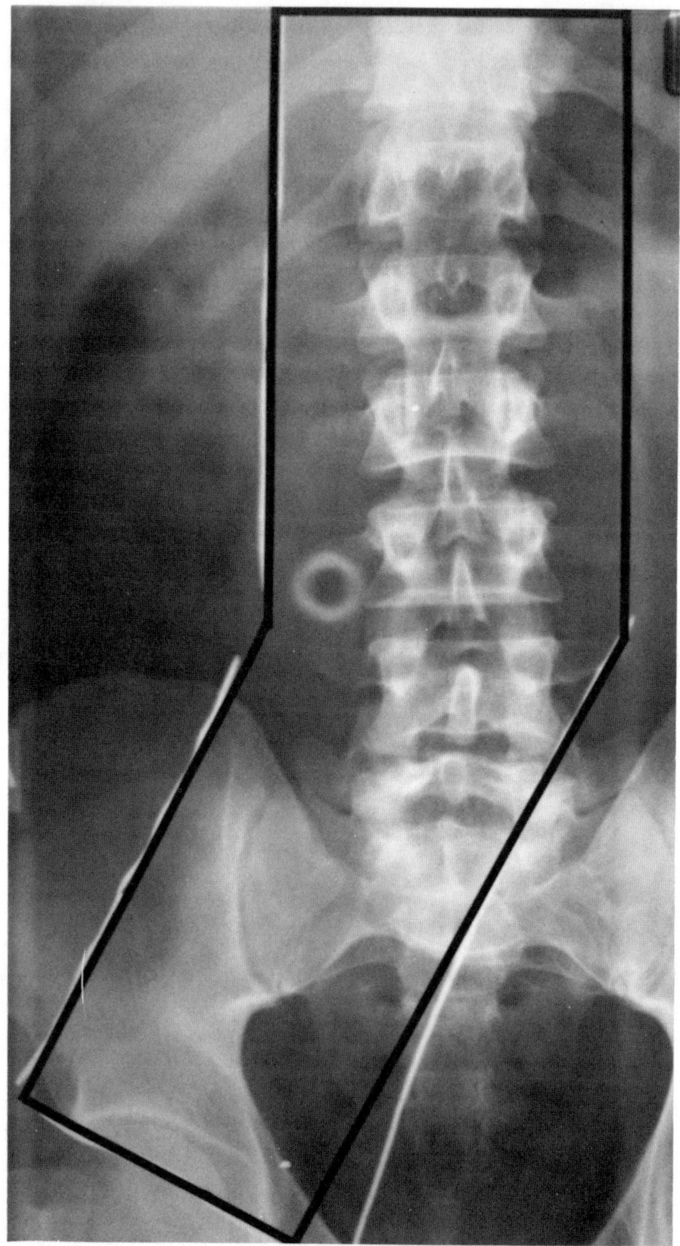

Figure 22.1 This is the simulator film for a patient with Stage I seminoma of the right testis-postop. He was treated with AP/PA portals.

mide, vinblastine, actinomycin D, bleomycin and cisplatin), developed at Memorial Hospital, NY and PVB (cisplatin ,vinblastine and bleomycin), developed at Indiana University.[21]

Early results from these institutions suggest that cure in 75% of patients with disseminated non-seminomatous disease should be possible. In Stage II non-seminomatous disease when chemotherapy is used as an adjuvant to surgery, the cure rate approaches 100%. Chemotherapy is also very effective in patients with disseminated seminoma.

CANCER OF THE PENIS

ETIOLOGY AND EPIDEMIOLOGY

Cancer of the penis is uncommon in the U.S. accounting for less than 1% of malignancies in males. In populations such as India where circumcision is not practiced and personal hygiene is sub-optimal, cancer of the penis accounts for 10% of malignancies in men.

PATHOLOGY

Most penile tumors are squamous cell carcinomas but malignant melanomas and sarcomas also occur. The primary mode of spread is to regional lymph nodes; 35-60% of patients have palpable inguinal adenopathy at presentation. Distant metastasis does not occur until late in the course of the disease.

TREATMENT

Surgery Surgical excision is usually the treatment of choice. Small tumors can be excised locally whereas larger tumors require partial or total penectomy. Inguinal lymphadenectomy is indicated in patients with inguinal lymph node metastasis.

Radiotherapy RT can be used for small squamous cell carcinomas. Small lesions can be treated with superficial x-rays or electrons (50 Gy in 3 weeks to 60 Gy in 5 weeks) or by interstitial implants with radium needles or iridium-192 wires or ribbons (60 Gy in 6 days).[22] External beam techniques are required for larger tumors since the entire shaft of the penis must be treated (65-70 Gy/5-7 weeks). [23]

Radiotherapy to the inguinal region may also be of value in selected patients. The inguinal regions can be treated electively (45-50 Gy) in patients at high-risk for occult metastasis or postoperatively (50-60 Gy) in patients who have extensive lymph node metastasis. The overall cure rate in patients treated by RT is about 65%; for early lesions (<2 cm) the cure rate is nearly 100%.

REFERENCES

1. Silverberg E, Boring CC, Squires TS. Cancer statistics, 1990, CA-A Cancer J for Clin 40:9-26, 1990.

2. Chapter 33, Kidney, In Manual for Staging of Cancer, Third Edition, Eds. Beahrs OH, Henson DE, Hutter RVP, Myers MH, J.B. Lippincott Company, Philadelphia, 1988, pp. 199-201.

3. Rosenberg SA, Lotze MT, Muul LM, et al. A progress report on the treatment of 157 patients with advanced cancer using lymphokine-activated killer cells and interleukin-2 or high dose interleukin-2 alone, N Engl J Med 316:889-, 1987.

4. Babaian RJ, Johnson DE, Chan RC. Combination nephroureterectomy and postoperative radiotherapy for infiltrative ureteral carcinoma, Int J Radiat Oncol Biol Phys 6:1229-1232, 1980.

5. Goodman GB, Hilsop TG, Elwood JM, Balfour J. Conservation of bladder function in patients with invasive bladder cancer treated by definitive irradiation and selective cystectomy, Int J Radiat Oncol Biol Phys 7:569-573, 1981.

6. Van der Werf-Messing B, Menon RS, Hop WCT. Cancer of the urinary bladder treated by interstitial implants: Second report, Int J Radiat Oncol Biol Phys 9:481-485, 1983.

7. Prout GR, Kaufman SD, Shipley WU, et al. Combined therapy in the treatment of patients with muscle-invading bladder cancer: A preliminary report of a bladder-sparing effort, J Urol 1339:268-. 1988.

8. Richie JP, Shipley WU, Yagoda A. Chapter 32, Cancer of the bladder, In Cancer-Principles & Practice of Oncology, 3rd Edition Eds. De Vita VT, Hellman S, Rosenberg SA, J.B. Lippincott Company, Philadelphia, 1989, pp 1008-1022.

9. Rifkin MD, Dahnert W, Kurtz AB. State of the art: Endorectal sonography of the prostate gland, AJR 154:691-700, 1990.

10. Drago JR. The role of new modalities in the early detection and diagnosis of prostate cancer, CA-A Cancer J for Clin 39:326-336, 1989.

11. Chapter 29, Prostate, In Manual for Staging of Cancer, Third Edition, Eds. Beahrs OH, Henson DE, Hutter RVP, Myers MH, J. B. Lippincott Company, Philadelphia, 1988, pp 177-179.

12. Fowler JE, Whitmore WF. The incidence and extent of pelvic lymph node metastasis in apparently localized prostatic cancer, Cancer 47:2941-2945, 1981.

13 Bagshaw MA, Cos RS, Ray GR. Status of radiation treatment of prostate cancer at Stanford University, NCI Monograph 7:47-60, 1988.

14. Pilepich MV, Perez CA, Walz BJ, Zivnuska FR. Complications of definitive radiotherapy for carcinoma of the prostate, Int J Radiat Oncol Biol Phys 7:1341-1348, 1984.

15. Asbell SO, Krall JM, Pilepich MV. Elective pelvic irradiation in Stage A2, B carcinoma of the prostate: Analysis of RTOG 77-06, Int J Radiat Oncol Biol Phys 15:1307-1316, 1988.

16. Whitmore WF, Hilaris B, Grabstald H. Retropubic implantation of iodine 125 in the treatment of prostatic cancer, J Urol 108:918-920 1972.

17. Kuban DA, El-Mahdi AM, Schellhammer PF. I-125 interstitial implantation for prostate cancer: What have we learned 10 years later?, Cancer 63:2415-2420, 1989.

18. Perez CA, Fair WR, Ihde DC. Chapter 33, Carcinoma of the prostate, In Cancer-Principles & Practice of Oncology, 3rd Edition, Eds. DeVita VT, Hallman S, Rosenberg SA, J.B. Lippincott Company, Philadelphia, 1989, pp 1023-1058.

19. Thomas GM, Rider WD, Dembo AJ, et al. Seminoma of the testis: Results of treatment and patterns of failure after radiation therapy, Int Radiat Oncol Biol Phys 8:165-174, 1982.

20. Clements JC, McLeod DG, Weisbaum GS, Stutzman RE. Radiation therapy for non-seminomatous cell tumors of the testis: A reappraisal, J Urol 126:490-492, 1981.

21. Einhorn LH, Crawford Ed, Shipley WU, Loehrer PJ, Williams SD. Chapter 35, Cancer of the testes, In Cancer-Principles & Practice of Oncology, 3rd Edition, Eds. DeVita VT, Hellman S, Rosenberg SA, J.B. Lippincott Company, Philadelphia, 1989, pp 1071-1098.

22. Daly NJ, Douchez J, Combes PF. Treatment of cancer of the penis by iridium-192 wire implant, In J Rad Oncol Biol Phys 8:1239-1243, 1982.

23. Sagerman RH, Yu WS, Chung CT, Puranik A. External-beam irradiation of carcinoma of the penis, Radiology 152:183-185, 1984.

Chapter 23

GYNECOLOGIC CANCER

CANCER OF THE CERVIX

ETIOLOGY AND EPIDEMIOLOGY

Invasive cancer of the cervix is the third most common malignant neoplasm of the female genitalia. In 1990, the disease was diagnosed in 13,500 women and was the cause of death in 6,000.[1] Mortality rates from cervix cancer have been decreasing over the past 40 years and the disease no longer ranks first as a cause of death from gynecologic cancer. The reasons for the decline in mortality are due to the success of population screening by cytology and improvements in therapy.

Epidemiologic studies have shown that cervix cancer is more common in women of low socioeconomic status who have coitus at an early age and are sexually promiscuous. The disease is rare among celibate women. These factors suggest that the disease is a sexually transmitted disease. There is evidence that herpes virus type 2 (HSV-2) may be etiologic in many patients. Also, human papillomavirus (HPB) has been shown to be associated with cervical intraepithelial neoplasia in many patients.

PATHOLOGY

Neoplasia of the cervix is a disease with a long natural history. The earliest lesion is mild dysplasia in which there is pleomorphism of many of the epithelial cells of the cervix. These have increased nuclear size and decreased cytoplasm and resemble carcinoma cells. These changes can progress to moderate dysplasia, severe dysplasia and carcinoma in-situ. The diagnosis of each of these lesions depends on the percentage of the thickness of the epithelium which is involved with the neoplastic changes.

An alternative schema which is widely used is the classification of cervical intraepithelial neoplasia (CIN). There are three grades of CIN: CIN I is equivalent to slight dysplasia; CIN II is severe dysplasia; CIN III is equivalent to carcinoma in-situ. Invasive carcinoma develops when the neoplastic process finally penetrates the basement membrane to invade the underlying stroma. A microinvasive carcinoma is one that has invaded the cervical stroma to a limited extent. If untreated, about 20% of dysplastic lesions will progress to invasive carcinoma in 5 years; 30% in 10 years; 40% in 20 years.

Eighty percent of invasive carcinomas are squamous cell carcinomas and 10% are adenocarcinomas. The remainder are a variety of adenocarcinoma patterns or mixtures. Twenty-five percent of squamous cell carcinomas are well-differentiated; 70% are moderately well-differentiated; 5% are small cell undifferentiated and have a worse prognosis than the others.

Cervical carcinomas spread predominately by local invasion and lymphatic metastasis. Local extension to the body of the uterus and upper vagina occurs early and invasion through the parametrium toward the pelvic wall is a characteristic feature. As the disease progresses, invasion of the ureters occurs leading to ureteral obstruction. Involvement of the bladder and/or rectum occurs late.

Lymphatic metastasis tends to occur in an orderly progression. The pelvic nodes are involved initially followed by the common iliac, para-aortic and finally the left supraclavicular nodes. Pelvic nodes are involved in 15-20% of Stage I cases, 25-40% in Stage II and 50%+ in Stage III. Hematogenous metastasis occurs late and the bones and lungs are frequently involved.

DIAGNOSIS

Symptoms Abnormal vaginal bleeding and discharge are the initial symptoms in 80-90% of patients with invasive cancer. Pelvic pain and urinary complaints are symptoms of advanced disease.

Pelvic examination The cervix may appear normal if the lesion is located in the cervical canal (endocervix) or if it is small. A visible lesion may be a fungating mass which bleeds easily or an ulcerating, destructive lesion. It may involve only the anterior or posterior lip or involve the entire cervix and there may be visible extension to the vaginal fornices or further down the vagina. Extension laterally into the parametria can be palpated and fixation indicates the tumor extends to the pelvic wall. The parametrial involvement may be unilateral or bilateral.

Vaginal cytology The Papanicolaou smear is the most important test for detecting preinvasive lesions. The false negative rate is 15%.

Colposcopy The major use of colposcopy is the evaluation of the patient with an abnormal Pap test when no gross lesion can be seen. The colposcope is a stereoscopic microscope which allows very small lesions to be visualized.

Biopsy Suspicious lesions seen at the time of speculum examination or colposcopy are biopsied. Endocervical curettage is used to obtain tissue from the endocervix in patients in whom no lesions are seen. In some patients a conization of the cervix is required to establish the diagnosis of invasive cancer.

STAGING

The staging system of the International Federation of Gynecology and Obstetrics (FIGO) is the most widely used classification (Table 23.1). Studies permitted in staging include biopsies, endocervical curettage, cystoscopy,

Table 23.1 FIGO staging system for carcinoma of the cervix[2]

Stage	Definition
0	Carcinoma in-situ
I	Cervical carcinoma confined to uterus
	Ia Preclinical invasive carcinoma diagnosed by microscopy
	Ia Minimal microscopic stromal invasion
	Ia Tumor with invasive component 5 mm or less in depth
	Ib Tumor larger than Ia
II	Cervical carcinoma invades beyond uterus but not to pelvic wall or lower third of vagina
	IIa Without parametrial invasion
	IIb With parametrial invasion
III	Carcinoma extends to the pelvic wall and/or lower third of vagina and/or causes hydronephrosis or non-functioning kidney
	IIIa Tumor involves lower third of vagina, no extension to pelvic wall
	IIIb Tumor extends to pelvic wall and/or causes hydronephrosis or non-functioning kidney
IVa	Tumor invades mucosa of bladder or rectum
IVb	Distant metastasis

proctoscopy, chest x-ray, skeletal x-rays and intravenous pyelography. Pelvic examination for the purpose of staging is usually carried out with the patient under general anesthesia.

In some institutions, surgical exploration with removal of common iliac and para-aortic lymph nodes for histologic examination is a part of the staging procedure. For example, in a study completed by the Gynecologic Oncology Group (GOG) involving patients who had operative staging, para-aortic lymph node metastasis was found in 5.6% of Stage Ib cases, 18.2% of Stage IIa, 32.8% in Stage IIb and 31.1% in Stage IIIb.[3]

TREATMENT

Surgery *Dysplasia and carcinoma in-situ* A number of techniques are available for the treatment of intraepithelial neoplasia.[4] The methods used include local excision, cryosurgery, laser surgery, electrocoagulation, conization and hysterectomy. In most clinics, patients with carcinoma in-situ who are over 35 and/or do not plan further childbearing are treated by total abdominal hysterectomy which entails removal of the uterus, upper vagina, tubes and ovaries.

Stage Ia Patients with microinvasive carcinoma are usually treated by simple extrafascial hysterectomy. However, if there is vascular space involvement, modified radical hysterectomy and pelvic lymphadenectomy are advised. Cases with more advanced disease are treated the same as Stage Ib cases.

Stages Ib and IIa In many institutions radical hysterectomy and bilateral pelvic lymphadenectomy is the preferred treatment for these Stages. In this operation the uterus, ovaries, fallopian tubes, upper vagina, the parametrial tissues and the pelvic lymph nodes are removed. The five year survival rate following surgery is 80-95%. Injury to the ureters is the most common complication seen in 2.5% of cases. The overall major complication rate is 10%. Surgery is particularly useful in young patients because the possible late effects of pelvic irradiation are avoided.

Stages IIb, IIIa and IIIb Patients in these Stages are not surgical candidates and are treated with RT.

Stage IVa and recurrent There are three operations used for selected patients with Stage IVa disease and some with locally recurrent disease postirradiation. Anterior exenteration involves removal of the uterus, ovaries, tubes, parametria and bladder. This procedure is used for patients with disease growing anteriorly into the bladder. In posterior exenteration the rectum is removed with the uterus and adnexal tissue and this operation is used for patients whose tumor extends into the rectum.

Total pelvic exenteration involves removal of the uterus, adnexa, bladder and rectum. It is indicated for patients whose tumor is so extensive that neither the bladder or rectum can be spared. The 5 year survival rate for patients undergoing pelvic exenteration is 20-25% and the surgical mortality rate is 10%.

Radiotherapy *Intracavitary brachytherapy* The first report of the successful use of radium for carcinoma of the cervix was by Margaret Cleaves in 1903. Initially, there was a shortage of radium which slowed its widespread use, but by the early 1920s many cases had been treated in Paris, Stockholm, New York and Baltimore to demonstrate that the method is potentially curative for many patients.

Two intracavitary systems, each initiated in the second decade of the century and perfected over many years, have been widely used throughout the world. In each system radioactive sources are placed in the uterus and the upper vagina. However, the two systems differ in one important respect. The Stockholm method, developed at the Radiumhemmet in Stockholm, employs a relatively large quantity of radium applied for a short time, whereas, in the Paris method, initiated at the Curie Foundation in Paris, smaller quantities of material are applied for a longer period of time. The Paris method has been widely used in the U.S.

The Paris technique was perfected in two other institutions. The basic dosimetry of the system was developed in the 1930s at the Christie Hospital in Manchester, England and further improvements were made at the M.D. Anderson Hospital in Houston, Texas between 1945 and 1965. [5,6]

Sources Radium or cesium-137 can be used. A stock of 10 mg, 15 mg, 20 mg and 25 mg sources should be available. The physical length of the sources is 2.0-2.2 cm and the active length is 1.5 cm. The diameter of the sources is 2-3 mm. Radium sources are usually filtered with 0.5 or 1.0 mm of platinum, whereas the cesium sources are filtered with 0.5 mm of stainless steel.

Applicators A number of suitable applicators are available. However, it is important that afterloading methods be used. In afterloading, the applicators are placed into the patient in the operating room and the sources are loaded into the applicators after the patient returns to her room. The most widely used applicators are the Fletcher-Suit afterloading tandem and colpostats designed at the M.D. Anderson Hospital (Figure 23.1).[7]

The main advantage of afterloading is that there is no radiation exposure to operating room personnel. Another important advantage of afterloading is that it allows the radiotherapist to choose appropriate applicators and loadings based

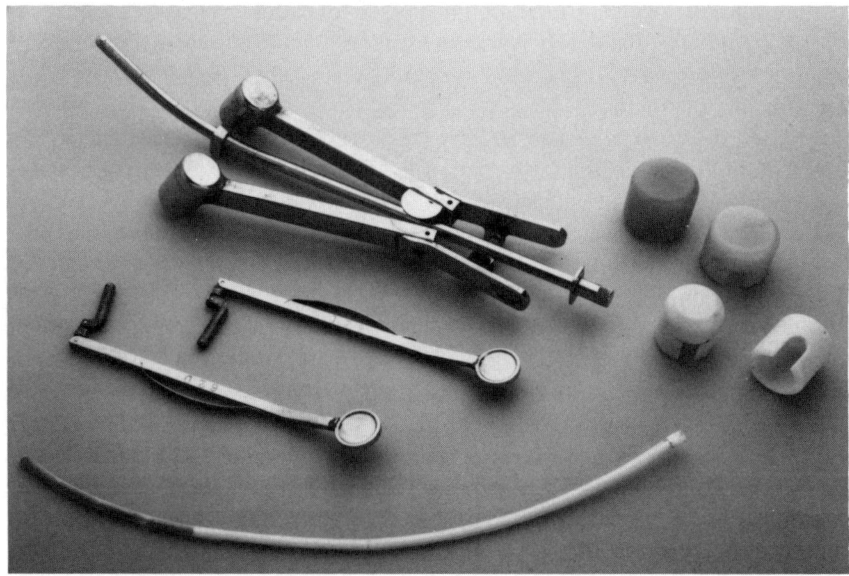

Figure 23.1 This is the Fletcher-Suit afterloading tandem and colpostat system. The tandem is shown in its proper position in relation to the colpostats. Also shown is the tandem insert containing four dummy sources, the two colpostat inserts and four colpostat covers. The covers are applied to the colpostats when medium-size or large colpostats are required.

on the clinical findings in the operating room and the appearance of the system on the post-application films.

The application In the operating room, the following procedures are carried out:

1) General anesthesia is administered
2) The patient is placed in the lithotomy position
3) A pelvic examination is carried out to assess the status of the tumor
4) The perineum and vagina are prepped and draped
5) A Foley catheter is placed into the bladder and the length of the uterine canal is measured with a uterine sound
6) The cervix is dilated
7) Stainless steel "seeds" are placed into the cervix at 12 and 6 o'clock to "mark" the position of the cervix for dosimetry films
8) The tandem is inserted into the uterus and colpostats into the vagina
9) Vaginal packing is used to hold the applicators in position

Loadings The standard loading for the tandem is 15-10-10 mg of radium or radium equivalents of cesium. The diameter of the colpostats can be varied according to the size of the vagina. The small colpostats, each 2.0 cm in diameter are loaded with 15 mg sources, the medium sized colpostats, 2.5 cm in diameter, are loaded with 20 mg sources; the large colpostats, 3.0 cm in diameter, are loaded with 25 mg sources.

Dose The dose is described in Gy at points A and B. Point A is located 2 cm up from the cervical os and 2 cm lateral to the cervical canal; point B is 3 cm lateral to point A. The basic protocol for combining external and intracavitary radiation is shown in Table 23.2. Two applications are carried out; each application is for 48 hours and each is separated by 2 weeks.

Table 23.2 Radiation doses for external and intracavitary therapy in cancer of the cervix

Stage	Whole pelvis dose (Gy)	Intracavitary (hours)	Point A (Gy)
Ib, IIa,IIb	40	48-2 weeks-48	40
IIIa, IIIb	50	48- 2 weeks-24-48	35
IVa	60	72	20-30
Massive	65-70	none	

Dosimetry Following the application, dummy sources are placed into the tandem and orthogonal films are taken (Figure 23.2). The adequacy of placement of the applicators in relation to the tumor is assessed. Contrast agents are placed into the bladder and rectum and the films are repeated. These films are used for preparation of computer generated isodose curves. From the isodose curves and films, the dose to points A and B (Figure 23.3) the bladder (point F),

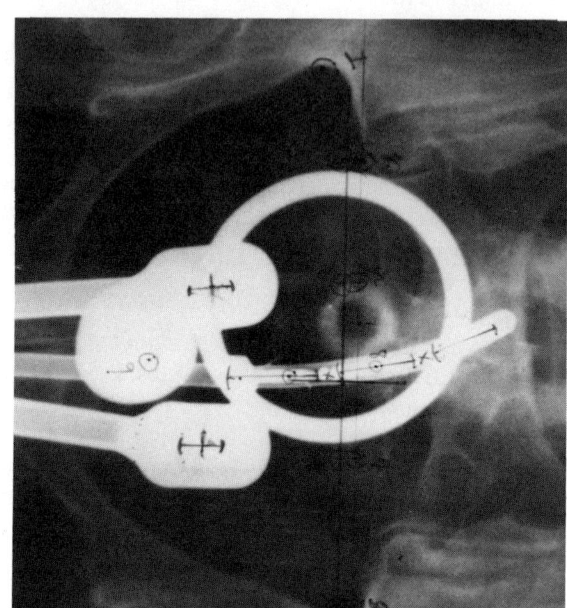

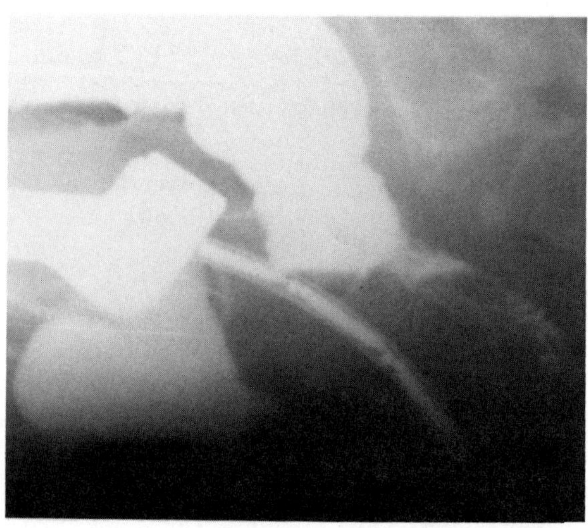

Figure 23.2 These orthogonal simulator films were taken following an intracavitary application for a patient with Stage II b carcinoma of the cervix. The film on the left is an anterior view showing the tandem containing 3 dummy sources and the colpostats. Also shown is a metal ring placed on the abdomen for film demagnification. The two small metallic seeds mark the position of the cervix. The lateral film on the right shows the tandem colpostat, the barium opacified rectum and the bladder with contrast material.

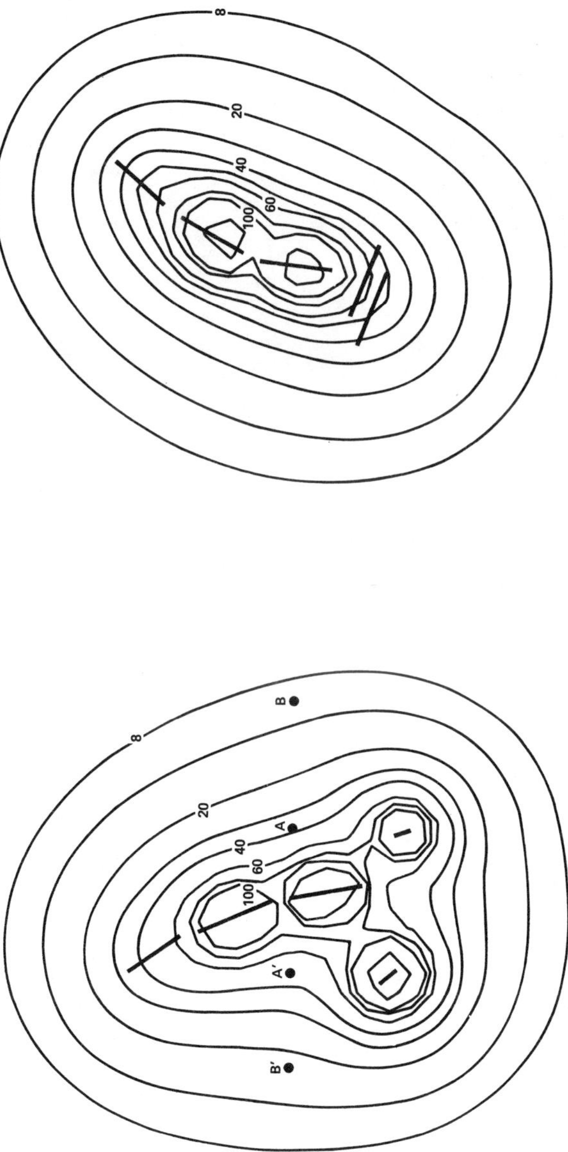

Figure 23.3 These are the isodose curves for the patient whose cesium films are shown in Figure 23.2. The dose at point A on the right was 22.27 Gy and at point 9, 7.87 Gy in 48 hours.

rectum (R1) and rectosigmoid (R2) are calculated (Figure 23.4).

<u>Patient care during implant</u>

1) The radiotherapist loads the sources in applicators and records time of start of application.

2) The physicist performs a survey of the patient's room and determines

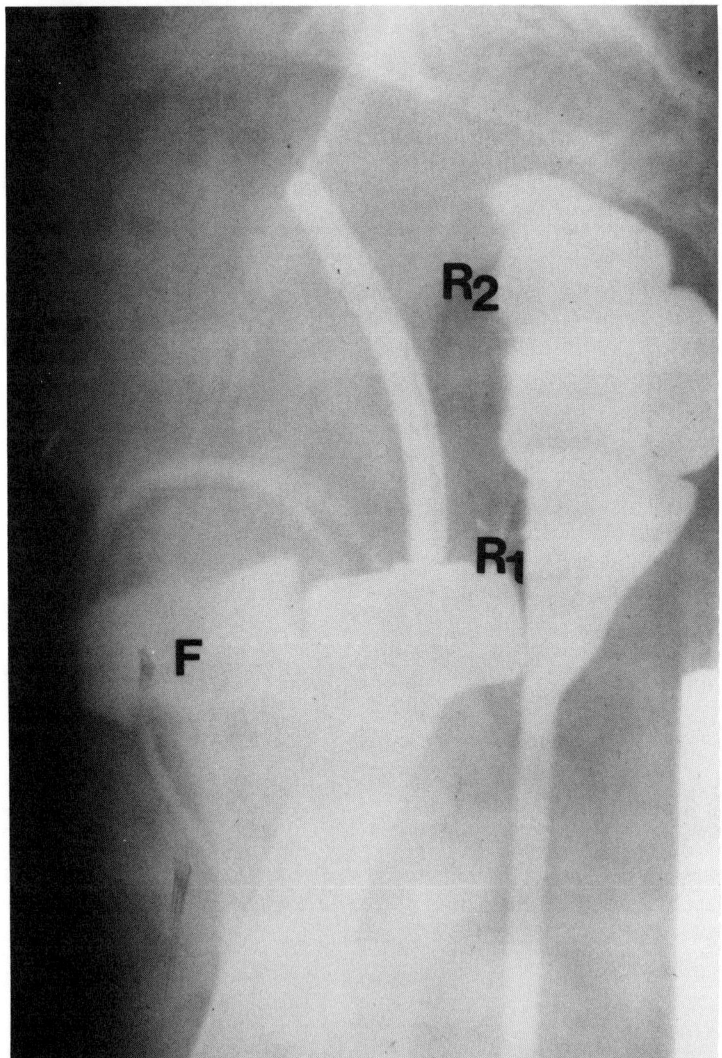

Figure 23.4 This lateral cesium simulator film demonstrates the F, R1 and R2 points used for calculation of the dose to bladder, rectum and rectosigmoid.

the time that nurses and visitors can safely remain in room.

3) The Foley catheter is allowed to drain continuously.
4) The patient is given heparin (anticoagulant) to prevent pulmonary emboli.
5) The patient remains supine during implant to prevent movement of applicators.
6) Temperatures and other vital signs are checked regularly. If the temperature becomes elevated to 39 degrees for 1-2 hours the applicators are removed.
7) At the completion of treatment sources and applicators are removed in the patients room. No anesthesia is required.

External whole pelvis irradiation In the 1920s it was realized that treatment results are superior if external beam therapy is added to the regimen. The external beam techniques in current use were worked out by Fletcher.[8] The portals cover the primary and upper vagina, the parametria and the external and common iliac lymph nodes (Figure 23.5). Radiation beams of 10-25 MV energy are used and isocentric techniques are preferred. Most patients can be treated with APPA portals but the four portal "box" technique is often used, particularly for large patients. All portals are treated each day.

Results Radiotherapy is potentially curative for patients in Stages Ib-IVa. Outstanding results have been reported from institutions throughout the world (Table 23.3).

Table 23.3 Survival in 1700 patients with cervical carcinoma treated with radiation at the M. D. Anderson Hospital

Stage	5 year survival (%)	10 year survival (%)
I	91.5	90.0
IIa	83.5	79.0
IIb	66.5	57.0
IIIa	45.0	39.5
IIIb	36.0	30.0
IVa	14.0	14.0

Extensive vaginal involvement Standard colpostats are unsuitable for patients with extensive vaginal involvement. Special lucite cylinders have been designed for this situation (Figure 23.6). One, two or three cylinders are placed on the tandem depending on the length of vagina involved and loaded with a line of sources.

Para-aortic metastasis When para-aortic lymph node metastasis are known to be present, the para-aortic region is irradiated in addition to the pelvis (45 Gy/

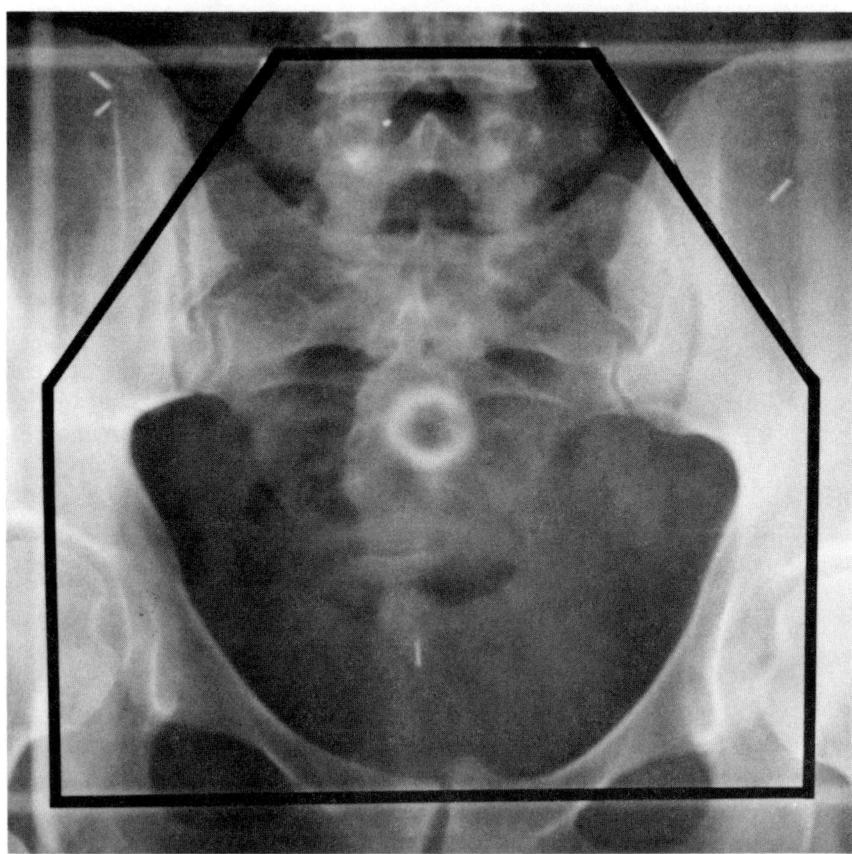

Figure 23.5 This simulator film demonstrates the volume treated in a patient with Stage IIB cancer. Opposing anterior and posterior portals were used. The metallic clips in the right and left upper corners of the film mark the position of the ovaries. The ovaries had been repositioned at the time of exploratory laparatomy to allow them to be shielded during RT. The metallic seed in the pelvis marks the position of the cervix.

5-6 weeks) (Figure 23.7). Thirty percent of patients with para-aortic metastasis survive at least 5 years following RT with the extended field technique.[9]

Postoperative radiotherapy A number of non-randomized studies suggest that treatment results are improved in patients found to have pelvic lymph node metastasis at the time of radical hysterectomy if postoperative whole pelvis RT (40-50 Gy/4-6 weeks) is given. Other pathologic findings, in addition to positive nodes, which are indications for postop RT are parametrial extension, positive resection margins, vascular invasion and deep invasion of the cervix to a depth of 70% or more of the cervical thickness.

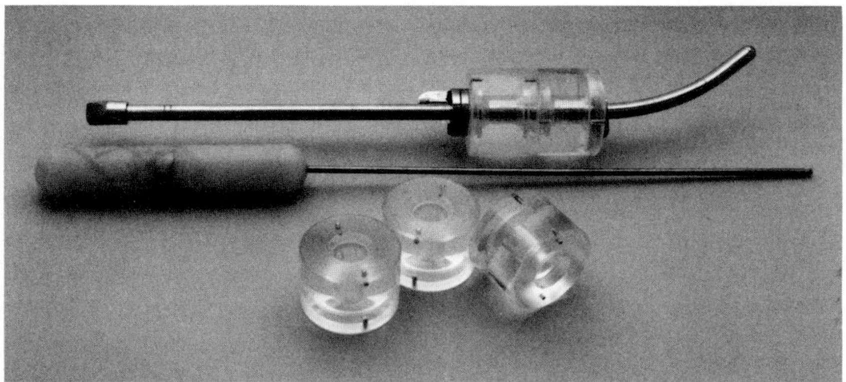

Figure 23.6 This is the Delclos afterloading tandem and vaginal cylinder system. It is used for patients whose disease extends down the vaginal walls.

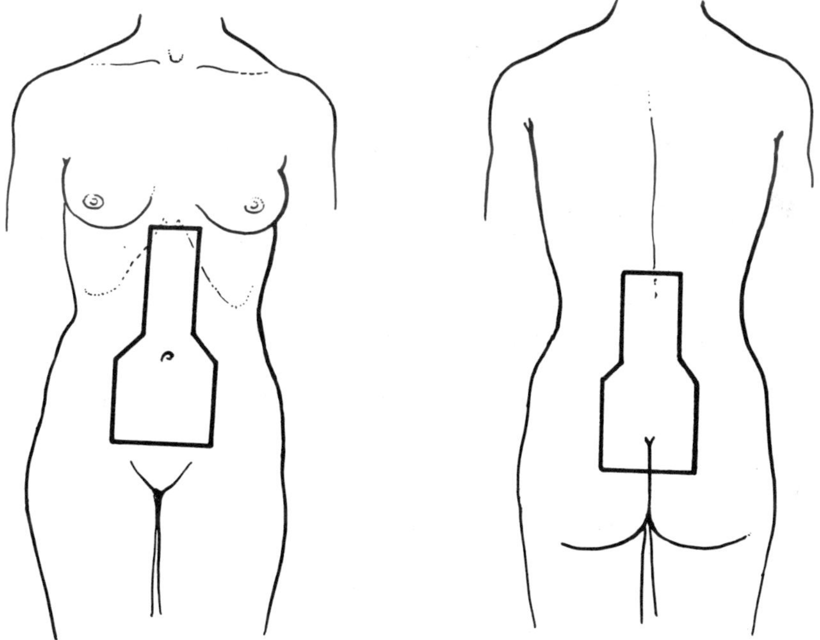

Figure 23.7 These are the portals for patients requiring RT to the pelvis and para-aortic region.

Supportive care <u>Vaginal hygiene</u> Douching with a solution of 1 tablespoonful of vinegar in a quart of warm water is prescribed during external therapy and following brachytherapy until the acute vaginal mucositis heals. After completion of treatment, sexual intercourse and daily use of a plastic vaginal dilator are prescribed to prevent vaginal adhesions.

<u>Diarrhea</u> Nearly all patients develop diarrhea after 2-3 weeks of external beam therapy due to the effect of radiation of the small bowel, large bowel and rectum. Lomotil, 1 or 2 tablet q 6 hours, is usually effective in controlling the symptoms.

<u>Nausea and vomiting</u> These symptoms are often seen during external beam therapy. Compazine 10 mg, 1 tid prn, is usually effective in controlling the symptoms.

<u>Dysuria</u> Acute radiation cystitis can cause burning and increased frequency of urination. These symptoms begin in the 2nd or 3rd weeks, but are usually not severe and can be controlled by encouraging fluid intake to produce dilution of urine.

<u>Nutrition</u> A well-balanced regular diet is recommended.

Complications of RT Curative RT for cervical carcinoma is a high dose technique carrying a significant risk of late complications. The severity of late effects are graded from 1-3.[10]

<u>Grade 1 injury</u>These cause minor symptoms responding to simple outpatient treatment. Mild radiation proctitis and cystitis are the most frequent grade 1 effects.

<u>Grade 2 injury</u> These cause symptoms with repeated occurrences often requiring hospitalization. Included are moderate radiation proctitis, rectal ulcer, chronic cystitis and partial small bowel obstruction.

<u>Grade 3 injury</u> These cause severe symptoms requiring surgery for correction. Included are rectovaginal fistula, bowel perforation, vesicovaginal fistula and hemorrhagic cystitis.

Ten per cent of patients develop grade 2 injury and 8% develop grade 3 injury.

Preservation of ovarian function In several centers, the ovaries are moved surgically to a lateral position in the pelvis (transposition) in young women with cervix carcinoma who are to undergo RT.[11] At the time of surgery, the new position of the ovaries is "marked" with metal clips. These can be seen by the radiotherapist on the simulator films allowing ovary shields to be made. In this way ovarian function is preserved following RT.

Interstitial brachytherapy Over the years, attempts to improve rates of local control and survival for patients with locally advanced disease through the use of interstitial implants have been made. The most popular current method involves the use of iridium-192 implanted transperineally through a specially designed template.[12]

Remote afterloading In a number of institutions, a machine called the Cathetron is used to deliver intracavitary treatment. This machine allows the uterine and vaginal sources to be loaded by remote control.[13] This greatly reduces radiation exposure to medical and nursing staff. Furthermore, the need for hospitalization is eliminated because high-intensity sources are used and therefore, the treatment time is reduced to only a few minutes.

Chemotherapy The results of chemotherapy for recurrent and disseminated carcinoma of the cervix are discouraging. Currently, the most active drug is cisplatin which produces responses of short duration in 50% of patients. Other active drugs are doxorubicin, bleomycin, vincristine, mitomycin C, methotrexate and cyclophosphamide. Combination chemotherapy is under investigation.

Chemotherapy has also been used in combination in attempt to improve local control rates in advanced disease. In a clinical trial as reported by the Gynecologic Oncology Group (GOG), the progression-free internal and survival were significantly improved in Stage IIIb and IVa cases treated with hydroxyurea combined with RT compared to RT alone.[14]

CANCER OF THE ENDOMETRIUM

ETIOLOGY AND EPIDEMIOLOGY

Endometrial carcinoma is the most common malignancy of the female genital tract. The disease was diagnosed in 1990 in 33,000 women and was the cause of death in 4,000. The incidence of the disease has been increasing since 1920. Endometrial cancer occurs primarily in postmenopausal women and the average age at diagnosis is 58 with a peak incidence at age 70.

Diseases associated with increased risk include obesity, hypertension, diabetes and infertility. An increasing amount of data suggests that estrogen stimulation of the endometrium is a major factor in etiology. Endometrial hyperplasia and cancer can be produced in experimental animals by estrogen administration. Furthermore, these diseases occur more commonly in women who take estrogen for contraception or postmenopausal symptoms.

PATHOLOGY

Most malignant tumors of the endometrium are adenocarcinomas, but adenosquamous, clear cell and squamous carcinomas and adenocanthomas also occur. Sarcomas of the uterus can arise from the endometrium or myometrium. Sarcomas of the myometrium are leiomyosarcomas, whereas, endometrial sarcomas can arise from endometrial stroma (stromal sarcoma) or a mixture of stromal and epithelial elements (mixed mesodermal sarcoma).

Adenocarcinomas evolve either from endometrial hyperplasia, an endometrial polyp or they may arise de novo. Hyperplasia of the endometrium is a spectrum of benign proliferative alterations in the epithelium which may eventually become malignant. The spectrum includes cystic hyperplasia, adenomatous hyperplasia and atypical hyperplasia. The risk of developing carcinoma increases respectively with each of these stages. The premalignant changes are reversible, but once carcinoma develops the process is no longer reversible.

Initially, adenocarcinomas grow slowly, producing a mass which fills the endometrial cavity but eventually invasion of the myometrium and extension to the cervix occurs. Metastasis to pelvic and para-aortic lymph nodes and the lungs is seen late in the course of the disease. Peritoneal metastasis by spread through the fallopian tubes or from uterine surface is also a late manifestation. Metastasis to the submucosal lymphatic vessels of the upper vagina is common.

The grade of the tumor is a major determinant in the biology of endometrial carcinoma. Grade 1 tumors are less likely to invade the myometrium or metastasize to regional lymph nodes, whereas grade 3 tumors frequently invade deeply into the myometrium and metastasize to regional lymph nodes. The tumor grade and depth of myometrial invasion correlate with prognosis and these two factors influence treatment.

DIAGNOSIS AND STAGING

Symptoms The presenting symptom in over 90% of cases is postmenopausal vaginal bleeding.

Pelvic examination The uterus may be enlarged.

Fractional curettage The usual method of obtaining tissue is by fractional curettage; tissue specimens are taken from the endocervical canal and the endometrial cavity and sent separately for histologic examination.

Staging The FIGO classification is seen in Table 23.4. The staging system is clinical and the findings at surgery cannot be used to change the Stage. Seventy-five percent of patients have clinical Stage I disease. The finding of cancer in the endocervical curettage puts the patient into Stage II. In Stage III there is involvement of the vagina or spread to the parametrium which can be detected at the time of pelvic examination.

The incidence of metastasis to pelvic and para-aortic lymph nodes increases with increasing penetration of tumor into the myometrium (Table 23.5) and with increasing stage.

TREATMENT

Surgery Standard treatment for the majority of patients with adenocarcinoma or sarcoma in clinical Stage I and II is total abdominal hysterectomy and bilateral salpingo-oophorectomy (TAH-BSO). This operation is performed through an abdominal incision. In some institutions, peritoneal cytology (collection of washings from the pelvis for cytology) and lymph node sampling (removal of

Table 23.4 FIGO staging classification for endometrial carcinoma[15]

Stage	Definition
0	Carcinoma in- situ
I	Tumor confined to corpus
	Ia Uterine cavity 8 cm or less in length
	Ib Uterine cavity more than 8 cm in length
II	Tumor invades cervix but does not extend beyond uterus
III	Tumor extends beyond uterus but not outside true pelvis
IVa	Tumor invades mucosa of bladder or rectum and/or extends beyond true pelvis
IVb	Distant metastasis

Table 23.5 Correlation of depth of myometrial penetration with incidence of lymph node metastasis in clinical Stage I[16]

Depth of invasion	%(+) pelvic nodes	%(+) para-aortic nodes
Endometrium only	1.3	1.7
Superficial muscle	2.7	0.6
Intermediate muscle	1.4	3.6
Deep muscle	28.4	17.1
Mean % of all cases	6.6	4.4

several pelvic and para-aortic lymph nodes for histologic study) is also carried out.

Radiotherapy in Stage I *RT alone* Outstanding results have been reported from the Radiumhemmet following intracavitary brachytherapy alone or combined with external beam therapy.[12] In the Stockholm method, metal capsules containing radium tubes are inserted into the endometrial cavity in a procedure known as the Heyman packing technique. Results obtained at the Radiumhemmet are shown in Table 23.6. The Heyman packing technique has not found wide acceptance in the U.S. because results of treatment by this method are inferior to those reported with surgery.

Postoperative RT The role of adjuvant RT in Stage I endometrial carcinoma is controversial. Evaluation of the possible benefits of RT is hampered by a lack of appropriate randomized trials. However, nonrandomized data suggest that adjuvant RT is of value primarily in grade 3 tumors and those deeply infiltrating the myometrium. Currently, one of the most popular techniques is postoperative whole pelvis irradiation.

The need for postop RT is based on a careful pathologic study of the surgical specimen. Whole pelvis RT (40-50 Gy/4-6 weeks) is recommended in

Stage I if: 1) the lesion is grade 3; 2) there is myometrial invasion to a depth of greater than 1/3 of the thickness of the myometrium; 3) there is extension to the cervix and 4) there is metastasis to tubes and/or ovaries. Retrospective studies suggest that the incidence of vaginal recurrence is <5% with postop RT, but have not shown that the survival rate is improved. [18]

Preop RT Treatment results are excellent with preop whole pelvis RT. In one study, the actuarial 12 year survival rate for Stage I cases was 95% following 35Gy to the whole pelvis followed in 1-2 weeks by surgery.[19]

Intracavitary brachytherapy In some institutions, intracavitary brachytherapy is preferred for adjuvant RT. Intracavitary treatment can be given pre-or postoperatively. If preop treatment is given, the Heyman packing technique or

Table 23.6 Radiotherapy alone for endometrial carcinoma at the Radiumhemmet [17]		
Stage	**No. Treated**	**5 year survival rate**
I	197	71%
II	105	53%
III	70	19%
IV	35	6%

afterloading tandem and colpostats are the methods most often used. If postop brachytherapy is preferred vaginal cylinders of afterloading colpostats can be used.

Radiotherapy in Stage II Preoperative RT is the standard treatment for patients with Stage II disease. Treatment consists of whole pelvis RT (40-50 Gy) plus 1 intracavitary tandem and colpostat application followed in 4-6 weeks by TAH-BSO. In one study, a 5 year survival rate of nearly 80% was achieved for patients with Stage II disease following preop RT and surgery.[20]

Radiotherapy in Stage III Patients found to have Stage II disease at the time of TAH-BSO usually receive whole pelvis RT. In one recent report, the 5 year survival rate was 44% for patients in Stage III following postop RT.[21]

Endocrine therapy Endometrial cancer is an endocrine responsive tumor. Progestational agents such as Provera, Megase and Delalutin are used in the treatment of patients with recurrent or advanced disease; 20-40% of patients experience an objective response. Endocrine therapy is ineffective in uterine sarcomas.

Chemotherapy Cytotoxic agents are used for patients who fail progesterone therapy. Doxorubicin is the most active agent producing objective responses in 35-40% of cases. Cyclophosphamide and 5-FU are also active. Combination chemotherapy is under study.

Uterine sarcomas Uterine sarcomas are rare and account for only 1-3% of uterine malignancies. Surgery is the initial treatment of choice. The role of RT is ill-defined, but recent studies suggest that postop whole pelvis RT improves 5 year local control and survival rates. The 5 year survival rate for Stage I cases treated by surgery and postop RT is about 60%.[22]

CANCER OF THE OVARY

ETIOLOGY AND EPIDEMIOLOGY

Cancer of the ovary is the fourth leading cause of death from cancer among women in the U.S. Approximately 20,500 new cases were diagnosed in 1990 and 12,400 patients died of ovarian cancer. The incidence has more than doubled since 1930. Mortality rates rise sharply after age 40 and the average age at diagnosis is 50. The disease is more common among unmarried women and married nulliparous women.

Among countries, the disease is uncommon in Japan and Chile and most common in the Scandinavian countries. The etiology of ovarian carcinoma is unknown and no environmental factors have been identified. Recent studies suggest that the use of oral contraceptives has a protective effect against the disease.

PATHOLOGY

Ovarian neoplasms are classified according to their tissue of origin. Ninety-five percent of malignant ovarian tumors are epithelial in origin and arise from the peritoneum of the ovary. Serous cystadenocarcinoma is the most commonly occurring carcinoma in this group. Germ cell tumors originate from oogonia or oocytes. Malignant teratoma and dysgerminoma are the most commonly occurring malignant germ cell tumors. Malignant tumors arising from the ovarian stroma include granulosa-theca cell tumors and other rare tumors. The common malignant ovarian tumors and their relative frequencies are shown in Table 23.7

Malignant ovarian tumors spread primarily by the transperitoneal route. Frequent sites of tumor cell implantation include the surfaces of the omentum, sigmoid colon, cecum and terminal ileum. Spread of tumor cells in peritoneal fluid of the undersurface of the diaphragm results in obstruction of lymphatic vessels of the diaphragm leading to ascites, a characteristic feature of ovarian cancer.

Lymphatic metastasis to para-aortic lymph nodes is common but hematogenous dissemination does not occur until late in the disease course. As abdominal metastases grow there is progressive interference with gastrointestinal function which leads to cachexia and bowel obstruction. In most patients, death occurs because of progressive intra-abdominal tumor growth.

DIAGNOSIS AND STAGING

Symptoms Ovarian cancer does not cause symptoms until the disease is

Table 23.7 Relative frequency of common cell types of malignant ovarian tumors

Cell type	Frequency (%)
Serous crystadenocarcinoma	40
Endometroid carcinoma	15
Undifferentiated adenoma	15
Mucinous cystadenocarcinoma	12
Clear cell carcinoma	6
Granulosa-theca cell	5
Metastatic carcinoma	5
Malignant teratoma	1
Dysgerminoma	1

advanced. Common symptoms include lower abdominal pain, abdominal distention and discovery of an abdominal mass.

Physical examination The presence of a palpable adnexal mass in a postmenopausal patient suggests ovarian cancer and demands investigation. Also, the presence of ascites and or abdominal masses suggest advanced malignancy.

Radiographic studies Ultrasonography and computed tomography can be helpful in distinguishing a simple cystic structure from a solid tumor.

Laparoscopy In this technique, a scope is inserted through a small abdominal incision. This allows the pelvic structures to be visualized. The method is useful in evaluating ovarian enlargement in patients suspected of having a mass on pelvic examination.

Laparotomy Most patients suspected of having a benign or malignant ovarian neoplasm have an exploratory laparotomy. The diagnosis is established by histologic study of removed tissue.

Staging The FIGO staging classification for ovarian cancer is shown in Table 23.8. Clinical studies used in staging include palpation, inspection, colposcopy, endometrial curettage, hysterography, hysteroscopy, cystoscopy, proctoscopy, intravenous pyelography, chest x-ray and skeletal x-rays. Laparoscopic findings can be used in patients who do not undergo laparotomy.

TREATMENT

Surgery There is a wide range of aggressiveness among ovarian carcinomas. Low-grade tumors of borderline malignant potential behave much less aggressively than frankly malignant tumors. This discussion concerns the treatment of aggressive ovarian carcinomas.

The findings at the time of exploratory laparotomy determine the operative

Table 23.8 FIGO staging classification for cancer of the ovary

Stage		Definition
I		Tumor limited to ovaries
	Ia	Tumor limited to one ovary; capsule intact, no tumor on ovarian surface
	Ib	Tumor limited to both ovaries; capsules intact, no tumor on ovarian surface
	Ic	Tumor limited to one or both ovaries with any of the following: capsule ruptured, tumor on ovarian surface, malignant cells in ascites or peritoneal washing
II		Tumor involves one or both ovaries with pelvic extension
	IIa	Extension and/or implants on uterus or tubes
	IIb	Extension to other pelvic tissues
	IIc	Pelvic extension with malignant cells in ascites or washings
III		Tumor involves one or both ovaries with microscopically confirmed peritoneal metastasis outside the pelvis and/or regional lymph node metastasis
	IIIa	Microscopic peritoneal metastasis
	IIIb	Macroscopic peritoneal metastasis 2 cm or less in diameter
	IIIc	Peritoneal metastasis more than 2 cm in diameter and/or regional lymph node metastasis
IV		Distant metastasis

procedure to be carried out. A systematic exploration of the abdomen by inspection and palpation is important in determining disease extent. Specimens are taken for cytologic study and suspicious lesions are biopsied.

The basic principle of surgery for ovarian cancer is primary and all metastasis should be removed if possible. A number of studies have shown that survival is best in patients in whom all, or nearly all, of possible tumor is removed. Therefore, surgeons must be aggressive in attempting to resect as much tumor as possible. Whenever possible, the involved ovary, the uterus, the fallopian tubes and the opposite ovary are removed.

"Second-look" laparotomy A small number of patients treated with chemotherapy for advanced ovarian carcinoma experience a complete response which is sustained for many months. In these, a "second-look" laparotomy is carried out. If no cancer is found chemotherapy is discontinued. If tumor is found, it can occasionally be removed. Five year survivals as high as 80% have been reported for patients having a negative "second-look".

Chemotherapy Ovarian carcinoma is responsive to chemotherapy and a small number of patients are cured by this treatment. For this reason, in many clinics chemotherapy has replaced radiotherapy as the primary treatment following surgery for patients in all stages. Alkylating agents such as melphalan, cyclophosphamide, chlorambucil and thiotepa are active drugs when used as single agents, but doxorubicin, cisplatin, 5-FU, and hexamethylmelamine also have significant activity.

Recent studies suggest that combination therapy is superior to single agents producing objective responses in 60-90% of cases. For example, a frequently used regimen, known as HexaCAF (Hexamethylmelamine, cyclosphosphamide, methotrexate and 5-FU) produces objective responses in 75% of cases.

Radiotherapy Postop RT has been used for many years in the management of epithelial cancers of the ovary. Unfortunately, the efficacy of RT has never been established in adequate clinical trials. Nevertheless, several techniques are used and these will be briefly described.

Whole pelvis RT In the past, pelvic RT (45 Gy/5 weeks) was considered to be adequate postop therapy for patients with Stage I ovarian carcinoma. However, a clinical trial completed by the GOG suggests that RT alone may not be adequate.[23] In this study, patients with Stage I disease were randomized to receive pelvic RT alone or RT + melphalan. With a median follow-up of 36 months, 30% of patients in the RT alone group had developed recurrence versus only 6% in the combined treatment group, a statistically significant difference.

Radionuclide therapy In some institutions, the policy is to place radionuclides into the abdominal cavity following surgery to treat the peritoneal surfaces in patients with epithelial carcinoma, Stages I and II. Radioactive colloidal gold-198 and phosphorus-32 are the agents used most frequently. P-32 is the isotope currently in favor.[24] Radioactive P-32 is a beta emitting isotope having a half-life of 14.3 days and a mean beta energy of 0.69 MeV.

External whole abdominal therapy with large, open portals. The entire abdomen can be irradiated with large opposing anterior and posterior portals. Thirty Gy in 5-6 weeks can be given if the liver and kidneys are adequately shielded. The kidneys are shielded with 2 half-value layers (HVL) of lead during treatment of the posterior portal and the right lobe of the liver with 1 HVL during treatment of the anterior and posterior portals. Additional treatment to the pelvis (20 Gy/2 weeks) is often given prior to or following whole abdominal irradiation.

Moving strip technique The second technique used for whole abdominal irradiation is the moving strip technique (Figure 23.8). This method was developed at the M.D. Anderson Hospital for use in ovarian cancer.[25] The technique allows delivery of a biologically more effective dose than is possible with the open field technique.

Transverse lines, 2.5 cm apart, are marked on the front and back of the

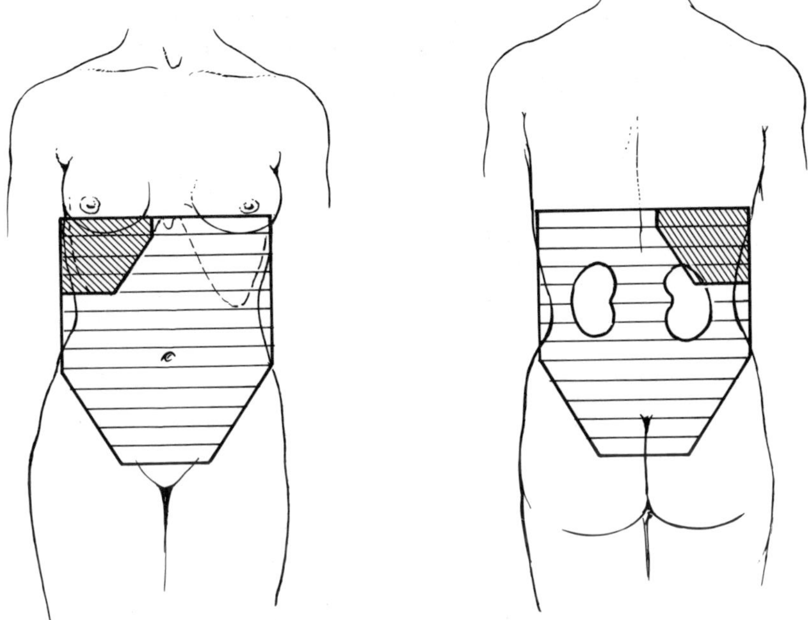

Figure 23.8 This is a diagrammatic illustration of the moving strip technique.

patient. On the first day, the lowest strip is irradiated and on subsequent days additional strips are added to the treatment volume until four strips (10 cm) are irradiated. Thereafter, the 10 cm strip is moved up by 2.5 cm each day until the final strip is reached. The volume is then reduced by one strip each day for the final four treatments. The kidneys are shielded from the posterior with 2 HVL of lead and the right lobe of the liver from the front and back with 1 HVL of lead.

Interest in whole abdominal irradiation for ovarian cancer waned for a number of years after two large clinical trials failed to show a survival advantage for patients treated with radiation compared to chemotherapy. In recent years, however, there has been a modest revival of interest in the moving strip technique, following the publication of the results of a clinical trial from the Princess Margaret Hospital in Toronto.[26]

Patients with Stage Ib, II and III disease received either moving strip irradiation (22.5 Gy) plus a pelvic boost (22.5 Gy) or whole pelvis irradiation (45 Gy) plus chemotherapy with chlorambucil. There was a significant survival benefit to the patients receiving the moving strip technique.

Combined modality therapy Recent reports involving small numbers of patients have evaluated combined modality therapy with surgery followed by chemotherapy and then second-look surgery followed by whole abdominal RT via the moving strip technique for patients with Stage I, II and III disease. [27]

Results Five year survival rates according to stage, for a large number of cases collected from a number of reports are shown in Table 23.9.

Table 23.9 Five year survival in ovarian carcinoma[28]

Stage	No. Patients	% 5 year survival
I	751	61
Ia	528	65
Ib	130	52
Ic	80	52
II	401	40
IIa	40	60
IIb	205	38
III	539	5
IV	101	3

Dysgerminoma This is a malignant germ cell tumor which deserves special consideration because of its marked radiosensitivity. Dysgerminomas occur predominantly in children and young women and account for only 1-2% of ovarian malignancies. Dysgerminomas are histologically similar to seminomas of the testis. In most cases the tumor is confined to one ovary, but about 10% of cases are bilateral and in 25% there is extension outside the ovary. Dysgerminomas differ from other ovarian malignancies in that they have a greater propensity to metastasize to regional lymph nodes and are less likely to spread intraperitoneally.

Dysgerminomas are treated by resection of the involved ovary, evaluation of the opposite ovary and careful palpation of pelvic and para-aortic lymph nodes.[29] Suspicious lymph nodes are biopsied. If the tumor is 10 cm in size or less and confined to one ovary no additional treatment is needed. In all other cases postop RT is indicated. Whenever possible, pelvic RT is limited to the hemipelvis on the side of the primary which allows the opposite ovary to be shielded.

The para-aortic lymph nodes are also irradiated and if para-aortic nodes are involved the mediastinal and left supraclavicular nodes are also irradiated. Tumor doses in the range of 20-25 Gy/2-3 weeks are sufficient with a boost of 5-10 Gy to sites of known lymph node metastasis or residual disease.

The prognosis depends on the extent of disease. Patients whose tumor is confined to the ovary have a 5 year survival rate of 90-95%. For those whose tumor has spread beyond the ovary the 5 year survival rate is 60-65%.

CARCINOMA OF THE VAGINA
ETIOLOGY AND EPIDEMIOLOGY

Primary malignant tumors of the vagina account for only 1-2% of gynecologic malignancies. The most common cell type, squamous cell carcinoma, occurs frequently in patients with a previous history of in-situ carcinoma of the cervix. In fact, squamous cell carcinomas of the cervix and vagina are epidemiologically similar in that they occur almost exclusively in sexually active women. The average age at onset is 62.

Epidemiologic studies have shown that adenocarcinomas of the vagina often develop in young women exposed in utero to diethylstilbestrol (DES). DES was given to the patients' mothers as treatment for vaginal bleeding during pregnancy. The average age at onset for DES related adenocarcinoma is 19.

PATHOLOGY

Ninety percent of primary vaginal cancers are squamous cell carcinomas, 5% are adenocarcinomas and 1% malignant melanomas. Tumors of the upper vagina metastasize primarily to pelvic lymph nodes, whereas those originating in the lower 1/3 metastasize to inguinal lymph nodes.

STAGING

The FIGO staging classification for vaginal cancer is shown in Table 23.10.

Table 23.10 FIGO staging of carcinoma of the vagina	
Stage	**Definition**
0	Carcinoma in-situ
I	Tumor confined to vagina
II	Tumor invades paravaginal tissue but not to pelvic wall
III	Tumor extends to pelvic wall
IVa	Tumor invades mucosa of bladder or rectum and/or exends beyond true pelvis
IV b	Distant metastasis

TREATMENT

Vaginal carcinomas are treated by RT.[30] In-situ carcinomas can be treated by intracavitary brachytherapy alone. Vaginal cylinders are used to deliver 50-60 Gy to the surface of the vagina. Invasive tumors require external beam therapy to the primary site and regional lymph nodes followed by intracavitary brachytherapy with vaginal cylinders or interstitial brachytherapy with iridium-192.

Five year survival rates following RT for squamous cell carcinomas of the vagina are good. For example, in one study, 5 year survival rates were as follows: Stage 0, 89%, Stage I, 69%, Stage II, 68.9%, Stage III, 27%, and Stage IV, 0%.[31]

CANCER OF THE VULVA

ETIOLOGY AND EPIDEMIOLOGY

Malignant tumors of the vulva account for 3-5% of gynecological malignancies. Squamous cell carcinoma, the most common histologic type, usually occurs in postmenopausal women and the mean age at diagnosis is 61. Carcinoma of the vulva is often seen in association with chronic diseases of the vulva such as leukoplakia, kraurosis, condyloma acuminata and lichen sclerosis.

PATHOLOGY

Ninety percent of vulvar carcinomas are squamous cell carcinomas. Basal cell carcinomas, adenocarcinomas of the Bartholin's ducts and glands, malignant melanomas, sarcomas and verrucous carcinomas occur rarely on the vulva. The labia majora is the most common site of origin followed by the labia minora and the clitoris.

Squamous cell carcinomas tend to spread to adjacent structures such as the vagina, urethra and anus. They metastasize to regional lymph nodes in 40% of cases; metastasis to superficial inguinal lymph nodes occurs early with subsequent spread to femoral, deep inguinal and deep pelvis nodes. Hematogenous dissemination does not occur until late in the disease.

STAGING

The FIGO staging system is shown in Table 23.11.

TREATMENT

The standard treatment for carcinoma of the vulva is radical vulvectomy and bilateral inguinal lymphadenectomy. RT has not found a role in the treatment of vulvar carcinoma because of the limited tolerance of the vulvar tissues to radiation. However, there is great interest in developing techniques for combining radiation and surgery.

For example, the GOG completed a randomized trial comparing RT to the inguinal and pelvic lymphatic regions following radical vulvectomy and bilateral inguinal lymphadenectomy and patients with proven inguinal metastasis versus radical vulvectomy and bilateral inguinal lymphadenectomy plus deep pelvic lymph node dissection. There was a statistically significant improvement in survival for patients in the RT group with no increased morbidity.[32] Therefore, deep pelvic lymph node dissection is not required in patients with positive inguinal lymph nodes if pelvic RT is given.

The 5 year survival rate for patients with squamous cell carcinoma is 70% in Stage I, 50% in Stage II, 30% in Stage III and 10% in Stage IV.

Table 23.11 FIGO classification of carcinoma of the vulva

Stage	Definition
O	Carcinoma in -situ
I	Tumor confined to the vulva; 2 cm or less in diameter. No clinically suspicious nodes.
II	Tumor confined to vulva; more than 2 cm; no clinically suspicious nodes
III	Tumor of any size with 1) spread to lower urethra and/or vagina, the perineum or the anus and/or 2) nodes in one or both groins clinically suspicious for metastasis
IV	Tumor of any size with 1) infiltration of bladder mucosa and/or upper urethra and/or rectum and/or 2) fixed to bone and/or 3) fixed or ulcerated nodes in one or both groins 4) distant metastasis

CARCINOMA OF THE FALLOPIAN TUBE

Primary cancer of the fallopian tube is a rare disease accounting for only 0.1% of gynecologic malignancies. The average age at diagnosis is 55. Most are adenocarcinomas. Hysterectomy and bilateral salpingo-oophorectomy is the treatment and postop RT to the pelvis is usually given. The 5 year survival rate for cases limited to the tube (Stage I) is 68%; for cases with extension to adjacent organs (Stage II), 39% and for cases with intra-abdominal spread (Stage III), 21%.[3]

CARCINOMA OF THE URETHRA

Primary carcinoma of the urethra is very rare accounting for less than 0.2% of gynecologic malignancies. Most carcinomas of the distal urethra are squamous cell carcinomas, whereas proximal urethral carcinomas are usually transitional cell or adenocarcinomas. Radiotherapy may have a role in treatment. A combination of external beam and interstitial techniques is usually required.[34]

TROPHOBLASTIC NEOPLASIA

ETIOLOGY AND EPIDEMIOLOGY

Gestational trophoblastic growth occurs in three forms; normal placenta, hydatidiform mole and choriocarcinoma.[30] Hydatidiform mole is an abnormal conceptus in which the villi develop abnormally as grape-like cystic structures without membranes or embryo. If there is associated anaplasia of the trophoblast and an absence of villi, the disease is called choriocarcinoma.

The incidence of hydatidiform mole in North American and Europe is 1 in 2,000 pregnancies. Only 10-20% of patients with hydatidiform mole develop trophoblastic neoplasia and, of these, only 3-5% develop choriocarcinoma.

The incidence of gestational trophoblastic neoplasia varies greatly throughout the world. The disease occurs 7-10 times more frequently in the Far East and Southeast Asia than in Europe and North America. The etiology of the disease is unknown but nutritional and socioeconomic factors may be involved in some cases. For example, in one epidemiologic study from the Philippines, poor women whose diet consisted mainly of fish and rice had a higher incidence of the disease than wealthier women who consumed greater quantities of red meat.

PATHOLOGY

Tumors of the placenta are unique in that they are derived from fetal tissues. There is a wide range of aggressiveness of trophoblastic growth. Three distinct clinical entities are recognized including hydatidiform mole, invasive mole and choriocarcinoma. The production of human chorionic gonadotropin (HCG) is a characteristic of each of them. In 5-10% of hydatidiform moles the abnormal villi invade into the myometrium and are called invasive mole. In about 3-5% of hydatidiform moles a highly malignant choriocarcinoma develops. Choriocarcinomas can also develop following normal pregnancy, abortion or ectopic pregnancy.

Choriocarcinomas have a great tendency to spread hematogenously and the lungs are the most common site. The brain, liver, ovary and vagina are also common sites.

DIAGNOSIS

Trophoblastic tumors can present with a wide range of symptoms and signs. Abnormal vaginal bleeding simulating threatened abortion is the most common sign. Occasionally, patients present with evidence of distant metastasis. The diagnosis is based on serum HCG determinations, radiographic studies such as pelvic ultrasound and histologic study of removed tissue.

TREATMENT

Hydatidiform moles are treated by evacuation of the uterine cavity by suction curettage. All patients with invasive mole and choroiocarcinoma are treated with chemotherapy. Choriocarcinoma was the first malignant tumor proven to be curable with chemotherapy. Methotrexate was the drug originally used but actinomycin D is equally effective.

Patients with favorable prognostic features include those with a history of a recent hydatidiform mole and a diagnosis of malignant trophoblastic disease based on perisistent HCG elevation, with no detectable tumor or with tumor confined to the pelvis and vagina or with only minimal metastatic disease in the lungs. A cure rate of nearly 100% can be expected in these patients following single agent chemotherapy with methotrexate or actinomycin D.

Patients with brain and/or liver metastasis are in the unfavorable group. They are treated with triple chemotherapy (methotrexate, actinomycin D and chlorambucil) + radiotherapy. The whole brain is given 30 Gy/3 weeks and the liver 20 Gy/2-3 weeks. Fifty percent of patients with brain and/or liver metastasis achieve a complete remission following chemotherapy and RT and the cure for patients in this unfavorable group is 75%.

REFERENCES

1. Silverberg E, Boring CC, Squires TS. Cancer statistics, 1990, CA-A Cancer J for Clinicians 40:9-26, 1990.

2. Chapter 24, Cervix uteri, In A Manual for Staging of Cancer, Third Edition, Eds.Beahrs OH, Henson DE, Hutter RVP, Myers MH. J.B. Lippincott Company, Philadelphia, 1988, pp 151-53.

3. Lagasse LD, Creasman WT, Singleton HM, et al. Results and complications of operative staging in cervical cancer: Experience of the Gynecologic Oncology Group. Gynecologic Oncology 9:90-98, 1980.

4. Di Saia, PJ, Crasman WT. Chapter 1, Preinvasive disease of the cervix, vagina, and vulva, In Clinical Gynecologic Oncology, Second Edition, The C.V. Mosby Company, St. Louis, 1984, pp 1-44.

5. Paterson R. Chapter 20, The uterine cervix, In Treatment of Malignant Disease by Radiotherapy, 2nd Edition, Williams & Wilkins, 1963, pp 331-359.

6. Fletcher GH. Cancer of the uterine cervix, Janeway lecture, 1970, Am J Roentgen 111:225-242, 1971.

7. Suit HE, Moore EB, Fletcher GH, Worsnop R. Modification of Fletcher ovoid system for afterloading standard-sized radium tubes, Radiology 81:126-1341, 1963.

8. Fletcher GH, Calderon R. Positioning of pelvic portals for external irradiation in carcinoma of the uterine cervix, Radiology 67:359-369, 1956.

9. Podczaski E, Stryker JA, Kaminski P, et al. Extended field radiation therapy for carcinoma of the cervix, Cancer 66:251-258, 1990.

10. Perez CA, Breaux S, Madoc-Jones H, et al. Radiotherapy alone in the treatment of carcinoma of the uterine cervix II. Analysis of complications, Cancer 54:235-246, 1984.

11. Husseinzadeh N, Nahhas WH, Velkley DE, et al. The preservation of ovarian function in young women undergoing pelvic radiation therapy, Gynecologic Oncol 18:373-379, 1984.

12. Gaddis O, Morrow CP, Klement V, et al. Treatment of cervical carcinoma employing a template for transperineal interstitial Ir [192] brachytherapy, Int J Radiat Oncol Biol Phys 9:819-827, 1982.

13. Newman H, Jur B, James KW, Smith CW. Treatment of cancer of the cervix with a high-dose-rate afterloading machine (The Cathetron), Int J Radiat Oncol Biol Phys 9:931-937, 1983.

14. Hreshchyshyn MM, Aron BS, Boronow RC, et al. Hydroxyurea or placebo combined with radiation to treat Stages IIB and IV cervical cancer confined to the pelvis, Int J Radiat Oncol Biol phys 5:317-322, 1979.

15. Chapter 25, Corpus uteri, In Manual for Staging of Cancer, Third Edition, Beahrs OIH, Henson DE, Hutter RVP, Myers MN. J. B. Lippincott Company, Philadelphia, 198, pp 157-159.

16. Lewis GC, Bundy B. Surgery for endometrial cancer, Cancer 48:568-574, 1981.

17. Joelsson I, Sondri A, Kottmeier HL, Carcinoma of the uterine corpus, Acta Radiol Supp 334, Stockholm, 1973.

18. Torrisi JR, Barnes WA, Popescu G, et al. Postoperative adjuvant external-beam radiotherapy in surgical Stage I endometrial carcinoma, Cancer 64:1414-1417, 1989.

19. Ritcher N, Lucas WE, Yon JL, Sanford FG. Preoperative whole pelvis external irradiation in Stage I endometrial cancer, Cancer 48:58-62, 1981.

20. Prempree T, Patanaphan V, Salazar OM, et al. Influence of treatment and tumor grade on the prognosis of Stage II carcinoma of the endometrium, Acta Radiol Oncol 21: (Fasc 4) 225-229, 1982.

21. Danoff BF, McDay J, Louka, M, et al. Stage III endometrial carcinoma: Analysis of patterns of failure and therapeutic implications, Int J Radiat Oncol Biol Phys 6:1491-1495, 1980.

22. Salazar OM, Dunne ME. The role of radiation therapy in the management of uterine sarcomas, Int J Radiat Oncol Biol Phys 6:899-902, 1980.

23. Hreshchyshyn MM, Park RC, Blessing JA, et al. The role of adjuvant therapy in Stage I ovarian cancer, Am J Obstet Gynecol 138:139-145, 1980.

24. Julian CG, Inalsingh CHA, Burnett LS, et al. Radioactive phosphorus and external radiation as an adjuvant to surgery for ovarian carcinomas, Obstet & gynecol 52:155-160, 1978.

25. Delclos L, Braun EJ, Herrara Jr, et al. Whole abdominal irraidiation by cobalt-60 moving strip technique, Radiology 81:632-641, 1963.

26. Bush RS, Allt WEC, Beale FA, et al. Treatment of epithelial carcinoma of the ovary: Operation, irradiation and chemotherapy, Am J Obstet and Gynecol 127:692-704, 1977.

27. Fuks Z, Rizel S. Anteby SO, et al. The multimodal approach to the treatment of Stage III ovarian carcinoma, Int J Radiat Oncol Biol Phys 8:903-908, 1982.

28. Tobias JS, Griffiths CT. Management of ovarian carcinoma, N Engl J Med 294:818-823; 855-882, 1976.

29. Weinblatt ME, Ortega JA. Treatment of children with dysgerminoma of the ovary, Cancer 49:2608-2611, 1982.

30. Hoskins WJ, Perez CA, Young RC. Chapter 36, Gynecologic tumors, In Cancer-Principles & Practice of Oncology, 3rd Edition, Eds. DeVita VT, Hellman S, Rosenberg SA. J. B. Lippincott Company, Philadelphia, 1979, pp 1099-1161.

31. Brown GR, Fletcher GH, Rutledge RN, et al. Irradiation of "in-situ" and invasive squamous cell carcinoma of the vagina, Cancer 28:1278-1283, 1971.

32. Homesley HD, Bundy BN, Sedlis A, Adcock L. Radiation therapy versus pelvic node resection for carcinoma of the vulva with positive groin nodes, Obstet & Gynecol 68:733-740, 1986.

33. Denham JW, MacLennon KA. The management of primary carcinoma of the fallopian tube, Cancer 53:166-172, 1984.

34. Prempree T, Amoremarn R, Patanaphan V. Radiation therapy in primary carcinoma of the female urethra, Cancer 54:729-733, 1984.

Chapter 24

LYMPHOMAS AND LEUKEMIA

HODGKIN'S DISEASE

ETIOLOGY AND EPIDEMIOLOGY

Hodgkin's disease is a malignant disease of lymph nodes which was identified in 1832 by the English pathologist Thomas Hodgkin. The etiology of the disease is unknown but some of the clinical features of the disease suggest an infectious cause. In 1990 there were 7,400 new cases diagnosed in the U.S. and 1,600 persons died of the disease.[1] The disease is slightly more common in males (4:3).

The incidence of Hodgkin's disease increases throughout life but there are two age peaks. One peak occurs between ages 15 and 34 and the second after age 50. The reason for the bimodal age-specific incidence curve is unknown but it is possible that there are two etiologic factors, one operative in younger age groups and the other in older age groups.

PATHOLOGY

The pathologic diagnosis of Hodgkin's disease depends on the identification of characteristic giant cells called Reed-Sternberg (RS) cells in biopsied lymph nodes or other tissue.[2] RS cells have double or multiple large nuclei containing large nucleoli. In addition, there are a wide range of associated histologic findings including an inflammatory type of cellular proliferation and varying degrees of necrosis and fibrosis.

The most widely used histopathologic classification of Hodgkin's disease was adopted at a conference in Rye, New York in 1965 (Table 24.1).

The anatomic distribution of sites of involvement, the clinical age, manner of spread and prognosis varies according to the histopathologic type. The lymphocyte predominate type tends to involve a single lymph node group in the neck, presents in Stage I or II, spreads contiguously from one lymph node group to another and has good prognosis.

The nodular sclerosing type tends to involve lymph nodes in the anterior-superior mediastinum, the supraclavicular region and the lower neck. Nodular sclerosis most often presents in Stage I or II, tends to spread contiguously from one lymph node group to another and has a good prognosis.

The mixed cellularity and lymphocyte depletion types are seldom confined to a single site or region. They are more likely to present in Stage III or IV and

Table 24.1 The Rye histopathologic classification of Hodgkin's disease

Type	Features	Frequency	5 yr surv.
Lymphocyte predominate	Abundant lymphocytes and/or histiocytes; no necrosis	15%	90%
Nodular sclerosis	Nodules of lymphoid tissue separated by bands of collagen; Reed-Sternberg cells in clear spaces (lacunae)	45%	85%
Mixed cellularity	Numerous RS cells and % atypical mononuclear cells with mixutre of eosinophils, lymphocytes and fibroblasts	30%	70%
Lymphocyte depletion	RS cells and mononuclear cells, few lymphocytes, diffuse fibrosis and necrosis	10%	45%

there is often noncontiguous involvement of lymph node groups. Furthermore, there is often hematogenous dissemination to liver, lungs and bone marrow.

DIAGNOSIS

Symptoms The presenting symptom in 90% of cases is an abnormal lump, or mass. The mass is usually in the neck but axillary and inguinal lymph nodes can be involved initially. The mass is not tender or painful.

Patients with Hodgkin's disease often have constitutional symptoms such as fever, night sweats and weight loss. These symptoms, when present, adversely influence prognosis. Generalized pruritus (itching) is present in 10% of cases and may be the presenting symptom. The presence of pruritus has no effect on prognosis.

Physical examination A complete physical examination is required in every patient; particular attention is given to examination of lymph nodes in neck, axillae and groin. Involved lymph nodes typically are enlarged and firm and have a rubbery consistency. Palpation of the upper abdomen is important to assess the size of the liver and spleen which may be enlarged.

Biopsy The diagnosis of Hodgkin's disease is confirmed by excisional biopsy and histopathologic study of an involved lymph node.

STAGING

The most widely used staging classification was adopted at a workshop held in Ann Arbor, Michigan in 1971 (Table 24.2). The staging workup in all patients consists of chest x-ray, complete blood count, urinalysis and liver function studies. Bone marrow biopsies from the iliac crests are a routine part of the workup. Furthermore, one or more of the following studies are required to evaluate the liver, spleen and retroperitoneal lymph nodes including lymphangiography, CT scanning of abdomen, gallium scanning and exploratory laparotomy.

Lymphangiography In this technique, a radiopaque contrast agent, Lipiodol, is injected into a lymph vessel on the dorsal aspect of each foot. The contrast material is taken up by the pelvic and retroperitoneal lymph nodes allowing assessment of the size and architecture of the lymph nodes. The presence of Hodgkin's disease causes enlargement and an alteration of the architecture of the involved lymph node. Experienced radiologists report an overall accuracy of 90% in the detection of disease in retroperitoneal lymph nodes.

Table 24.2 Ann Arbor clinical staging classification of Hodgkin's disease

Stage	Definition
I	Involvement of a single lymph node region (I) or a single extralymphatic organ or site (I_E)
II	Involvement of two or more lymph node regions on the same side of the diaphragm (II) or localized involvement of an extralymphatic organ or site and one or more lymph node reigons on the same side of the diaphragm (II_E)
III	Involvement of lymph node regions on both sides of the diaphragm (II) which may be accompanied by involvement of the spleen (III_S) or by localized involvement of an extralymphatic organ or site (III_E) or both (III_{SE})
IV	Diffuse or disseminated involvement of one or more extralymphatic organs or tissues with or without associated lymph node involvement
	The presence or absence of fever, night sweats and/or unexplained loss of 10% or more of body weight in the six months preceding admission are noted by suffix letter B. If these symptoms are not present, the suffix letter A is used.

CT scanning This technique has become an important method for evaluating the liver, spleen and retroperitoneal lymph nodes in Hodgkin's disease. However, CT scanning is not as sensitive or as accurate as lymphangiography in detecting retroperitoneal lymph node involvement.

Gallium Scanning It has been shown that gallium-67 citrate is often taken up by lymph nodes involved with Hodgkin's disease. Therefore, gallium scanning is often useful in detecting disease in the chest and/or abdomen. However, this test is not as sensitive as lymphangiography in detecting retroperitoneal node involvement.

Staging laparotomy At the Stanford University Medical Center between 1961 and 1968, 65 patients with Hodgkin's disease underwent exploratory laparotomy and splenectomy. It was found that the spleen was involved in 1/3 of cases when splenic enlargement had not been detected clinically. A systematic study was then carried out in which liver biopsy, splenectomy, bone marrow biopsy and biopsies of retroperitoneal lymph node were performed on a consecutive series of patients. The findings of the original study were confirmed.

Exploratory laparotomy with splenectomy has become an accepted and widely practiced technique for evaluation of the abdomen in Hodgkin's disease. The findings are especially useful when clinical studies suggest early disease and consideration is being given to treating the patient with RT alone.

TREATMENT

Surgery Surgical resection is not a standard form of treatment for Hodgkin's disease. However, surgeons have a major role in preparing patients for treatment by performing biopsy in all patients and staging laparotomy in selected patients. In female patients who are to receive RT to the pelvis, surgeons perform oophoropexy. In this technique, which is usually performed at the time of staging laparotomy, the ovaries are moved from their normal position to a location behind the uterus or to a lateral position outside the pelvis. Oophoropexy allows the ovaries to be shielded during the RT thus preserving endocrine and reproductive function.

Chemotherapy An important milestone in cancer treatment was the development of combination chemotherapy for the curative treatment of Hodgkin's disease. The most successful and widely used combination was developed at the National Cancer Institute and is known as MOPP (mechlorethamine, vincristine, procarbazine and prednisone).[3] These agents are given in 2 week courses for 6 months with a 2 week rest interval between each course. Eighty percent of patients with Stage III and IV disease achieve a complete remission and of those achieving a complete remission, 68% are disease-free at 10 years.

A regimen which is equally effective is known as ABVD (doxorubicin, bleomycin, vinblastine and DTIC). This regimen, which was developed in Milan, Italy, produces complete remission in up to 60% of MOPP failures. Data from Milan suggests that superior results are seen with alternating courses of MOPP and ABVD in Stages III and IV than with either regimen alone.[4]

Radiotherapy It was known since the early 1900s that Hodgkin's disease is a radiosensitive tumor. Modern RT for the disease began in 1925 with the work of Gilbert (Geneva, Switzerland) who advocated large treatment portals covering lymph node groups and adjacent uninvolved areas. However, it was not until 1950, when Peters (Toronto, Canada) reported her data for patients treated with high doses, that the curative potential of RT was recognized. [5]

Finally, in the 1960s, Kaplan demonstrated that with modern megavoltage equipment curative doses could be administered to all potentially involved lymph node areas on both sides of the diaphragm.

The mantle technique This technique is used to irradiate the nodal regions above the diaphragm. The lymph nodes in both sides of the neck, both axillae and the mediastinum are irradiated with large opposing anterior and posterior portals. The lungs and most of the heart are shielded with individually con-structed shielding devices. The stops in treatment planning of the mantle are as follows:

1) The patient is placed in the supine position on the simulation table with hands on hips and chin extended.

2) The central axis of the beam is located at the suprasternal notch and the portal sizes are set to cover both sides of the neck, both axillae and the mediastinum. The portal size is 30 to 40 cm at a source skin distance of 100 to 120 cm. The upper border falls at the ear lobes and includes most of the mandible. The lower border falls at the xiphoid process of the sternum.

3) A simulator film is taken

4) The radiotherapist draws on the simulator film the outline of the lung shields (Figure 24.1).

5) The thickness of the tissue at the following points for use in computer dosimetry is measured: the right and left upper and lower neck, the right and left supraclavicular area, the right and left axillae, the SSD point and the upper, middle and lower mediastinum.

6) The above procedures are repeated with the patient in the prone position.

7) The dosimetrist prepares styrofoam templates for the lung shields (Figure 24.2).

8) Cerrobend is poured into the template (Figure 24.3) and allowed to cool (Figure 24.4).

9) The patient returns to the simulator room the next day. The lung shields are placed on the shadow tray and placed in position with the aid of the previous days simulation films.

10) The patient is placed in the treatment position and a film is taken to confirm the proper location of the shields. The skin is marked for the lung shields and for the shields for the larynx and humeral heads.

Inverted "Y" technique This technique is used to irradiate the lymph node regions below the diaphragm. The para-aortic, iliac, inguinal and femoral lymph nodes are irradiated with large opposing anterior and posterior inverted "Y" shaped portals. If the spleen requires irradiation, it is included in the treatment volume.

The inverted "Y" can be treated with large portals covering the a para-aortic, iliac, inguinal and femoral nodes or the treatment volume can be divided and

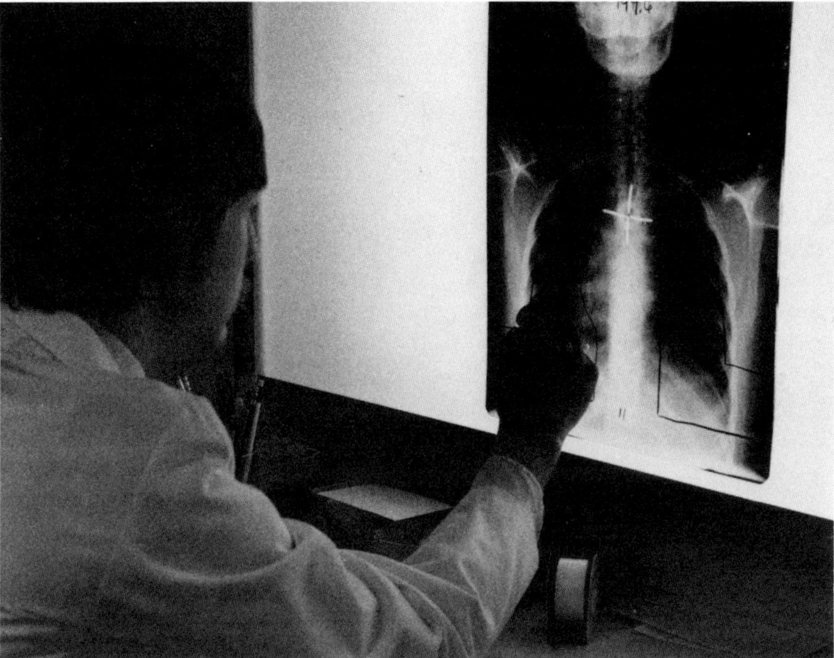

Figure 24.1 The radiotherapist outlines the lung shields on the simulator

treated in two separate courses. In this case, the para-aortic and splenic areas are treated initially followed by a 2 to 4 week rest before the pelvic lymph nodes are treated

Extended field technique This technique is used to irradiate the lymph node groups superior to the diaphragm (mantle) and the para-aortic lymph node+/- the spleen. Initially, the mantle is irradiated and following a 2 to 4 week rest, the para-aortic region, the splenic hilum and the spleen if present, are treated.

Total lymphoid technique This technique is used to irradiate all potentially involved lymph nodes on both sides of the diaphragm. Initially, the mantle is irradiated and, following a rest, the inverted "Y" is treated.

"Gap" calculation At the junction of the mantle and para-aortic portals in the extended field and total lymphoid techniques, it is important that there be a gap on the skin between the adjacent portals to prevent overlap on the spinal cord. The length of the required gap is calculated using the following formula: $s_1 = 1/2L_1$ (d/SSD); $s_2 = 1/2l_2$ (d/SSD; S. = $s_1 + s_2$ where s_1 and s_2 = portal "half-separation", S = portal separation, L_1 and L_2 = portal lengths, d = the specified depth beneath the skin at which the junction between the portals is to occur (usually the midline) and SSD = source-skin distance.[6]

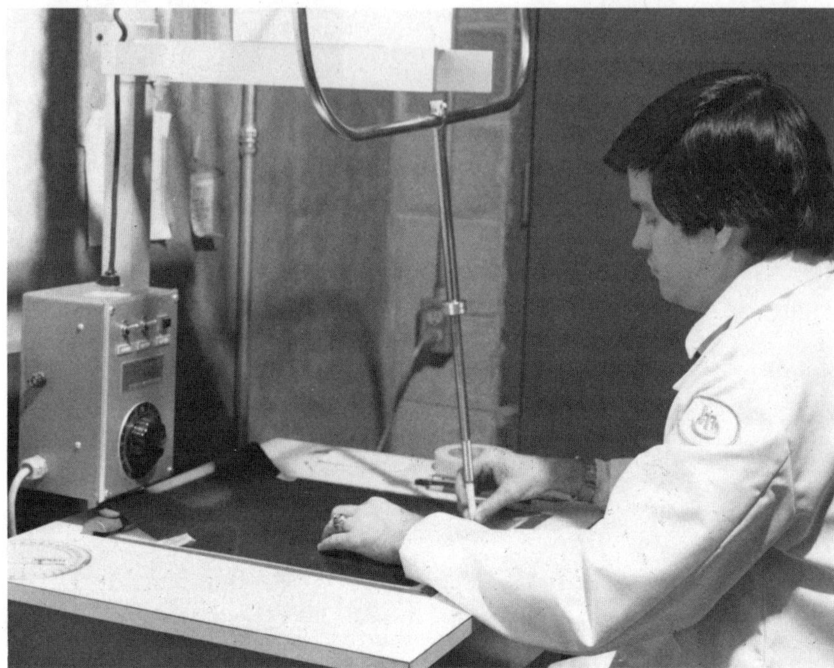

Figure 24.2 The dosimetrist uses a hot wire to cut a template in styrofoam.

Involved field technique In this technique, RT is given only to areas known to be involved with Hodgkin's disease. This technique is often used in combination with chemotherapy.

Dose Tumor masses to be treated with RT alone are given 40 to 44 Gy, whereas areas irradiated for microscopic disease receive 30 to 35 Gy. Daily tumor doses in the range of 1.5 to 2.2 Gy for 5 fractions per week are effective. When RT is given to involved portals, doses in the range of 25 to 30 Gy are sufficient.

Indications for various techniques Most authorities agree that extended field RT alone is the treatment of choice for the majority of patients in Stages IA and IIA. However, patients with large mediastinal masses occupying more than 1/3 of the transverse diameter of the chest have a high-risk of recurrence following RT alone. Therefore, these patients are given chemotherapy initially followed by involved field RT to the mediastinum.

Patients in Stages IB or IIB can be treated with extended field or total lymphoid RT alone or with chemotherapy + involved field RT. Stage IIIA associated can be treated with total lymphoid RT alone, or with chemotherapy + involved field RT. Stage IIIA cases are treated with total lymphoid RT alone,

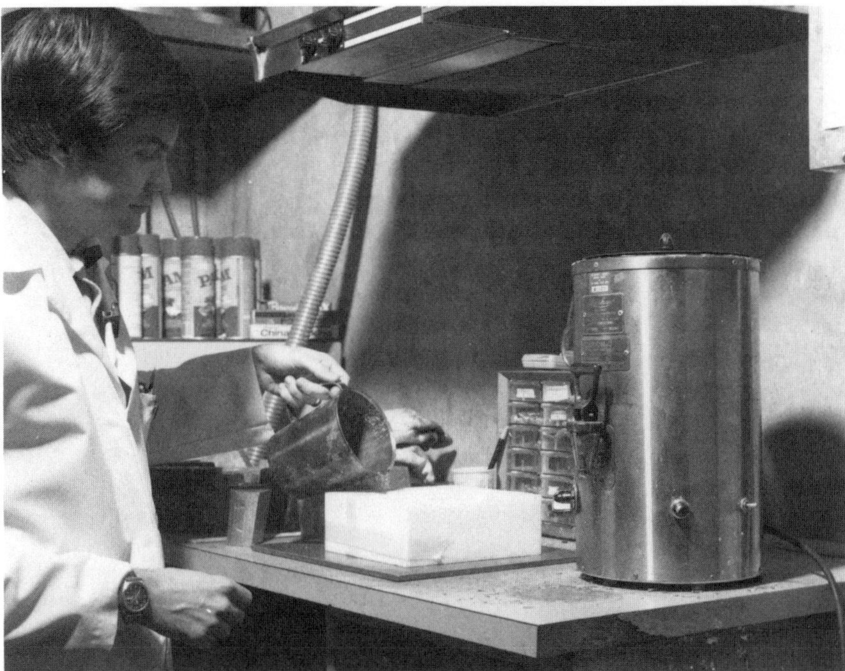

Figure 24.3 A low melting-point alloy of lead, called cerrobend, is poured into the template.

chemotherapy alone or chemotherapy and involved field RT. Patients in Stages IIIB, IVA or IVB usually receive chemotherapy alone.

Side-effects of RT <u>Mantle</u> Side-effects are commonly experienced by patients undergoing treatment to the mantle. Anorexia and fatigue are seen in all patients and many experience nausea and vomiting. Dryness of the mouth due to radiation effect on the salivary glands is often seen. For this reason patients should be evaluated by a dentist prior to the RT. The teeth should be in optimum condition and daily fluoride applications to prevent caries may be initiated.

Loss of taste develops in most patients due to the effect of radiation on the taste buds. Dysphagia develops in most patients after 2-3 weeks as a result of radiation esophagitis and pharyngitis. Mild pain medication and/or xylocaine viscous 2%, to be gargled and swallowed prior to meals is effective in relieving these symptoms.

All patients experience hair loss in the occipital area of the scalp and in the axillae. Erythema of the skin usually occurs in the neck near the completion of mantle RT.

<u>Extended fields and inverted "Y"</u> Anorexia, nausea and vomiting are

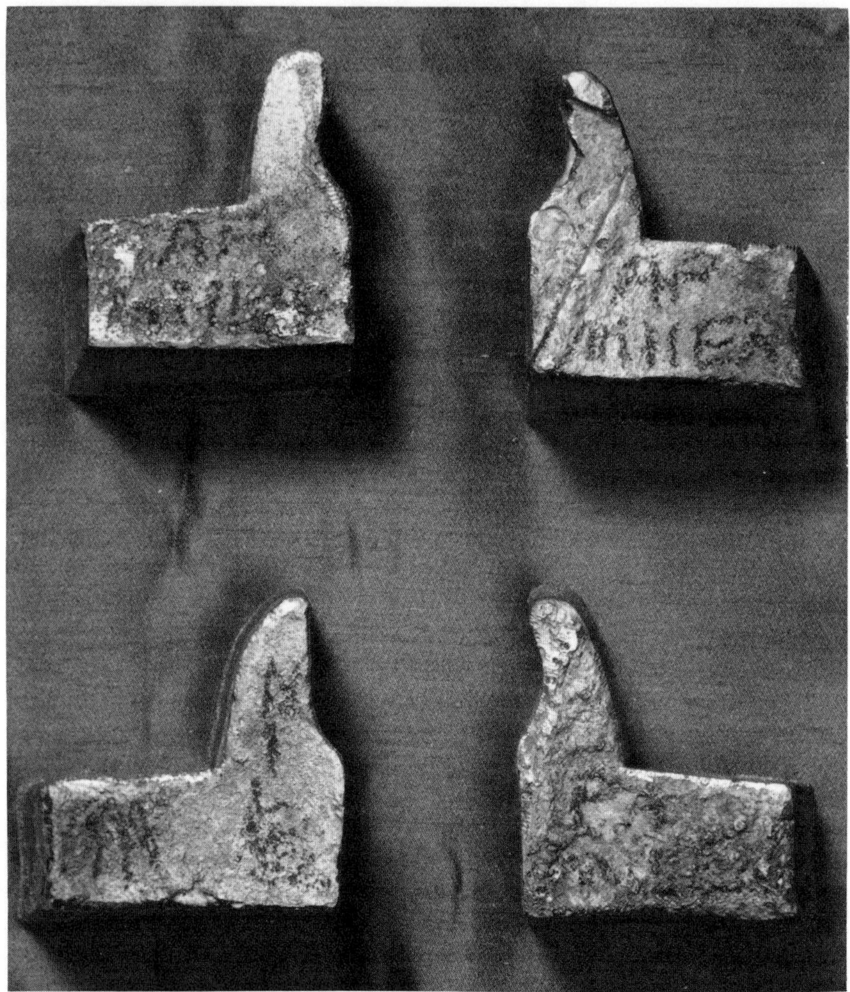

Figure 24.4 The lung shields for both anterior and posterior are ready for use.

common and diarrhea is seen when the pelvis is irradiated. Leukopenia can occur in patients undergoing total lymphoid RT. Interruption of RT is considered when the WBC falls below 2,000 and the platelet count below 50,000.

Late effects of RT <u>Radiation pneumonitis</u> The incidence of radiation pneumonitis following mantle treatment depends on the volume of lung irradiated and the dose. A higher incidence is seen following irradiation of large mediastinal masses. The incidence of severe lung reactions is <5%. The complication can usually be prevented with careful treatment technique. Severe cases are treated by systemic steroids.

<u>Radiation-induced heart disease</u> The spectrum of radiation-induced heart disease includes acute and chronic pericarditis, fibrosis of the myocardium and coronary artery disease with myocardial infarction. The incidence is related to the volume of heart irradiated and the dose. The incidence of severe pericarditis requiring surgery is <5%. The incidence can be minimized by shielding as much of the heart as possible during mantle irradiation.

Particular care must be exercised when combining doxorubicin and radiation. The incidence of treatment related disease is increased when doxorubicin is administered prior to, during, or following RT to the heart. Therefore, when the two modalities must be used, the dose of each is reduced and as much of the heart is shielded as possible.

<u>Injury to spinal cord</u> The most common neurologic manifestation of radiation injury to the spinal cord is known as Lhermitte's syndrome. The syndrome occasionally develops a few months following mantle treatment and is manifest by "electric" shock-like sensations down the back and/or arms and/or legs when the patient flexes the neck. The cause of the syndrome is unknown but the symptoms are transient and usually subside within 6 months.

Radiation myelopathy should not be seen with proper techniques. However, following overlap of the para-aortic portal on the spinal cord previously irradiated by the mantel, this complication might occur. Irreversible loss of strength in the lower extremities and loss of bowel and/or bladder function would be seen in this complication.

<u>Hypothyroidism</u> Reduced function of the thyroid gland following mantle therapy is common and overt clinical hypothyroidism is seen in 10% of cases. In addition thyroid nodules and cancer may occur following mantle irradiation. Therefore, patients should be followed indefinitely post-treatment for early detection of hypothyroidism and thyroid cancer.

<u>Leukemia</u> The occurrence of acute leukemia following treatment for Hodgkin's disease is an important complication. In one study, the incidence of acute leukemia 5 years after treatment for Hodgkin's disease was 4 % and at 9 years the incidence was 10%.[7] However, no patient treated with RT alone developed acute leukemia. All patients had been treated either with chemotherapy alone or RT+chemotherapy.

<u>Gonadal function</u> Reduced gonadal function is seen in nearly all patients who receive RT to the pelvis but not in patients receiving treatment to the para-aortic region only. In males, reduced spermatogenesis is seen following pelvic RT but recovery eventually occurs. In females who have had oophoropexy, 70% maintain or regain menstrual function and many later prove to be fertile.[8]

<u>Immune function</u> Immune status can be evaluated using delayed-type hypersensitivity tests to common recall antigens, counting T and B lymphocytes

in the peripheral blood, with in vitro tests of immune responsiveness to mitogen, antigens and allogenic lymphocytes and measuring serum levels of immunoglobulin. These tests indicate that severe impairment of immune status is observed following RT, but significant evidence of repair occurs in the months and years post-treatment.[9]

Results The prognosis for patients with Hodgkin's disease has continued to improve. In the Stanford series, the 5 year survival rate for 363 patients with all stages treated between 1968 and 1974 was 86% and 66% were in the first remission. For patients treated between 1974 and 1980, the 5 year survival rate was 89% and 77% were in their first remission.[10]

At the Joint Center for Radiation Therapy in Boston, 192 patients were treated with RT alone for Stages IA and IIA between 1969 and 1978. The actuarial 8 year survival rate for these patients was 95% for Stage IA and 92% for Stage IIA.[11]

Hodgkin's disease during pregnancy Abortion is recommended for patients who develop Hodgkin's disease early in pregnancy. During the latter half of pregnancy, asymptomatic disease can be followed without treatment but early delivery is recommended.[12] Patients with symptomatic disease above the diaphragm can be treated with RT, but single agent chemotherapy is preferred for symptomatic abdominal disease.

Hodgkin's disease in children The major limitation of RT in children with Hodgkin's is the marked impairment of bone growth seen following high-dose treatment of large volumes of tissue. For this reason, current protocols for children combine MOPP chemotherapy with low-dose (15-25 Gy) RT to involved fields. In one report from Stanford, 96% of 46 children treated in this way were surviving 3 to 10 years post-treatment.[13]

NON-HODGKIN'S LYMPHOMAS

ETIOLOGY AND EPIDEMIOLOGY

Non-Hodgkin's lymphomas were diagnosed in 35,600 people in the U.S. in 1990 and 18,200 died of the disease. The diseases are slightly more common in males. The mean age at diagnosis is 42 but in the U.S. there is a steady increase in age-specific incidence from childhood through age 80.[14] The incidence rates show marked variations from country to country. For example, in Africa Burkitt's lymphoma is very common, whereas in the U.S. this lymphoma is very rare.

The etiology of the disease is unknown but evidence is growing that, at least some lymphomas, are caused by viruses. For example, type C RNA virus have been isolated from cultured large cell lymphoma cell lines and from certain T cell lymphoma cell lines. Furthermore, Burkitt's lymphoma in African children has been associated elevated serum antibody levels against the herpes-like DNA virus known as Epstein-Barr (EBV).

The incidence of malignant lymphoma is markedly increased in diseases or conditions associated with immune deficiency. Examples include AIDS, ataxia telangiectasia syndrome, Wiscott-Aldrich syndrome, and Swiss-type agammaglobulinemia. Also, the disease occurs with increased frequency in patients undergoing treatment with immunosuppressive drugs such as renal transplant recipients.

PATHOLOGY

There are numerous pathologic classifications of non-Hodgkin's lymphoma in use around the world. The one currently used most frequently in the U.S. is the Working Formulation of Non-Hodgkin's Lymphoma (Table 24.3).

In follicular (also called nodular) lymphomas, the neoplastic cells grow in circumscribed aggregations which microscopically resemble germinal centers of lymph nodes. In fact, follicular lymphomas arise from follicular B lymphocytes.

In diffuse lymphomas, the cells grow in a diffuse pattern. They may grow in a diffuse pattern throughout their natural history or undergo transition from a follicular to a diffuse growth pattern. Most diffuse lymphoma arise from B lymphocytes but some arise from T lymphocytes.

Non-Hodgkin's' lymphomas differ from Hodgkin's disease in a number of ways. Non-Hodgkin's lymphomas present as an extranodal tumor in 50% of cases versus <10% for Hodgkin's cases. The extranodal sites most frequently involved are Waldeyer's ring and the GI tract. Hematogenous dissemination to bone marrow, liver, CNS and other sites occurs more frequently in non-Hodgkin's lymphoma and exhibit a non-contiguous pattern of spread, whereas in Hodgkin's disease the pattern of spread is usually contiguous from one nodal group to an adjacent nodal group.

DIAGNOSIS AND STAGING

Symptoms The discovery of an enlarged lymph node by the patient is the most common presenting complaint. However, in 1/3 of the cases a symptom related to an extranodal lesion is the presenting complaint. Weight loss, loss of appetite and fatigue are the presenting complaints in 10% of cases.

Biopsy The diagnosis is established by removal of an involved lymph node or other tissue for histologic study.

Staging The Ann Arbor staging classification is used and the staging workup is similar to that employed for Hodgkin's disease. However, laparotomy is usually not routinely used in the staging of non-Hodgkin's lymphoma. Most patients have Stage III or IV disease at diagnosis. A major problem in staging of patients with non-Hodgkin's lymphoma is that the patients are often elderly and

---

Table 24.3 A working formulation of non-Hodgkin's lymphoma for clinical usage

Low grade

A.   Malignant lymphoma, small lymphocytic - consistent with chronic lymphocytic leukemia

B.   Malignant lymphoma, follicular, predominately small cleaved cell

C.   Malignant lymphoma, follicular mixed, small cleaved and large cell

Intermediate grade

D.   Malignant lymphoma, follicular - predominately large cell

E.   Malignant lymphoma, diffuse small, cleaved cell

F.   Malignant lymphoma, diffuse mixed, small and large cell sclerosis

G.   Malignant lymphoma, diffuse

      Large Cell

      Cleaved cell

      Non-cleaved cell

      Sclerosis

High Grade

H.   Malignant lymphoma large cell, immunoblastic

I.   Malignant lymphoma lymphoblastic

J.   Malignant lymphoma small noncleaved cell

---

have associated medical problems which preclude invasive diagnostic studies. Nevertheless, bone marrow biopsies are obtained on all patients and are frequently positive. Lymphangiography is the most accurate technique for evaluating para-aortic lymph nodes but other techniques such as CT scanning are more frequently used. Gallium scanning is a useful non-invasive test which is positive in many patients.

TREATMENT

Surgery The major role of surgery in the treatment of lymphomas is for tumors originating in the GI tract. Most patients undergo a laparotomy and, if possible, a resection of the involved segment of bowel is carried out.

Chemotherapy Combination chemotherapy is the standard treatment for patients in Stages III and IV. Chemotherapy is also used alone or with local RT for most patients in Stages I and II. CHOP (cyclophosphamide, doxorubicin, vincristine and prednisone) is currently the most popular regimen producing remissions in 70% of patients with aggressive diffuse lymphomas.

New chemotherapy regimens are under investigation for patients with diffuse aggressive lymphomas. For example, a regimen developed at the NCI called Pro-MACE-MOPP used 8 different drugs in combination including cyclophosphamide, doxorubicin, etoposide, methotrexate and prednisone plus nitrogen mustard, vincristine, procarbazine, and prednisone.

Chemotherapy protocols such as ProMACE-MOPP are able to induce complete remissions in 80% of cases; 50% remain relapse-free for at least 2 years and many appear to have been cured.

Follicular lymphomas have a longer natural history than the aggressive lymphomas and the average survival for some subtypes exceeds 5 years. For this reason, some authorities recommend withholding treatment until symptoms develop. Combination chemotherapy yields complete responses in 50% of patients with follicular lymphoma, but it has not been shown that chemotherapy yields improved overall survival.

Radiotherapy *Stages I and II* If adequate staging is carried out on each patient, only a small number have localized disease and these are candidates for RT alone or combined with chemotherapy.

<u>Head and neck</u> Tumors confined to Waldeyer's ring with or without lymph node involvement, are treated with opposing lateral portals which cover Waldeyer's ring and the upper neck. The lower neck is irradiated with an anterior portal. Most lymphocytic tumors are controlled with 30 Gy/3 weeks, but some aggressive large cell lymphomas may require doses as great as 40-50 Gy/4-5 weeks.

<u>Abdomen</u> Patients with a GI tract lymphoma who have gross disease removed usually receive RT to large portals covering the tumor bed and regional lymph nodes. Opposing anterior and posterior portals are used and daily tumor doses in the range of 1.5 to 2.0 Gy are tolerated. Care must exercised to prevent excessive doses to the kidneys and liver. A sophisticated technique for irradiation of the whole abdomen has been described by the Stanford group.[15]

<u>Extended field irradiation</u> A small number of patients (10) with Stage I diffuse aggressive lymphomas were treated by Leavitt with extended field irradiaiton with excellent results.[16] All 10 were surviving without evidence of disease 19-102 months following RT. However, all of the patients had a staging laparotomy. Since most institutions do not employ laparotomy in non-Hodgkin's lymphoma, this method of treatment has not found wide acceptance.

<u>Chemotherapy +RT</u> Several clinical trials involving patients with localized aggressive lymphomas have shown treatment results which are superior in patients treated with combination chemotherapy+RT compared to those with RT alone. Therefore, most patients with Stage I and II disease are currently treated with chemotherapy combined with local RT.

In Stage I and II disease it is possible to achieve long-term relapse-free survival in more than 80% of patients with initial CHOP therapy followed by local RT.[17]

Stages III and IV <u>Total lymphoid irradiation</u> RT alone has never found a role in curative treatment of patients with advanced disease. However, a number of patients with Stage III follicular lymphoma have been treated with total lymphoid irradiaton. Cox et al, reported a 5 year survival rate of 78% for 29 patients treated with TLI.[18] Hematologists are reluctant to refer patients for this form of treatment because they are concerned that the radiation dose to the large volume of bone marrow would compromise future chemotherapy.

<u>Total body radiation (TBI)</u> Another technique which has been used for patients with advanced disease is TBI.[19] Doses of 0.1 to 0.15 Gy administered 2 times weekly for a total of 1.5-3.0 Gy are capable of producing complete responses and 5 year survivors in patients with Stage III or IV follicular lymphoma. This method has never found wide acceptance because the treatment results are not superior to those seen with chemotherapy.

NON-HODGKIN'S LYMPHOMA IN CHILDHOOD

Non-Hodgkin's lymphomas in children are uncommon. They differ from those seen in adults in a number of important ways: Follicular lymphomas are rare in children; the histologic types seen in children differ and include: 1) diffuse undifferentiated lymphoma, Burkitt's type; 2) diffuse undifferentiated lymphoma, non-Burkitt's type; 3) diffuse lymphoblastic lymphoma and; 4) diffuse large cell lymphoma. The biologic behavior of lymphomas in children is characterized by rapid growth, early dissemination and a high incidence of involvement of bone marow and CNS.

The primary modality of treatment for childhood lymphomas is chemotherapy. Spectacular improvements in treatment results have been seen with aggressive protocols. For example, a protocol known as $LSA_2\text{-}L_2$, developed at Memorial Sloan-Kettering Cancer Center, New York, employs 10 different drugs administered in a complex regimen during induction, consolidation and maintenance phases, plus low-dose RT to involved areas plus CNS prophylaxis with intrathecal methotrexate.[20] Approximately 75% of patients treated with this protocol are surviving disease-free 9 years post-treatment.

LYMPHOMAS OF SKIN

Mycosis fungoides and Sezary syndrome are cutaneous T cell lymphomas. Sezary syndrome is thought to be a leukemic form of mycosis fungoides. The skin involvement in both conditions consists of infiltrates of neoplastic lymphoid cells in the upper dermis which tend to migrate into the epidermis producing the characteristic Pautrier microabscess. Initially, the disease is limited to the skin but lymph nodes and visceral organs eventually become involved. In Sezary syndrome abnormal cells called Sezary cells are found in the peripheral blood.

Mycosis fungoides is a radiosensitive tumor and RT may have a role in treatment. Electron beam therapy to the total skin surface of the body is a technique that was developed to treat the entire skin surface with low energy electrons in an attempt to cure the disease.[21] However, few patients were cured with this technique and therefore, topical chemotherapy with nitrogen mustard is currently the most popular treatment. Nevertheless, local electron beam therapy has an important palliative role in this disease.

All cell types of lymphoma can involve the skin at some time during the course of the disease. Diffuse large cell lymphoma is the most common type to involve the skin. Electron beam therapy can provide useful palliation for these patients.

ACUTE LEUKEMIA
ETIOLOGY AND EPIDEMIOLOGY

The acute leukemias are malignant diseases of the bloodforming organs characterized by the proliferation of immature lymphoid or myeloid cells called blasts in the bone marrow, peripheral blood and other tissues. The blasts progressively replace the normal bone marrow cells leading to diminished production of normal blood cells, resulting eventually in anemia, infection and hemorrhage.

There are two main forms of acute leukemia, acute lymphoblastic (ALL) and acute myelogenous (AML). Each, if untreated, causes death within one year.

The incidence of ALL increases rapidly and peaks before age 5 and decreases thereafter. The incidence of AML is constant through age 10; there is a small peak in late adolescence after which the incidence remains constant through age 55, then rises to peak at age 75. Eighty percent of children with acute leukemia have ALL whereas 80% of adult cases are AML.

Ionizing radiation is the most documented etiologic factor for acute leukemia in man. RNA viruses (retroviruses) can induce leukemia in animals and may cause the disease in humans. Many chemicals have been implicated as etiologic factors. For example, workers exposed to benzene have an increased risk of AML; also cancer patients treated with alkylating agents have an increased risk of AML.

Finally, there is evidence that genetic factors play a role: if one of a pair of identical twins develops acute leukemia, the chance of the other twin developing the disease is 20%.

DIAGNOSIS

Signs and symptoms Pallor, headache and shortness of breath are signs of anemia; bloody nose, bleeding gums, easy bruising, GI bleeding and hematuria are signs of thrombocytopenia; infections that persist in spite of treatment are signs of granulocytopenia. These symptoms are common presenting complaints in patients with leukemia.

The liver, spleen and lymph nodes are commonly involved and these organs may be enlarged. Bone pain due to infiltration of the periosteum by blast cells is a common presenting symptom. Involvement of the meninges of the brain can cause increased intracranial pressure resulting in headaches, nausea, vomiting and papilledema. CNS involvement is not usually seen at presentation but is commonly the first site of recurrence.

Laboratory findings Anemia, abnormal leukocyte and differential cell counts and thrombocytopenia are common findings in the peripheral blood. Blast cells are often easily detectable in the peripheral blood, but the diagnosis of acute leukemia usually depends on the identification of increased number of blast cells in the bone marrow.

TREATMENT

The mainstay of therapy for acute leukemia is chemotherapy. The initial goal is the induction of a complete remission which is defined as the reduction of leukemic cells to undetectable levels. This includes a return of the bone marrow to normal (<5% blasts) and a return of the peripheral blood counts to normal.

ALL There are three phases of treatment: remission induction, CNS prophylaxis and maintenance therapy. The most effective drug combination is vincristine and prednisone which produces complete remissions in 90% of children and 50% of adults.

After remission induction, CNS prophylaxis is given for the purpose of killing leukemic cells which may be present in the brain and meninges. Three methods for CNS prophylaxis are available: RT alone to the entire brain and spinal axis (24 Gy), cranial irradiation (18-24 Gy) (Figure 24.5) combined with methotrexate administered intrathecally, and intrathecal methotrexate alone.

Following CNS prophylaxis, the maintenance phase begins. Methotrexate and 6-mercaptopurine are the drugs most commonly used. Maintenance therapy continues for 2.5 to 5 years.

Favorable prognostic factors in ALL include age 2-10 years, white race, female sex and a white count of <20,000 cells per microliter. Sixty percent of patients in the favorable group remain in continuous complete remission for 5 years or more after diagnosis. Unfavorable prognostic factors include age less than 2 or greater than 10, male sex, the presence of a mediastinal mass and a markedly elevated white count.

AML The combination of cytosine arabinoside (Ara-C) and daunorubicin

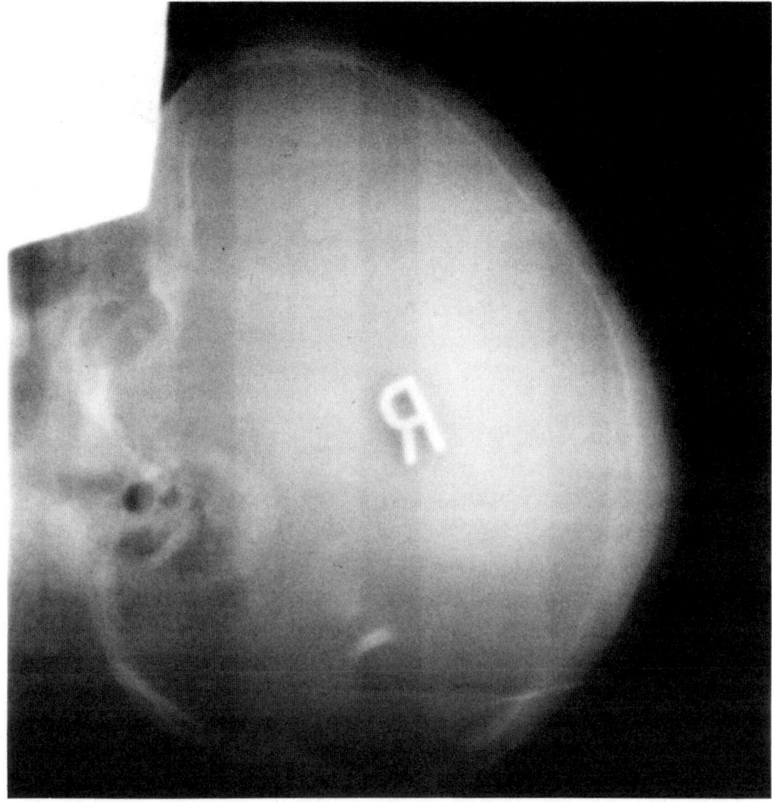

Figure 24.5 This is the lateral port film for a patient with ALL in remission who received CNS prophylaxis with cranial irradiation and intrathecal ARA-C. Opposing lateral portals were used.

or doxorubicin is successful in inducing remission in 50-85% of patients. The combination of Ara-C and 6-thioguanine is used for maintenance therapy. The role of CNS prophylaxis is controversial. CNS leukemia is less common in AML and, although treatment reduces the incidence of CNS relapse, it does not improve prognosis. Only 10-20% of patients remain in remission for 5 years or longer.

Bone marrow transplantation An alternative form of treatment for acute leukemia is allogeneic (the donor and recipient are of different genetic origins) bone marrow transplantation. To prepare a patient for bone marrow transplantation, the immune system and the leukemic cells must be destroyed. This is accomplished by administration of massive doses of cyclophosphamide or TIB or a combination of the two. The donor marrow is then infused intravenously.

Within 2-4 weeks, marrow cellularity increases and the peripheral blood count rises. All hematopoietic and immune cells of the recipient have originated from those of the donor.

The most serious problem which may develop in transplanted patients is graft-versus-host disease (GVHD). Acute GVHD disease involves the skin, GI tract and/or the liver, whereas chronic GVHD causes skin, eye, GI tract, lung and liver lesions and generalized wasting. Chemotherapeutic drugs such as methotrexate, corticosteroid and immunosuppressive drugs such as cyclosporine are used in the treatment of GVHD disease.

Bone marrow transplantation has been most successful in acute leukemia when performed early in the course of the disease. For example, in the Seattle series, 53% of AML patients transplanted during the first remission were surviving and, in ALL, 36% of patients transplanted in the second or subsequent remission were surviving.[22]

Autologous bone marrow transplantation is under investigation in a number of centers for disease such as leukemia, Hodgkin's disease, non-Hodgkin's lymphoma, breast cancer, lung cancer, testicular tumors, ovarian cancer and pediatric tumors such as neuroblastoma and Ewing's sarcoma. In this technique, the patient's own marrow is removed and saved, high-dose chemotherapy is administered, and then the patient's own stored marrow is infused.

CHRONIC LYMPHOCYTIC LEUKEMIA (CLL)

Etiology and epidemiology CLL is a tumor of slowly proliferating B lymphocytes which are immunologically defective. The disease accounts for 25% of all cases of leukemia and is the most common form of chronic leukemia in the U.S. CLL occurs primarily in the elderly and the mean age at onset is 60. The etiology is unknown, but the incidence is higher among family members than the general population, suggesting that there is a genetic predisposition in some cases.

Diagnosis *Signs and symptoms* In about 25% of cases there are no symptoms and the diagnosis is made by discovery of an elevated lymphocyte count in the peripheral blood. However, as the disease advances patients experience malaise, fatigue, poor appetite, weight loss, fever, night sweats and susceptibility to infection. Easy bruising, epistaxis and other bleeding are seen in advanced cases. The physical examination may be normal initially, but eventually enlargement of lymph nodes and of the liver and spleen are seen.

Laboratory findings The diagnosis of CLL depends on the finding of an increased number of small lymphocytes in the peripheral blood.

Treatment No treatment is required early in the disease. When symptoms develop chemotherapy is given which usually causes a reduction in the lymphocyte count and decrease in the size of lymph nodes and spleen. Low-dose RT (10-

15 Gy) to enlarged lymph nodes may be helpful in patients with massively enlarged lymph nodes. Also, low-dose RT to the spleen (2.5 Gy in 10 treatments) can reduce spleen size and result in elevation of the hemoglobin and a reaction in the WBC.

Prognosis CLL has a variable natural history wth survival times ranging from 1 to 20 years. Common causes of death include infection, bleeding and progressive infiltration of vital tissues by leukemic cells.

CHRONIC MYELOGENOUS LEUKEMIA (CML)

Etiology and epidemiology CML is a chronic form of leukemia originating from primitive stem cells which have the capacity to differentiate and retain the function of normal blood cells. Later in the course of the disease the leukemic cells lose their capacity to differentiate and they become more malignant. In CML all leukemic cells have a chromosome abnormality known as the Philadelphia chromosome.

CML accounts for 15% of all cases of leukemia. The disease occurs primarily in adults and the peak incidence is in the third and fourth decades. The etiology is unknown but several etiologic factors have been identified including ionizing radiation, benzene and alkylating agents used in cancer therapy.

Diagnosis *Signs and symptoms* Common early symptoms include fatigue, reduced exercise tolerance, weight loss, poor appetite, fullness in the upper abdomen due to splenic enlargement, headaches, fever, sweating and bleeding. The most common physical finding is splenic enlargement.

Laboratory findings The most common abnormality is leukocytosis. The Philadelphia chromosome is found in bone marrow cells.

Treatment In early cases, no treatment is needed. Chemotherapy with alkylating agents such as busulfan, cyclophosphamide and melphalan is used in symptomatic cases. Low-dose splenic irradiation (2.5 Gy 10 treatments) is effective in reducing spleen size and the WBC. Splenectomy may be needed for patients who develop massive splenic enlargement. Bone marrow transplantation is associated with long-term disease-free survival in 70% of patients.

Eventually a transition in the disease from the chronic phase to an accelerated phase occurs. During this phase the disease becomes progressively unresponsive to treatment. The accelerated phase is followed by the blast phase when an increase in the number of blast cells is seen in the peripheral blood and marrow.

The median survival of patients with CML is about 3 years with a range of 1 to 10 years. Survival in the accelerated phase is less than 1 year and the blast phase a few months.

REFERENCES

1. Silverberg E, Boring CC, Squires TS. Cancer statistics, 1990, CA-A Cancer J for Clinicians 40:9-26, 1990.

2. Kaplan HS. Hodgkin's disease, Second Edition, Harvard University Press, Cambridge, MA, 1980.

3. DeVita VT, Serpick AA, Carbone PP. Combination chemotherapy in the treatment of advanced Hodgkin's disease, Ann Int Med 73:881-895, 1970.

4. Santoro A, Bonadona G, Bonfaite V, Valagussa P. Alternating drug combinations in the treatment of advanced Hodgkin's disease, N Engl J Med 306:770-775, 1982.

5. Peters MV. A study of survival in Hodgkin's disease treated radiologically, Am J Roentgenol 63:299-311, 1950.

6. Hopfan S, Reid A, Simpson L, Ager PJ. Clinical complications arising from overlapping of adjacent fields-physical and technical considerations, Int J Radiat Oncol Biol Phys 2:801-808, 1977.

7. Pedersen-Bjergaard J, Larsen SO. Incidence of acute nonlymphocytic leukemia, preleukemia and acute myeloproliferative syndrome up to 10 years after treatment for Hodgkin's disease, N Engl J Med 307:965-971, 1982.

8. Horning SJ, Hoppe RT, Kaplan HS, Rosenberg SA. Female reproductive potential after treatment for Hodgkin's disease, N Engl J Med 304:1377-1382, 1981.

9. Van Rijswijk REN, Sybesma JP, Kater L. A prospective study of the changes in immune status following radiotherapy for Hodgkin's disease, Cancer 53:62-69, 1984.

10. Rosenberg SA. Chapter 20-6, Hodgkin's disease, In Cancer Medicine, 2nd Edition, Eds. Holland J, Frei E, Lea and Febiger, Philadelphia, 1982, pp 1478-1502.

11. Mauch P, Lewis A, Hellman S. Chapter 26, The role of radiation therapy in the treatment of Stage I and II Hodgkin's disease, In Malignant Lymphomas: Etiology, Immunology, Pathology, Treatment, Eds. Rosenberg SA, Kaplan HS, Academic Press New York, 1982, pp 453-467.

12. Jacobs C, Donaldson SS, Rosenberg SA, Kaplan HS. Management of the pregnant patient with Hodgkin's disease, Ann Int Med 95:669-675, 1981.

13. Donaldson SS, Kaplan HS, Chapter 34, A survey of pediatric Hodgkin's disease at Stanford University: Results of therapy and quality of survival, In malignant Lymphomas: Etiology, Immunology, Pathology, Treatment, Eds. Rosenberg SA, Kaplan HS, Academic Press, New York, 1982, pp 503-512.

14. DeVita VT, Jaffe ES, Mauch P, Longo DL Chapter 50, Lymphocytic lymphomas In Cancer-Principles & Practice of Oncology, 3rd Edition Eds. DeVita VT, Hellman S, Rosenberg SA, J.B. Lippincott Company, Philadelphia, 1989, pp 1741-1798.

15. Goffinet DR, et al. Abdominal irradiation in non-Hodgkin's lymphomas, Cancer 37:2797-2805, 1976.

16. Leavitt S, Bloomfield CD, Frizzera G, Lee CKK, Curative radiotherapy for localized diffuse histiocytic lymphoma, Cancer Treatment Reports 64:175-177, 1980.

17. Miller TP, Jones SE. Initial chemotherapy for clinically localized lymphomas of unfavorable histology, Blood 62:413-418, 1983.

18. Cox JD, et al. Stage III nodular lymphoreticular tumors (non-Hodgkin's lymphoma): Results of central lymphatic irradiation, Cancer 47:2247-2252, 1981.

19. Loeffler RK. Therapeutic use of fractionated total body and subtotal body irradiation, Cancer 47:2253-2258, 1981.

20. Wollner N. Chapter 36, LSA$_2$-L$_2$ in childhood non-Hodgkin's lymphoma, In Malignant Lympohmas: Etiologoy, Immunology, Pathology, Treatment, Eds. Rosenberg SA, Kaplan HS, Academic Press, New York, 1982, pp 603-626.

21. Hoppe RT, Cox RS, Fuks ZY, et al. Electron beam therapy in the treatment of mycosis fungoides: The Stanford experience, Cancer Treat Rep 63:691-, 1979.

22. Thomas ED. Chapter 299, Bone marrow transplantation, In Harrison's Principles of Internal Medicine, Twelfth Edition Eds. Wilson JD, Braunwald E, Isselbacher KJ, et al, McGraw-Hill, Inc., New York, 1991, pp 1571-1575.

Chapter 25

BONE AND SOFT TISSUE TUMORS

MALIGNANT BONE TUMORS
OSTEOGENIC SARCOMA

ETIOLOGY AND EPIDEMIOLOGY

Osteogenic sarcoma is an uncommon tumor, but except for multiple myeloma, it is the most frequent occurring primary malignant bone tumor. The disease usually occurs in the second decade of life and males are affected more often than females (2:1).

The etiology of osteogenic sarcoma is unknown but the disease tends to occur during the period of rapid adolescent growth. In older patients, osteogenic sarcoma can arise in association with Paget's disease of the bone. The disease can also occur as a complication of radiation therapy; osteogenic sarcomas can develop in irradiated tissues 10 to 20 years following RT for another malignant tumor.

Viruses can induce osteosarcomas in mice and chickens and extracts of human osteosarcomas can induce osteosarcomas in hamsters.

PATHOLOGY

Osteogenic sarcomas are malignant spindle cell sarcomas which arise from bone-forming mesenchyme that produces neoplastic osteoid. They often involve the metaphysics of long bones and the majority arise in the knee area: the distal femur is the most common site followed by the proximal tibia and the proximal humerus. The vertebral column is the primary site in only 1% of cases. Most osteosarcomas are high-grade, aggressive tumors. They tend to metastasize early to the lungs.

DIAGNOSIS

Symptoms Pain at the site of the primary is the most common presenting symptom and there is usually an associated mass.

Radiographic appearance The appearance is characteristic, consisting of a destructive metaphyseal tumor with indistinct margins and extension to soft tissues. There is usually new bone formation and periosteal reaction. Bone scans, CT scans, MRI and angiography are used in preoperative assessment of disease extent.

Biopsy Great care must be exercised in choosing the site and technique for biopsy. The biopsy is made by the surgeon who will be responsible for the decision about the operative procedures.[1] Needle and trephine or core biopsies are favored techniques. Frozen-section analysis is obtained on all specimens.

TREATMENT

Surgery Limb-sparing operations can spare many patients amputation. Chemotherapy is given prior to surgery to induce tumor sterilization and reduce tumor size. Limb salvage surgery is possible if an adequate surgical margin can be obtained while preserving enough tissue to maintain a functional limb. Cadaver bone grafts or metallic prostheses are used to fill bone defects. Surgical resection is also used in combination with chemotherapy for lung metastasis.

Chemotherapy Exciting improvements in cure rates for patients with osteosarcoma have been seen in recent years due to developments in chemotherapy. The initial breakthrough occurred in 1972 when high dose methotrexate with citrovorum rescue was introduced by Jaffee and Djerassi.[2] A response of 43% was seen in a group of patients with metastatic disease treated with this regimen.

Chemotherapy has an important role as adjuvant therapy for patients with localized disease. In one protocol, the patients received high-dose methotrexate and citrovorum factor rescue, doxorubicin, bleomycin, cyclophosphamide and dactinomycin prior to surgery.[3] Chemotherapy is continued postoperatively. This protocol produced a disease-free survival rate of 90% at 3 years post-treatment.

Radiotherapy RT has not found a significant role in this tumor because of radioresistance. However, occasional patients with disease located in surgically inaccessible sites require palliative RT.

EWING'S SARCOMA

Etiology and epidemiology Ewing's sarcoma, although a rare disease, is the second most common primary bone tumor in children and young adults. The disease occurs most frequently in the second decade of life and is seen more frequently in males (1.5:1). The etiology is unknown.

Pathology Ewing's sarcoma is a tumor of small, round anaplastic cells. The pelvis is the most common site followed by the femur, tibia, humerus and ribs. The tumor tends to originate in the diaphysis of long bones. Extensive involvement of the medullary cavity of the affected bone is seen and the tumor tends to grow through the cortex into the soft tissues producing a soft tissue mass. Distant metastasis to lungs and bone marrow is common.

Diagnosis *Symptoms* Pain and swelling at the affected site is the usual presenting symptom. Fever, weight loss and fatigue are also frequent complaints.

Radiographic appearance The lesion is usually seen as a diffuse, destructive "moth eaten" diaphyseal tumor. Extension to soft tissue is common and there is often a periosteal reaction which produces an "onion skin" appearance. Radionuclide bone scans, CT scans and MRI have a role in evaluating the primary site and searching for bone and/or lung metastasis.

Treatment *Surgery* Tumors of the ribs, clavicle, foot and fibula are best treated by surgical resection and postoperative irradiation. Also, distal lower extremity tumors in young patients are managed surgically since RT would cause marked shortening of bone. Limb-sparing surgery combined with RT is often used for tumors at other sites.

Radiotherapy Ewing's sarcoma is a radiosensitive tumor and RT has been the standard treatment for the primary for many years. The entire affected bone must be irradiated because of the tendency of the tumor to permeate the marrow cavity. Fifty Gy is given to the entire bone followed by a boost to the main tumor mass to bring the total tumor dose to the primary site to 60 Gy.

For extremity tumors, a strip of tissue on the lateral aspect of the irradiated limb is shielded to prevent post-irradiation complications such as lymphedema. Local control rates in the range of 80% are seen with this dose, whereas lower doses are often associated with local recurrence.

Chemotherapy Striking improvements in treatment results have occurred with chemotherapy given in combination with surgery and/or RT to the primary.[4] VAC (vincristine, dactinomycin and cytoxan) and VACA (VAC + doxorubicin) are the regimens most commonly used. Chemotherapy is usually initiated prior to surgery and/or RT.

Autologous bone marrow transplantation combined with chemotherapy and TBI has shown promise in treatment of patients with metastastic Ewing's sarcoma.[5]

MULTIPLE MYELOMA

Etiology and epidemiology Multiple myeloma is a disseminated malignant bone tumor in which a clone of malignant cells proliferates in the bone marrow producing extensive skeletal destruction, anemia, impaired renal function, immunodeficiency, increased susceptibility to infection and an M-protein.

In 1990 there were 11,800 new cases and 8,900 deaths from multiple myeloma, making it the most common primary malignant bone tumor in the U.S.[6] The disease occurs predominantly in middle and old age and the incidence is slightly higher in males. The etiology is unknown.

Diagnosis *Symptoms* The disease may remain asymptomatic for many years but eventually sever bone pain, weakness, weight loss and repeated infections occur.

Skeletal roentgenography The most common abnormality seen on skeletal x-rays is multiple osteolytic lesions in the vertebrae, ribs, skull, pelvis and long bones.

Bone marrow In the bone marrow, 10-90% of the cells are plasma cells.

M-protein An M-protein can be demonstrated and measured in the serum or urine in 99% of patients by electrophoresis.

Bence-Jones protein At least 70% of patients develop proteinuria. Initially the urine protein consists of low molecular weight fragments of immunoglobulin called Bence-Jones proteins. Renal failure is a frequent complication in patients who excrete Bence-Jones protein in the urine because the protein tends to precipitate in the renal tubules leading to tubular obstruction.

Treatment Multiple myeloma has a chronic phase which can last for 1 to 10 years and during this time response to treatment is good. However, during the terminal phase, which is usually of short duration, the disease is unresponsive to treatment.

Chemotherapy Melphalan, cyclophosphamide, chlorambucil and BCNU can produce objective improvement in 30-50% of patients The addition of prednisone improves the response rate. Interferon is under investigation as an agent which can prolong response to chemotherapy.

Patients responding to treatment experience a reduction in their bone pain and an improved sense of well-being. Objectively there is a fall in the M-protein impairment in renal function and in 10% of patients there is radiographic evidence of healing of bone lesions. Patients who show objective improvement have a median survival of nearly 40 months whereas non-responders have a median survival of only 10 months.

Radiotherapy RT is often required for palliation of painful bone lesions. Doses of 20-30 Gy in 2-3 weeks are usually effective in providing pain relief.

SOLITARY PLASMACYTOMA

Occasionally, a plasma cell tumor appears to be localized to a single skeletal site. These solitary lesions often disappear completely following local treatment. In most cases, however, there is reappearance of the tumor, years later as multiple myeloma. Solitary plasmacytomas are classified as solitary plasmacytoma of bone or extramedullary plasmacytoma (i.e., nasopharynx, nose, sinuses). Local RT is the treatment of choice for both types and 40-50 Gy in 4-5 weeks is the recommended dose.[7]

CHONDROSARCOMA

This is an uncommon primary bone malignancy. The disease occurs usually in the 4th, 5th and 6th decades of life. Two-thirds of cases occur in males. The pelvis is the most common primary site followed by the femur, humerus, shoulder and ribs. The majority of chondrosarcomas are low to moderate grade, tend to remain localized and have a long natural history. Surgery is the only known treatment and RT and chemotherapy have limited value.

GIANT CELL TUMOR OF BONE

This is a rare malignant tumor which occurs most commonly in the 3rd and 4th decades of life. The tumor originates in the knee in 50% of cases, but the proximal humerus, proximal femur, sacrum and pelvis are common sites. It tends to be low-grade and does not often metastasize. Total excision is the treatment of choice but the recurrence rate is high. RT is used for lesions that cannot be removed.

NON-HODGKIN'S LYMPHOMA OF BONE

Lymphoma of bone is a rare tumor accounting for only 5% of primary bone tumors. The peak incidence is age 50-60. The femur and the pelvis are the most common sites. Most cases are treated by a combination of RT and chemotherapy. Cure rates as high as 50% have been reported for patients with localized disease.

BONE METASTASIS

Painful bone metastasis is one of the most common indications for RT. Although the symptomatic result for RT is usually considered satisfactory, very few critical studies have appeared assessing the frequency and quality of response to RT. The literature suggests that there is no optimal dose-time-fraction schedule for symptomatic RT of bone metastasis. Therefore, short treatment courses should be used. The most popular regimen appears to be 30 Gy/ 10 treatments over 2 weeks.

EOSINOPHILIC GRANULOMA OF BONE

This is an uncommon benign lesion which usually occurs in persons under age 20 but can occur at any age. The lesions are radiosensitive and local control is achieved with fractionated doses in the range of 4.5-12 Gy.[8]

HETEROTOPIC BONE FORMATION

Significant functional impairment is seen in patients who develop radio-graphically visible bone in the soft tissues around the hip joint in the months and years following hip arthroplasty. This condition, called heterotopic ossification (HO), occurs following hip arthroplasty in 15-30% of patients.

Patients at high-risk for HO include those with pre-existing heterotopic bone, those suffering from hypertrophic osteoarthritis or ankylosing spondylitis and patients who have had multiple surgical procedures to the hip.

Post-operative RT to the hip joint can prevent HO. Fractionated doses (10-20 Gy/1-2 weeks) and single doses (6-7 Gy) have been used.[9] Treatment is initiated as soon as possible following hip surgery. In our institution, 7 Gy is given to the hip joint in a single fraction the day after surgery.

SOFT TISSUE SARCOMAS

ETIOLOGY AND EPIDEMIOLOGY

Soft tissue sarcomas account for less than 1% of all malignant tumors. They develop in all age groups and occur with equal frequency in males and females. The etiology is unknown. Direct trauma has often been claimed in medicolegal cases to be the cause of soft tissue sarcomas, but a single acute trauma has never been shown to be capable of inducing sarcomas.

Recent evidence suggests that viruses may be an etiologic factor in some cases because type C RNA viruses have been found in sarcomas in chickens, mice and cats and also in humans. Chemical carcinogens are known to cause soft tissue sarcomas in experimental animals and one epidemiologic study suggested that exposure to phenoxyacetic acid (a class of herbicide) and chlorphenol (wood preservative) is associated with an increased incidence of the disease in humans.

PATHOLOGY

Soft tissue sarcomas can arise anywhere in the body. About 40% arise on the lower extremity, 30% on the trunk, 15% on the upper extremity and 15% in the head and neck. The percent of trunk cases arise in the retroperitoneal tissues and the remainder on the abdominal or chest wall.

Each type of soft tissue can undergo malignant transformation. The tissues of origin, the malignant tumors arising from each tissue and the incidence among all types is shown in Table 25.1.

Soft tissue sarcomas are graded from 1 to 3; the grade determines the metastatic aggressiveness of the tumor and the prognosis. Soft tissue sarcomas

Table 25.1 Pathologic classification of soft tissue sarcoma

Tissue of origin	Malignant tumor	Incidence
Fibrous	Fibrosarcoma	24.0%
Adipose	Liposarcoma	19.0%
Striated muscle	Rhabdomyosarcoma	15.0%
Uncertain	Alveolar soft-part sarcoma	12.5%
Histiocyte	Malignant fibrous histiocytoma	7.0%
Synovial	Synovial sarcoma	6.5%
Smooth muscle	Leimayosarcoma	5.0%
Nerve	Neurofibrosarcoma	4.5%
Vascualr &	Angiosarcoma	1.5%
lymphatic	Lymphangiosarcoma	
	Kaposi's sarcoma	
	Malignant hemangiopericytoma	

tend to invade locally along nerve fibers, muscle bundles, fascial planes and blood vessels. Lymph node metastasis is not common, but hematogenous dissemination is common and the lungs are the most frequent metastatic site.

DIAGNOSIS

Soft tissue sarcomas usually present as a painless mass. Radiographic studies such as CT scans, MRI and arteriography are important in assessing the local disease extent. CT scans of the chest and radionuclide bone scans are used to search for metastatic lesions. Biopsy of the mass for histologic study yields the diagnosis.

TREATMENT

Multimodality therapy Recent studies suggest that adjuvant chemotherapy combined with surgery alone or with RT, yields improved survival rates for patients with soft tissue sarcoma of the extremities. Rosenberg, et al, at the NCI did a randomized study in which patients with high-grade sarcomas received local therapy plus doxorubicin, cyclophosphamide and high-dose methotrexate.[10]

The chemotherapy was initiated in the immediate post-operative period. The continuous disease-free survival rate at 3 years was 90% in the combined treatment group versus only 60% in the local treatment group. The authors conclude that adjuvant chemotherapy should be part of the treatment of the adults with soft tissue sarcoma of the extremities.

Limb-sparing surgery combined with RT Surgical resection is the treatment of choice for the primary. Extensive resections are required because of the tendency of sarcomas to invade locally. However, amputations are avoided whenever possible by combining surgery with RT and chemotherapy.

The operations most commonly used are wide excision (removal of the tumor and a wide margin of normal tissue) and radical local resection (removal of the tumor and the entire anatomic compartments occupied by the tumor).

A number of radiotherapy techniques have been used including post-operative external beam therapy,[11] surgical resection combined with interstitial brachytherapy[12], and preoperative external beam therapy combined with surgery and intraoperative radiation.[13]

External beam techniques In adults, the doses and treatment techniques are the same for all histologies. Treatment techniques must be individualized according to tumor site and local disease extent. Large fields are employed initially to encompass the tumor and all surrounding normal tissues which could potentially be involved with micrometastasis. However, for extremity tumors, the entire circumference of the extremity is never irradiated and a strip of tissue is shielded along at least one margin of the treatment volume.

In addition, to ensure dose homogeneity, when extremity tumors are treated, molds, cradles or casts are constructed to immobilize the part to be irradiated.[14] Computerized treatment plans are generated for all patients; wedged and compensating filters are used frequently.

Results Lindberg reported on 300 adults with soft tissue sarcoma treated at the M.D. Anderson Hospital between 1963-1977.[15] The patients were treated by conservative surgical excision and postop RT (60-70 Gy/6-7 weeks). The 2 year and 5 year disease-free survival rates were 74% and 61% respectively. The overall local recurrence rate was 22%. The combination of conservative surgery and postop RT maintained a functional limb in 85% of patients with extremity tumors.

REFERENCES

1. Malawer MM, Link MP, Donaldson SS. Chapter 42, Sarcomas of bone, In Cancer-Principles & Practice of Oncology, 3rd Edition, Eds. DeVita VT, Hellman S, Rosenberg SA, .J.B. Lippincott Company, Philadelphia, 1989, pp 1418-1468.

2. Jaffe N. Recent advances in the chemotherapy of metastatic osteogenic sarcoma, Cancer 30:1627-1631, 1972.

3. Rosen G, Caparros B, Huvos AG, et al .Preoperative chemotherapy for osteogenic sarcoma: Selection of postoperative adjuvant chemotherapy based on the response of the primary tumor to preoperative therapy, Cancer 49:1221-1230, 1982.

4. Rosen G, Caparos B, Nirenberg A, et al. Ewing's sarcoma: Ten year experience with adjuvant chemotherapy, Cancer 47:2204-2213, 1981.

5. Kinsella TJ, Glaubiger DF, Disseroth A, et al. Intensive combined modality therapy including low-dose TBI in high-risk Ewing's sarcoma patients, In J Radiat Oncol Biol Phys 9:1955-1960, 1983.

6. Silverberg E, Boring CC, Squires TS. Cancer statistics, 1990, CA-A Cancer J for Clinicians 40:9-26, 1990.

7. Mendenahall CM, Thar TL, Million RR. Solitary plasmacytoma of bone and soft tissue, Int J Radiat Oncol Biol Phys 6:1497-1501, 1980.

8. Pereslegin IA, Ustinova VF, Podlyaschuk EL. Radiotherapy for eosinophilic granuloma of bone, Int Radiat Oncol Biol Phys 7:317-321, 1981.

9. MacLennan I, Keys HM, Evarts CM, Rubin P. Usefulness of postoperative hip irradiation in the prevention of heterotopic bone formation in a high risk group of patients, Int J Radiat Oncol Biol Phys 10:49-53, 1984.

10. Rosenberg SA, Tepper J, Glatstein E, et al. Prospective randomized evaluation of adjuvant chemotherapy in adults with soft tissue sarcomas of the extremities, Cancer 42:424-434, 1983.

11. Leibel SA, Tranbaugh RF, Wara WM, et al. Soft tissue sarcomas of the extremities, Cancer 50:1076-1083, 1982.

12. Shiu MH, Turnbull AD, Nori D, et al. Control of locally advanced extremity soft tissue sarcomas by function-saving resection and brachytherapy, Cancer 53:1385-1392, 1984.

13. Suit HD, Mankin HJ, Wood WC, Proppe KH, Preoperative, intraoperative and postoperative radiation in the treatment of primary soft tissue sarcoma, Cancer 55:2659-2667, 1985.

14. Tepper J, Rosenberg SA, Glatstein E. Radiation therapy technique in soft tissue sarcomas of the extremity-policies of treatment at the National Cancer Institute, Int J Radiat Oncol Biol Phys 8:263-273, 1982.

15. Lindberg RD, Martin RG, Romsdahl M Barkley HT. Conservative surgery and postoperative radiotherapy in 300 adults with soft-tissue sarcomas, Cancer 47:2391-2397, 1981.

Chapter 26

PEDIATRIC NEOPLASMS

Neoplastic diseases are the second leading cause of death in children. The yearly incidence of the various malignancies is shown in Table 26.1. The major difference between adult and pediatric radiotherapy is that retardation or arrest of bone and soft tissue growth in irradiated tissues in children leads to body asymmetry.[2] In addition, children are more likely than adults to develop radiation-induced malignancy.

Table 26.1 Cancer incidence by site for children under 15, SEER Program 1973-1976

Rank	Site	Number of Cases	% of total
1	Leukemia	664	30.0%
2	CNS	409	18.5%
3	Lymphoma	298	12.5%
4	Neuroblastoma	170	8.0%
5	Rhabdomyosarcoma	141	6.5%
6	Wilms' tumor	135	6.0%
7	Osteogenic sarcoma	101	4.5%
8	Retinoblastoma	58	3.0%
9	Liver	26	1.0%
	All others	195	10.0%

Therefore, radiotherapists have become more conservative and many patients, who in past years would have been treated with radiation, are now treated with surgery and/or chemotherapy. In fact, a desire to avoid late effects has led to modifications of classical treatment methods by all oncologists; surgical procedures are more conservative, radiation portals are smaller and doses lower, and the number of cycles of chemotherapy have been reduced.

This conservatism combined with an increased awareness among oncologists of the strengths and weaknesses of each modality and an increased understanding of how each modality can be utilized most effectively in combination, has led to an improved quality of life for the patients and an increase in cure rates.

WILMS' TUMOR

ETIOLOGY AND EPIDEMIOLOGY

Wilms' tumor is the most common renal tumor in children and the second most common pediatric abdominal tumor. The peak age at diagnosis is 1-3 years and 90% of cases are less than 7. The incidence is equal between the sexes. The etiology is unknown but 40% of cases are thought to be hereditary. In hereditary cases, the disease is transmitted as an autosomal dominant disorder. Hereditary cases occur in younger patients and can be bilateral and multiple.

Wilms' tumor is often associated with congenital anomalies such as aniridia (complete or partial absence of the iris), hemihypertrophy (congenital overgrowth of one side of the body), and genitourinary abnormalities.

PATHOLOGY

Wilms' tumor is thought to arise from the embryonic metanephric blastema. The tumor is usually a single expanding renal mass, but there may be multiple sites and about 5% of cases are bilateral. The tumor tends to infiltrate through the renal capsule into adjacent structures and there is often extension to the renal pelvis, ureter, renal vein and vena cava. Metastasis to regional lymph nodes is common. Metastasis to the lungs is common.

Microscopically, Wilms' tumor contains both mesenchymal and epithelial elements and the tumor resembles embryonic renal tissue. In about 10% of cases there are histological findings which are associated with an unfavorable prognosis such as anaplastic or sarcoma-like changes. The relapse rate is 75% in patients having unfavorable histology.

DIAGNOSIS AND STAGING

Symptoms The discovery by the parent or physician of an abdominal mass is the usual presenting complaint. Abdominal pain, fever and hematuria are also occasionally seen.

Radiographic studies The intravenous pyelogram is the most important initial study. This demonstrates a mass distorting the calices and displacing the kidney. Ultrasonography is used to evaluate the vena cava for possible tumor extension; CT scans and angiography are of value in selected cases. Chest x-rays and tomograms are indicated in all patients.

Staging The National Wilms' Tumor Study classification is shown in Table 26.2.

TREATMENT

Surgery Surgical removal of the involved kidney is carried out in all patients. The abdominal cavity is inspected and suspicious lesions are biopsied.

Table 26.2 National Wlims' Tumor Study staging classifciation

Stage I   Tumor limited to the kidney and completely excised; the surface of the kidney is intact. The tumor was not ruptured during removal. There is no apparent tumor beyond the margins of excision.

Stage II   Tumor extends beyond the kidney but is completely excised. There is local extension of tumor, i.e. penetration through renal capsule into perirenal soft tissues, or para-aortic lymph node metastasis. The renal vessels otuside the kidney may be involved. There is no known residual tumor.

Stage III   Residual tumor confined to the abdomen, any of the following may be present:

    1)   The tumor has been biopsied or ruptured before or during surgery

    2)   There are implants on peritoneal surfaces

    3)   There are involved lymph nodes beyond the para-aortic region

    4)   The tumor is not completely removed because of extension to vital structure

Stage IV   Distant metastasis to lung, liver, bone or brain

Stage V   Bilateral renal involvement

If a lesion in the opposite kidney is found, a heminephrectory is carried out. Bilateral nephrectomy and renal transplantation is only rarely required.

Chemotherapy Dactinomycin, vincristine and doxorubicin are the drugs used. Stage I cases with favorable or unfavorable histology and Stage II cases with favorable histology receive dactinomycin and vincristine. RT is not needed in Stage I cases and may not be needed in Stage II cases with favorable histology.[3]

Stage III and IV cases with favorable histology and Stage II, III and IV cases with unfavorable histology receive chemotherapy with dactinomycin, vincristine, and doxorubicin plus postop RT.

Radiotherapy RT portals should be tailored to the extent of disease found at the time of surgery. Residual disease or lymph node involvement requires tumor bed irradiation. The hemiabdomen is treated, including the tumor bed and para-aortic regions, with parallel opposing portals. The treatment portals cover the entire width of the vertebral bodies to prevent unequal growth arrest in the growth centers of the irradiated vertebrae. Twenty Gy/1.5 Gy per fraction 2 1/2-3 weeks is the usual tumor dose. The opposite kidney must be shielded completely.

Radiotherapy to the whole abdomen is required only in cases in which the tumor was ruptured and spilled into the abdomen at the time of surgery. Patients with lung metastasis who require renal bed irradiation receive 12-15 Gy/1.5 Gy per fraction to the entire thorax and renal fossa plus a boost of 10 Gy to the renal fossa (Figure 26.1).

Prognosis The current overall cure rate is almost 90%. The 2 year survival rate in Stage I cases with favorable histology is 98%.

NEUROBLASTOMA

ETIOLOGY AND EPIDEMIOLOGY

This is the most common malignant solid tumor of childhood except for brain tumors. Twenty-five percent of cases are diagnosed in the first year of life, but 50% are diagnosed after age 2. The peak incidence is age 2. The etiology of neuroblastoma is unknown, but the disease occurs with increased frequency in von Recklinghausen's disease and occasional instances of multiple cases in families have been reported suggesting a hereditary basis in some cases.

PATHOLOGY

Neuroblastoma is a malignant tumor of neural crest origin. They usually arise in the adrenal gland but may originate in sympathetic nerve tissue in any location; 70% of cases originate in the abdomen, 20% in the thorax or neck and 5% in the pelvis.

Neuroblastomas tend to infiltrate locally along tissue planes and around major vessels making surgical removal difficult. Regional lymph node metastasis is common and widespread metastasis via the blood steam occurs early; the bone marrow, liver and skin are common distant sites.

DIAGNOSIS AND STAGING

Symptoms The discovery by the parents of an abdominal mass is the most common presentation. However, there is a wide variety of possible presenting signs and symptoms and patients often present with distant metastasis. Bone pain and neurological complaints such as weakness and paralysis due to spinal cord compression are not uncommon.

Radiographic studies Routine studies include chest x-ray, IVP, radionuclide bone scans, abdominal ultrasound and CT scans.

Laboratory Seventy percent of patients excrete vanilmandelic acid (VMA) or homovanillic acid (HVA) or both. Elevations can be quantified with 24 hour urine collections. Bone marrow aspsiration is routine.

Staging The classification is shown in Table 26.3.

TREATMENT

Surgery The primary tumor is removed whenever possible. Even in patients whose tumor cannot be totally removed, as much tumor is removed as possible.

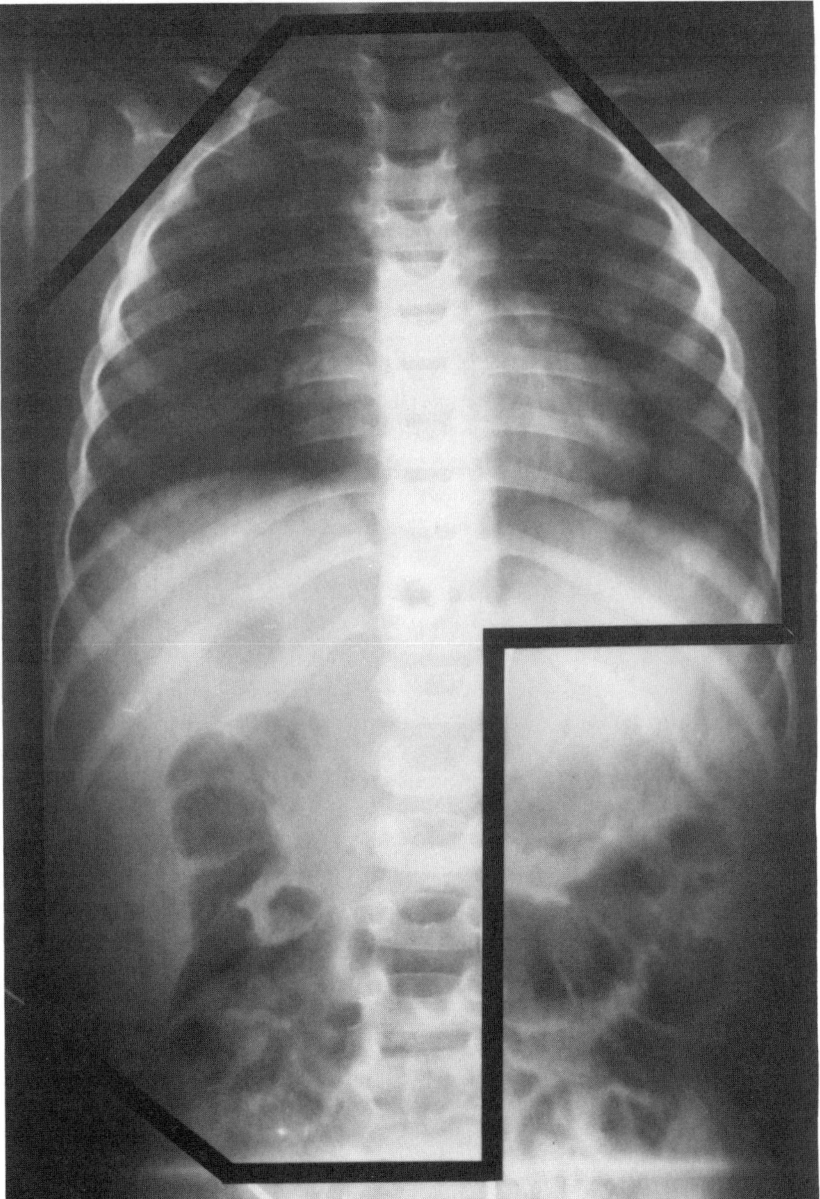

Figure 26.1 This is the simulator film for a patient with Stage IV Wilms' tumor. The renal bed and thorax was irradiated with opposing AP-PA portals (12 Gy/8 treatments). The renal bed was boosted (8Gy/5 fractions). Dactinomycin, doxorubicin and vincristine were also given.

<table>
<tr><td colspan="2" align="center">Table 26.3 Evans Staging System for neuroblastoma[4]</td></tr>
<tr><td>Stage I</td><td>Tumor confined to the organ or structure of origin</td></tr>
<tr><td>Stage II</td><td>Tumor extends beyond the organ or structure of origin but does not cross the midline of the body. Regional lymph nodes on the side of the primary may be involved.</td></tr>
<tr><td>Stage III</td><td>Tumor extends beyond the midline. Lymph nodes may be involved on both sides of the midline.</td></tr>
<tr><td>Stage IV</td><td>Distant metastasis</td></tr>
<tr><td>Stagve IVS</td><td>Local Stage I or II with distant metastasis to liver, skin and/or bone marrow</td></tr>
</table>

Chemotherapy There are a variety of agents that are effective in neuroblastoma. Cyclophosphamide is the most effective single agent followed by doxorubicin and cisplatin. Combination chemotherapy is more effective than single. There is no evidence that adjuvant chemotherapy improves overall cure rates for patients in Stages I-III.[4] In Stage IV, chemotherapy can produce responses in 70% of patients.

Radiotherapy This is a radiosensitive tumor but the role of RT is ill-defined. RT has not contributed to improving cure rates except in Stage III.[5] In general, patients with neuroblastoma who are under 12 months of age are not treated with RT. In Stage I, for children in the 12-14 month age group, RT is not required; in Stage I, areas of known postop residual are usually irradiated (20-25 Gy). In Stage III, the patients are treated initially with chemotherapy followed by "second-look" surgery; if there is known residual, RT is given. Stage IV cases receive RT for palliation only.

Children aged 24 months or more receive postop RT in Stage I if the surgical margins are inadequate; Stage II cases usually are given RT (20-30 Gy); in Stage III, RT is combined with surgery and chemotherapy and in Stage IV, RT may be of value for treatment of lymph node metastasis.

Stage IVS Patients with Stage IVS are infants with a small primary and metastasis in the liver, bone marrow and skin. These children have a good prognosis and survival rates as high as 80% have been reported in this special group. In Stage IVS the disease tends to undergo spontaneous remission and no treatment is given unless symptoms and signs necessitate treatment.

Bone marrow transplantation This method is used for patients with recurrent metastatic disease.[6] The patients receive local RT, high-dose chemotherapy, TBI and infusion of either allogenic or autologous marrow. Early results suggest that metastatic neuroblastoma can be controlled with high-dose chemotherapy and TBI and bone marrow rescue.

Prognosis The age of the child has an important influence on prognosis. In one series, 93% of children diagnosed at less than 1 year of age were surviving disease-free 2-12 years post -treatment, whereas only 40% of children diagnosed when over age 1 were surviving.[5] The overall survival at 2-12 years in this series was nearly 60%.

RHABDOMYOSARCOMA

ETIOLOGY AND EPIDEMIOLOGY

This is the most common soft tissue sarcoma in the pediatric age group accounting for 5-10% of malignant childhood tumors. There are two age peaks; one between ages 2 and 6 and the second in the mid-teens. The tumors in the younger group tend to be of the embryonal type and usually occur in the head and neck or genitourinary regions, whereas the older patients tend to have alveolar or undifferentiated histologic types which originate on the trunk or extremities.

PATHOLOGY

These tumors are derived from undifferentiated mesodermal tissue. Nearly 40% originate in the head and neck region and the orbit is the most frequent site. One third of cases occur in the GU region and the remainder on the trunk or extremities.

The histologic types are embryonal, alveolar and undifferentiated or pleomorphic. Sarcoma botryoides is a form of embryonal rhabdomyosarcoma which presents as a vaginal mass having the appearance of clusters of grapes. Rhabdomyosarcomas spread by local extension, regional lymph node metastasis and distant metastasis to lungs.

TREATMENT

Surgery The role of surgery varies with the location, size and extent of disease. Surgical removal is performed if it can be accomplished without causing functional disability.

Chemotherapy Cure rates have improved markedly with VAC (vincristine, doxorubicin and cyclophosphamide). This regimen is used as an adjuvant for localized disease and for metastatic disease.

Radiotherapy The majority of patients require RT for control of the primary. Large portals are required to cover gross tumor masses and potential areas of microscopic disease. Local control is achieved in a high percentage of cases with doses of 55 Gy and microscopic disease with 40 Gy.

SACROCOCCYGEAL TERATOMA

In childhood, germ cell tumors develop in the sacrococcygeal region, the testis, ovary, retroperitoneum and mediastinum. Sacrococcygeal teratomas are the most common germ cell tumors in children and 75% occur in females.

Seventy-five percent are found on the first day of life. They originate at the coccyx and present as an obvious external mass. Forty percent are malignant.

Histologically, the tumor may contain skin, nerve, intestine, lung, fat, cartilage, bone and muscle. The malignant component is usually the infantile type of embryonal carcinoma (yolk sac tumor), but seminoma, adult embryonal carcinoma and choriocarcinoma are also seen.

Surgical removal is the main treatment, malignant teratomas also receive adjuvant VAC. RT is needed for patients having an incomplete removal and for recurrence. The prognosis depends on the histology of the tumor; most patients with benign teratoma are cured by surgery; very few malignant teratomas are cured.

HISTIOCYTOSIS X

The histiocytosis syndromes are a spectrum of diseases of unknown etiology referred to as histiocytosis X. The diseases are eosinophilic granuloma, Hand-Schuller -Christian disease and Letterer-Siwe disease. Histological examination of biopsy specimens from all three disorders reveals a diffuse proliferation of histiocytes, some eosinophils and an occasional granuloma.

Eosinophilic granuloma This lesion is seen primarily in older children. The disease presents with the patient complaining of tenderness and swelling over single or multiple lytic bone lesions. Treatment consists of surgical curettage or local RT. The lesions are very radiosensitive and respond to fractionated doses of 4.5-9 Gy.The prognosis is good.

Hand-Schuller-Christian disease This disease occurs in children older than 2. Presenting symptoms include tenderness and swelling over multiple skeletal lesions, exophthalmos, diabetes insipidius, chronic otitis media and dental lesions. Low-dose RT (4.5-9 Gy) is used to control skeletal lesions causing pain, visual loss or diabetes insipidus. The disease follows a chronic and fluctuating course.

Letterer-Siwe disease This disease is seen primarily in children less than 2. Presenting symptoms include skin rash, anorexia and failure to thrive. There is usually enlargement of the liver, spleen and lymph nodes. Hemorrhages may occur at various sites. Death from infection of organs is possible. Chemotherapy is usually required; 30% to 80% of patients respond and treatment appears to improve survival.

REFERENCES

1. Silverberg E. Cancer statistics, 1982, CA-A Cancer J for Clinicians 32:15-31, 1982.

2. Pizzo PA, Horowitz ME, Poplack DG, et al. Chapter 48, Solid tumors of childhood, In Cancer-Principles & Practice of Oncology, 3rd Edition, Eds. De Vita VT, Hellman S, Rosenberg SA, J.B. Lippincott Company, Philadelphia, 1989, pp 1612-1670.

3. D'Angio GJ, Beckwith JB, Breslow NE, et al. Wilms' tumor: An update, Cancer 45:1791-1798, 1980.

4. Evans AE. Staging and treatment of neuroblastoma, Cancer 45:1799-1982, 1980.

5. August CS, Serta KT, Koch PA, et al. Treatment of advanced neuroblastoma with supralethal chemotherapy, radiation and allogeneic or autologous marrow reconstitution, J Clin Oncol 2:609-616,1984.

6. Rosen EM, Cassady JR, Frantz CN, et al. Neuroblastoma: The Joint Center for Radiation Therapy/Dana-Farber Cancer Institute/Children's Hospital experience, J Clin Oncol 2:719-732, 1984.

Chapter 27

EMOTIONAL RESPONSE
TO CANCER

The emotional impact of cancer on the patient and his or her family is profound. The patient's emotional response to the early symptoms of cancer and to its diagnosis and treatment can have a major influence on the clinical course of the disease. An important determinant of the patient's emotional response is the meaning that he or she associates with the disease such as pain, disfigurement, hospitalization, debts, inability to care for family and possible death. The emotional response of the family, the members of the medical treatment team and the social contacts of the patient can also influence outcome.

SOCIAL ATTITUDES TOWARD CANCER

Cancer has been known for centuries as an incurable disease. In earlier times patients were sent home to die and were never told the diagnosis. Neither the patient or the family could discuss their feelings openly. The victim may have been considered dirty or unclean because of foul smelling ulcerations. The disease was also feared because of the pain and body wasting which still occurs today. Guilt was usually a part of the psychologic response because it was thought that cancer developed as punishment for an immoral act. For these reasons cancer carried a horror far beyond that of other diseases. Fortunately, a more rational and hopeful approach has developed in recent years due to improvements in diagnosis and treatment. However, many of these old emotions remain in the public and naturally have an impact on the emotional response of patients to cancer.

FEAR OF CANCER AND DELAY IN DIAGNOSIS

Many persons, when they discover a mass or develop abnormal bleeding or other symptoms, suspect that they may have cancer. Some seek medical help immediately but others wait. The reasons for delay vary but, for most, fear is the underlying cause. They may be afraid of physicians, hospitals, surgery, anesthesia, radiation, chemotherapy, the response of family and friends, and death.

Whatever the reason, delay is a serious problem in cancer therapy because some patients delay until there is no hope for cure. Nevertheless, when the patient finally does seek medical help, we should not express disapproval of the patient's actions because this will add to their burden of guilt. Calm acceptance of the facts is the most appropriate response coupled with reassurance that others have experienced the same problem.

THE DIAGNOSIS OF CANCER
INFORMING THE PATIENT

Physicians' attitudes toward informing the patient of the diagnosis of cancer have undergone a complete reversal in the past 20 years. This change has taken place because people are better educated about health matters and want to know the diagnosis and what to expect. Also, the increased involvement of the legal profession in medicine has led to the realization that patients have a legal right to know and that treatment must not be undertaken without the patient's informed consent.

COPING WITH CANCER

Each patient must develop ways of coping with the emotional problems associated with the illness. The patient must:

1. Deal with pain and incapacitation.
2. Deal with the hospital environment and treatment procedures.
3. Develop adequate relationships with the professional staff.
4. Preserve a reasonable emotional balance.
5. Preserve a satisfactory self image.
6 Preserve relationships with family and friends.
7. Prepare for an uncertain future.

Some of the ways that patients cope with the emotional pain are carried out unconsciously. A defense is a mechanism of adaptation that is used unconsciously to manage anxiety, hostility, resentment and frustration. These are a few examples of defense mechanisms:

1. Denial is a common defense mechanism in which the seriousness of the illness is minimized or denied. Some denial is healthy and necessary to assist them and the family to deal with the disease and its treatment.

2. Projection is attributing to another what one is feeling oneself. Finding fault with the doctors, the nursing care or the food are examples of projection. Often anger is projected onto someone close such as the spouse rather than onto the professional staff because this is more socially acceptable.

3. Distortion is changing reality to protect against emotional distress. For example, the patient, after being told of the diagnosis of malignancy, might say that he is happy because it is only a benign tumor and not cancer. Distortion is unhealthy because it causes misunderstanding.

OTHER WAYS PATIENTS DEAL WITH EMOTIONS

There are other examples of ways that patients and their families can deal with the emotional impact of cancer to give them a sense of control over the situation:

1.   Learning illness related procedures such as colostomy care and help to reaffirm the patient's confidence and independence.

2.   Seeking information, such as reading material about cancer, can provide intellectual mastery over the situation which assists in dealing with helpless feelings.

3.   Requesting comfort, reassurance, and emotional support from family, friends, professional staff and from community support groups can help to relieve emotional tensions.

4.   Setting goals such as going away for the weekend or going back to work gives patients something to look forward to and gives them a sense of achievement when the goal is completed.

DEPRESSION

Depression is a common response for patients and their families. Symptoms such as weight loss, poor appetite and insomnia are often a manifestation of depression. Tranquilizers and antidepressant medications can be helpful in relieving anger and depression and in allowing the patient to sleep. Open discussion of depressed and angry feelings can also help.

HOSTILITY AND ANGER

Hostility is a very common emotion in patients who have cancer and it can appear in many ways. It is important for the professional staff to realize this when statements by the patient and family convey hostile feelings toward the staff. Members of the staff must not take this personally because behind the anger are feelings of sadness and loss. The correct response requires an awareness of the patient's and one's own hostility and an attempt to allow the patient and family to recognize the sadness and loss.

ANXIETY

Anxiety is always present in patients and their families. Acceptance of the patient's anxiety as normal by the staff is important. Discussing the anxiety with the physician can help the patient to master feelings, but if the anxiety is interfering with daily functioning, medication may be required.

DEATH

Patients pass through stages of dying as described by Kübler-Ross. These are denial, anger, bargaining and acceptance. These are a sequence of coping methods to handle the stress involved. This is a time when religious beliefs help to maintain emotional balance with a sense of purpose, meaning and love.

EMOTIONS AND SURGERY

Patients often become angry, resentful, depressed, anxious and panicked about the prospect of surgery. The underlying cause of these reactions is fear. Many patients are afraid that they might die on the operating table. They are apprehensive about anesthesia and loss of consciousness which they equate with helplessness and loss of control. They also fear the pain that they might experience afterward and they fear the mutilation that is often associated with cancer surgery. The members of the surgical team can help to alleviate the patient's concerns through preoperative counseling.

EMOTIONS AND RADIOTHERAPY

Patients may have misconceptions and apprehensions about radiotherapy. The prospect of receiving invisible treatment from a large machine in a closed room is often frightening. Furthermore, they often associate radiotherapy with far advanced cancer and may view the procedure as hopeless. They may also believe that they will be burned or disfigured and they may be worried about other effects including loss of sexuality and sterility. Many also believe they will be radioactive after treatment. An assessment by the radiotherapist of the patient's knowledge of the disease and radiotherapy can be helpful in determining the extent of his misconceptions.

In all cases, however, extensive counseling is needed prior to treatment and the patient should receive instruction about the objectives of radiotherapy, the function of the equipment, the effects of radiation on tissues and tumors, the side effects of treatment and what can be done to prevent or treat them, the prognosis, alternative forms of treatment and what to expect from department routines such as skin markings, treatment planning, treatment times.

The radiotherapy nurses and technologists are an important source of information and counseling. Also, written materials should be given to the patient for further education and reinforcement. A brief tour of the department at the initial visit may help to lessen some of the fears of the equipment.

EMOTIONS AND CHEMOTHERAPY

Most patients have considerable fear of chemotherapy. Many have known or heard about other patients who became ill following chemotherapy and may associate chemotherapy with end stage cancer. The nausea and vomiting are the primary concerns, but loss of hair is a problem for many. All patients require a great deal of information and counseling from all members of the oncology team prior to and during treatment.

CANCER IN THE YOUNG

Cancer in children is associated with intense emotional responses affecting each family member and each member of the oncology team. Each member of the team must be aware of the special problems faced by the child and family. Members of the team include pediatric oncologists, radiotherapists, radiation therapy technologists, psychiatrists, psychologists, nurses, social workers, play therapists, rehabilitation specialists, chaplains and teachers. Other parents whose children have had cancer and also support organizations can provide emotional support.

COPING BY THE HEALTH PROFESSIONAL

Health professionals are subject to the same emotions and fears that their patients experience and they deal with the emotions and fears in much the same way through denial, anger, depression and avoidance of the problem. If these defense mechanisms are carried to the extreme, isolation of the professional from his or her patients and co-workers can result.

In addition, the constant giving and caring is an emotional and physical drain which can lead to burnout. He or she may seem irritable, quick to anger and frustration and suspicious. Burnout can lead to such harmful effects as ulcers, migraine, drug and alcohol abuse, marital problems, mental illness. Its effects can be seen in low employee morale, absenteeism and high job turnover.

In response to his intolerable situation he or she may leave the field altogether or assume an administrative position which eliminates patient care. Therefore, the health professional must develop ways to remain remote enough to think and function, but close enough to relate to the patients and co-workers. Reducing the number of patients that the worker is responsible for, reducing the number of work hours and alternating patient care with other duties are helpful in reducing stress.

Also, the professional should develop relationships with others outside the work setting, take regular vacations, take time to attend conferences and seek emotional support from family members. Regular exercise can help relieve tension and encourage sleep. Regularly scheduled staff meetings can promote a supportive environment where the professional can air his or her feelings, tell about lessons learned and develop insight into his or her feelings about cancer.

Such meetings can also be the time for a pat on the back and/or constructive criticism so that the technologist gains an idea of what he or she is doing right and where improvement is needed. Most importantly he or she learns that emotions are an acceptable response to the pressure of caring for cancer patients.

SUPPORT PROGRAMS AVAILABLE TO CANCER PATIENTS

People with common problems tend to unite for their common good. Support groups and national and regional programs to assist cancer patients are available. Some are listed here:

Leukemia Society of America Financial assistance and consultation for adults and children.

Make Today Count For patients with incurable disease, 200 chapters nationwide.

United Cancer Council A federation of voluntary cancer agencies seeking control of cancer through service, education and research. Funded through the United Way.

United Ostomy Association 500 chapters nationwide. Provides support following removal of bowel and bladder.

Can Surmount Designated a national program by the American Cancer Society. Volunteers, who are themselves cancer patients, are trained to visit cancer patients and families to provide support and education.

I Can Cope Designated a national program by the American Cancer Society. A course taught by health professionals to address the educational and emotional needs of cancer patients.

International Association of Laryngectomies Sponsored by the American Cancer Society. 225 local clubs which support the rehabilitation of patients following removal of the larynx.

Reach to Recovery Programs of American Cancer Society to support women following mastectomy by trained volunteers who have had mastectomy.

The American Cancer Society A national voluntary organization of health professionals and laymen with programs in education, research, patient services and rehabilitation.

Candlelighters 110 chapters in 40 states-family support groups for children with cancer.

Ronald McDonald Houses Lodging for out-of-town families during treatment of their children.

The National Hospice Organization Care for terminally ill patients and their families. The concept originated in England, particularly St. Christopher's Hospice. The primary objective is to provide comprehensive management of physical symptoms, particularly pain. The goal is to keep patients comfortable but alert. Home care is emphasized but inpatient facilities are available in some programs.

REFERENCES

1. U.S. Department of Health and Human Services. Public Health Service, National Institutes of Health: Coping with Cancer-A Resource for the Health Professional, NIH Publication No. 80-2080, National Cancer Institute, Bethesda, MD, 1980.